Expert Praise for the *PDR® Family Guide* Series of Personal Health Handbooks

"A great resource for the patient in his or her dialogue with the physician."
Joseph R. Cruse, MD
Founding Medical Director
The Betty Ford Center

"The premier professional drug reference now gives consumers their best guide to medical problems and the medications prescribed for them. . . . Clear, readable, comprehensive."
Barrie R. Cassileth, PhD
Adjunct Professor
University of North Carolina and
Duke University Medical Center

"Comprehensive, easy to understand. . . . Sorts out fact from fantasy in a lucid, interesting style."
Stephen Brunton, MD
Clinical Professor
Department of Family Medicine
University of California at Irvine

"Superbly written and understandable by those we wish to help—our patients and their families."
Edwin C. Cadman, MD
Ensign Professor and Chairman
Department of Internal Medicine
Yale University School of Medicine

"A valuable and timely adjunct in this age of consumer education, patient rights, and quality health care for all."
Roberta S. Abruzzese, EdD, RN, FAAN
Editor, *Decubitus: The Journal of Skin Ulcers*

Published by Ballantine Books:

THE PDR® FAMILY GUIDE TO OVER-THE-COUNTER
    DRUGS™
THE PDR® FAMILY GUIDE ENCYCLOPEDIA OF MEDICAL
    CARE™
THE PDR® FAMILY GUIDE TO COMMON AILMENTS™

THE PDR®
FAMILY GUIDE
TO COMMON AILMENTS ™

BALLANTINE BOOKS • NEW YORK

PHYSICIANS' DESK REFERENCE®, PDR®, PDR for Ophthalmology®,
Pocket PDR®, and The PDR® Family Guide to Prescription Drugs® are registered
trademarks used herein under license. PDR for Nonprescription Drugs and
Dietary Supplements™, PDR Companion Guide™, PDR® for Herbal
Medicines™, PDR® Medical Dictionary™, PDR® Nurse's Handbook™, PDR®
Nurse's Dictionary™, The PDR® Family Guide to Common Ailments™, The
PDR® Family Guide Encyclopedia of Medical Care™, The PDR® Family Guide
to Over-the-Counter Drugs™, The PDR® Family Guide to Natural Medicines
and Healing Therapies™, and PDR® Electronic Library™ are trademarks used
herein under license.

Officers of Medical Economics Company: *President and Chief Executive
Officer:* Curtis B. Allen; *Vice President, New Media:* L. Suzanne BeDell; *Vice
President, Corporate Human Resources:* Pamela M. Bilash; *Vice President
and Chief Information Officer:* Steven M. Bressler; *Chief Financial Officer:*
Christopher Caridi; *Vice President, Finance:* Claudia Flowers; *Vice President and
Controller:* Barry Gray; *Vice President, Directory Services:* Paul Walsh; *Vice
President, New Business Planning:* Linda G. Hope; *Executive Vice President,
Healthcare Publishing and Communications:* Thomas J. Kelly; *Senior Vice
President, Primary Care:* Frank B. Lederer; *Executive Vice President, Magazine
Publishing:* Lee A. Maniscalco; *Vice President, Allied Healthcare:* Terrence W.
Meacock; *Vice President, Business Integration:* David A. Pitler; *Vice President,
Specialty & Medical Education:* Thomas C. Pizor; *Vice President, Healthcare
Publishing Business Management:* Donna Santarpia; *Vice President, Magazine
Business Management:* Eric Schlett; *Senior Vice President, Operations:* John R.
Ware; *Senior Vice President, Internet Strategies:* Raymond Zoeller

Contents

Disease Overviews

The PDR® Family Guide to Common Ailments™

Editor-in-Chief: David W. Sifton
Director of Professional Services: Mukesh Mehta, R Ph
Art Director: Robert Hartman

Senior Associate Editor: Lori Murray

Assistant Editors: Paula Benus; Gwynned L. Kelly

Writers: Nancy K. Bannon; Janette V. Carlucci; Lisa A. Maher; Kathleen Rodgers, R Ph

Editorial Production: *Director of Production:* Carrie Williams; *Manager of Production:* Kimberly H. Vivas; *Senior Production Coordinator:* Amy B. Brooks; *Electronic Publishing Designer:* Robert K. Grossman

Medical Economics Company

Senior Vice President, Directory Services: Paul Walsh
Director of Product Management: Mark A. Friedman
Associate Product Manager: Bill Shaughnessy
Director of Sales: Dikran N. Barsamian
National Sales Manager, Medical Economics
Trade Sales: Bill Gaffney

Publisher's Note

How to Use This Book

Are you getting the best treatment available?

No matter what your medical problem, that's no longer an easy question to answer. Science is progressing so rapidly that new and better remedies are appearing almost daily. At the same time, doctors are learning more about the potent benefits of nutrition and rediscovering the value of certain natural herbs. Some physicians are even beginning to experiment with a variety of alternative therapies that offer some hope of relief when other treatments fail. The bottom line: To solve any kind of health problem, your range of choices has never been greater.

To help you take advantage of *all* your options, this book aims to provide you with a snapshot of the leading remedies for a broad selection of the most common ailments. It doesn't attempt to give all the details (which would take up a small library). It merely serves as a "heads up" on the possibilities to consider. Drawing on the immense database of healthcare information maintained by *Physicians' Desk Reference,* it offers you a checklist of the measures you can take on your own—and the array of treatments you can discuss with your doctor.

So that you can quickly locate the specific facts you need, each disease overview in the book is divided into ten standard sections, covering every concern from cause to cure. Here's a closer look at what you'll find in each section.

The Basics. Here you'll find a quick summary of the problem, including its cause, the most likely victims, the way it's spread, how long it takes to clear up, and its telltale signs and symptoms. Because totally different diseases sometimes produce remarkably similar symptoms, this information won't provide you with a definite diagnosis. For that, there's no substitute for a medical exam and testing. However, this section can give you a fairly reliable idea of what you may be facing.

Call Your Doctor If . . . If you develop any of the symptoms listed under this heading, it's a signal to contact your doctor. Chances are that you will need additional treatment or care. The problems shown here are not necessarily dangerous . . . but they can't be ignored, either.

Seek Care Immediately If . . . The symptoms itemized here are emergencies that should send you to the ER or Urgent Care Center *as soon as possible*. They are *not* problems that can wait for a doctor's appointment. If you experience such symptoms, don't hesitate to call 911 or the operator for help.

What You Can Do. In this section you'll find a set of tips for easing your symptoms, speeding recovery, and preventing an encore. Depending on the nature of the illness, you may also encounter some strategies for avoiding the problem in the first place.

What Your Doctor Can Do. Here you'll get a brief recap of conventional treatment options and the circumstances under which each is typically used. Included are the key diagnostic tests to expect, types of medication and therapy that may be prescribed, and—for serious problems—the surgical procedures that may be needed. Advanced and experimental operations—clearly labeled as such—are sometimes included as well. This information is designed to give you a general idea of your major alternatives. It does not include every specialized technique or describe special measures that vary from case to case. Every patient is unique, and so is every treatment plan. So, although your doctor's recommendations may be similar to one of the approaches seen here, you shouldn't expect them to be identical.

Prescription Drugs. This section provides you with a list of options to explore with your doctor if your current prescription fails to do the job. Included are all major medications approved for the ailment by the U.S. Food and Drug Administration. When talking with your doctor, remember that many prescription medications are *not* suitable for certain patients with specific medical conditions or complications. Hence, not every drug on the list may be a viable option in your case. The drugs are listed by both generic name and the names of the leading brands. You can find additional information on most of these drugs—including warnings, side effects, and standard dosage—in *The PDR® Family Guide to Prescription Drugs™.*

Over-the-Counter Drugs. Shown here are the remedies you can get without a visit to the doctor. Such nonprescription medicines typically do an excellent job of easing your symptoms, but rarely cure the under-lying problem (over-the-counter yeast medications are one of the notable exceptions). When considering an over-the-counter drug, re-member that it might interact badly with any prescription medicines you may be taking. For more information on such interactions, as well as other precautions to observe, turn to *The PDR* *Family Guide to Over-the-Counter Drugs™.*

Herbal Remedies. So many claims are made for a seemingly endless list of botanicals that you may have despaired of ever sorting out the genuine remedies from the bogus nostrums. In this section, however, you'll find only those herbs that have been deemed truly effective by an advisory commission of the German Regulatory Authority. (Our own Food and Drug Administration does not review herbs for safety and efficacy.) Like other over-the-counter products, herbs rarely can correct an underlying disorder, but you may find some of them surpris-ingly effective for symptomatic relief. You can find a detailed discus-sion of each herb listed here in *The PDR* *Family Guide to Natural Medicines and Healing Therapies™.*

Nutritional Support. Diet plays a significant role in a surprising vari-ety of illnesses. This section offers you tips on the vitamins, minerals, and foods that will help you combat the illness—and warns you of ones to avoid. The information is based on the current expert consen-sus regarding the role of nutrition in health.

Alternative Treatments. With unconventional treatments that range from acupuncture to yoga, the field of alternative therapy is unques-tionably the most controversial area in medicine today. For each suc-cessful trial of an alternative treatment, there's another that claims to debunk it. Listed in this section are only those unconventional thera-pies that have demonstrated a significant chance of providing lasting relief. If a purported remedy isn't listed here, it's because the proce-dure either hasn't undergone any scientific tests or has failed in the trials it has entered. For a thorough review of all forms of alternative therapy—proven and otherwise—turn to *The PDR* *Family Guide to Natural Medicines and Healing Therapies™.*

The Doctor-Patient Partnership

Today's sophisticated nutritional supplements, herbal extracts, and nonprescription drugs give all of us new power to maintain and enhance our health. But when something goes seriously wrong, there's still no substitute for a visit to the doctor. Only a doctor can weigh all aspects of your condition and choose the treatment most likely to meet your needs.

Likewise, books such as this one can suggest alternatives that merit further investigation, but only your doctor can decide whether a particular option makes sense for you. We hope that this book suggests some beneficial avenues to explore with your doctor, even if some turn out to be the wrong choice for you. Most of all, we hope it helps in some small way to keep all your illnesses as mild and brief as possible—and to make every recovery speedy and complete.

Alzheimer's Disease

The Basics

Alzheimer's has a well-deserved reputation as the disease that destroys memory. But that's only the beginning of the story. This progressive, degenerative disorder causes physical changes in the brain that eventually lead to disorientation, emotional instability, and loss of muscular control.

The chances of developing Alzheimer's increase dramatically with age. One in 10 persons over age 65 and nearly half of those over 85 have the disease. So far the only known risk factor other than age is a family history of the problem, although it is likely that other forces are at work. Researchers hope to find contributing factors so that people will someday be able to take steps to prevent the disease. In the meantime, doctors are emphasizing symptom control through medication and lifestyle changes to improve the quality of life for patients and their families.

The course of Alzheimer's can run anywhere from 3 to 20 years, although the average is about 8 years. Once it begins, the disease typically becomes well advanced within 2 to 3 years. However, the speed of progression and the types and extent of impairments that result vary greatly from person to person.

Symptoms may begin with misplacing things or fear of venturing out. The disease may then progress to forgetfulness about recent events or daily tasks, followed by confusion, combativeness, and mood and behavior problems. Subsequently, there is often a decline in judgment and decision-making abilities. In the late stages, physical problems usually emerge, including loss of coordination, lack of personal hygiene, and incontinence. Some people even lose the ability to walk and/or swallow. Eventually, all people with Alzheimer's lose their ability to function and must be cared for.

Call Your Doctor If . . .

Minor memory lapses and momentary disorientation are normal, but if memory loss starts to affect daily life, it's time to check with your doctor. Other symptoms that should prompt a consultation include:

■ Loss of recent memory affecting job performance
■ Difficulty performing familiar tasks
■ Problems with language

- Disorientation toward time and place
- Poor or decreased judgment
- Problems with abstract thinking
- Misplacing things
- Changes in mood or behavior
- Changes in personality
- Loss of initiative

Seek Care Immediately If . . .

A person with Alzheimer's becomes a danger to himself or others, is seriously injured, or has a serious reaction to medication.

What You Can Do

There is growing appreciation of the role the environment can play in relieving symptoms of Alzheimer's. If you are caring for an Alzheimer's patient at home, your goal should be to keep him or her as active and engaged as possible. It is important for people with Alzheimer's to continue the same social activities and hobbies they enjoyed before becoming ill, making adjustments as the disease progresses. Keep family members and friends informed so that they know what to expect in terms of the patient's abilities and level of interaction. Remember that hobbies requiring tools, toxic substances, or machinery will eventually become a threat to the patient. When they do, replace dangerous aspects of the hobby with creative, safe alternatives so that the patient can continue doing what he or she enjoys for as long as possible.

Also, encourage Alzheimer's patients to remain physically active. Some physicians believe regular exercise can help to halt deterioration of motor function. It also serves as an outlet for anxiety and tension, relieves constipation, and stimulates appetite in poor eaters.

Finally, as the patient's physical abilities decline, keep the living area as safe as possible. Eliminate clutter and loose electrical wires that may cause a fall. Also, beware of home appliances and nonfood items, such as cleansers, that could be dangerous if ingested.

Eventually all people with Alzheimer's deteriorate physically and emotionally to the point where they require part- or full-time professional care. When that time arrives, there is an array of options available, including licensed home professionals, adult day care facilities, respite care, assisted living housing, life care facilities, and nursing homes.

What Your Doctor Can Do

Treatable disorders such as depression or drug reactions can easily be confused with Alzheimer's, so it's important to seek an accurate diagnosis. The doctor will begin by endeavoring to rule out all other possible causes of the symptoms. This requires a complete physical exam and a thorough medical history. In addition, the doctor will probably perform tests of coordination, balance, mental functioning, and sensory abilities. He is likely to ask family and friends for feedback about the patient's ability to perform daily tasks, and will probably order blood and urine analyses. Brain imaging such as computerized tomography (CT) scanning, magnetic resonance imaging (MRI), or positron emission tomography (PET) scanning may also be used to detect abnormalities in the brain.

Once a diagnosis is made, your doctor may suggest starting the patient on one of the two prescription medications mentioned below. In addition to those medications, doctors often can treat some symptoms of Alzheimer's disease, such as depression, agitation, anxiety, and sleeplessness, by prescribing mood-altering drugs, such as antidepressants. These drugs must be used with caution, however, since they have side effects such as memory loss, confusion, incontinence, and drowsiness that can actually make the Alzheimer's seem worse.

Prescription Drugs

There are two drugs that can provide some relief from the symptoms of early Alzheimer's disease: Aricept (donepezil hydrochloride) and Cognex (tacrine hydrochloride). Both can temporarily improve brain function in some (but not all) Alzheimer's sufferers, but neither can cure the disease. Both drugs may produce certain side effects and seem to have a better chance of working when given as early as possible in the course of the disease.

Over-the-Counter Drugs

There are no over-the-counter remedies that will reverse the effects of Alzheimer's disease. However, a number of products may prove useful when dealing with certain related symptoms. Over-the-counter sleep aids, for example, may help with insomnia. Always check with your doctor, however, before giving a nonprescription remedy.

Herbal Remedies

Only one herb—ginkgo—has shown any ability to relieve symptoms of senility. Ginkgo improves circulation, discourages clot formation, reinforces the walls of the capillaries, and protects nerve cells from harm when deprived of oxygen. The ingredients in ginkgo also appear to have an antioxidant effect, sparing brain tissue from the damage caused by free radicals.

Ginkgo has not been found to halt or reverse the progress of Alzheimer's, but given the lack of reliable alternatives, it may be worth a try. Because the active ingredients are limited to minute quantities in natural ginkgo leaves, only concentrated ginkgo extract is really effective.

Nutritional Support

There are no specific foods that will prevent or cure Alzheimer's disease, but a healthy diet remains important. People with Alzheimer's, like everyone else, are apt to feel better when they eat well and remain physically fit.

Alternative Treatments

Although there are few studies to support the use of nondrug techniques, some people have found that relaxation exercises, yoga, visualization, and meditation can calm people with Alzheimer's.

Faced with a disease like Alzheimer's, it's natural to want to try anything that promises a cure, but beware of quacks selling worthless and potentially harmful "remedies." Also beware of chelation therapy, a process that pulls certain metals out of the body. It has not been proven helpful and may cause serious harm.

Angina

The Basics

Five million people in the U.S. suffer from angina pectoris, chest pain caused by a shortfall in the supply of oxygen-rich blood reaching the muscle of the heart. The pain of angina usually strikes during periods of increased demand, such as unusual exertion or emotional excitement. Ordinarily, the coronary arteries expand during such periods to deliver more blood to the heart muscle. But arteries clogged with fatty plaque eventually become rigid, fail to dilate, and can't meet the extra demand. Although angina usually subsides when the exertion stops, some people suffer pain even when resting. Angina is often the first symptom of more serious heart problems to come, and should never be ignored.

Stable angina is the most common form. The chest pain may feel crushing, tight, or heavy, or may burn like a case of indigestion. The pain commonly starts below the breastbone and on the left side of the body. It may spread into your arm or up into your jaw or shoulder blade. It typically starts slowly and lasts only a few minutes.

Unstable angina is pain that comes back often and hurts more every time it returns. It can start even while you're resting. If it starts during exercise, it may continue when you rest.

Call Your Doctor If . . .

■ Your chest pain:
- Is more painful each time you have it, or is returning more frequently.
- Lasts longer than 10 to 15 minutes even after you rest.
- Does not go away after taking your nitroglycerin or other medicine as directed.
- Wakes you from sleep.
- Occurs during exercise and doesn't go away with rest.

■ Your medicine is making you light-headed or dizzy, sweaty, or nauseated.

Seek Care Immediately If . . .

■ You have chest pain that spreads to your arms, jaw, or back, and you start sweating, become nauseous, and have trouble breathing. These are signs of a heart attack. **This is an emergency. Call 911 or 0 (operator)** to get to the nearest hospital or clinic. **Do not drive yourself.**

■ You have any of the problems listed under "Call If," but live in an area remote from a hospital and ambulance service.

■ You feel dizzy or faint.

What You Can Do

■ If you feel that your prescribed medication isn't helping, call your doctor, but do not stop taking it on your own.

■ If your doctor prescribes nitroglycerin, you may find that it gives you a headache or makes you feel a little dizzy. It's best to take it while sitting or lying down.

■ To prevent further damage to your arteries, follow a diet low in fat and cholesterol.

■ If you smoke, you had better quit; it puts extra stress on the heart. If you have trouble quitting, your doctor can prescribe aids such as the drug Zyban or a nicotine patch, inhaler, or gum.

■ Ask your doctor about an exercise program. Daily exercise helps strengthen the heart.

■ Excess weight makes the heart work harder. If you are overweight, talk to your doctor about a plan to shed pounds.

■ Since it is hard to avoid stress, you must try to control it. Try some of the techniques listed under "Alternative Treatments."

What Your Doctor Can Do

Stable angina can usually be treated with medicines that open up the arteries to the heart and lower the amount of oxygen it needs. These medicines should reduce your pain and the frequency of your attacks.

For unstable angina, you'll probably need to go to the hospital. You may be given a stress test (to gauge your heart's ability to cope with exercise) or a cardiac catheterization (to examine the arteries in your heart). Depending on the results of the tests, your doctor may recommend an angioplasty (in which a tube is snaked into an affected artery to remove the blockage) or surgery to bypass arteries that are severely blocked.

Prescription Drugs

One of the most commonly prescribed drugs for angina is nitroglycerin. This medication increases the heart's oxygen supply by relaxing the walls of the arteries and veins, allowing them to expand and carry more blood to the heart muscle.

Nitroglycerin is available in a variety of forms. As a patch or ointment applied to the skin, it helps to *prevent* chest pain, as does swallowing it in capsule or tablet form. In the form of sublingual (held under the tongue) or buccal (held in the cheek) tablets, or in an oral spray (sprayed on or under the tongue), it is used to *relieve* chest pain that is already underway. Leading brands of nitroglycerin include Nitro-Bid, Nitro-Dur, Nitrolingual Spray, Nitrostat Tablets, and Transderm-Nitro.

Beta-blockers, such as propranolol (Inderal), atenolol (Tenormin), metoprolol (Lopressor), and nadolol (Corgard), are also often used to treat angina. They work by blocking some of the nerve impulses that stimulate the heart. This decreases the force and rate of the heartbeat and lowers blood pressure, thus reducing the heart muscle's demand for oxygen.

Calcium-channel blockers are another option. They work by reducing the amount of calcium entering the muscle cells in the heart. With less calcium available, the muscle contracts less forcefully and the coronary arteries relax and expand. This has the effect of simultaneously reducing the heart's demand for oxygen while increasing its supply. This group of drugs includes verapamil (Isoptin, Calan), amlodipine (Norvasc), nifedipine (Procardia, Adalat), and diltiazem (Cardizem, Dilacor XR).

If the doctor finds that you have high cholesterol levels, which often foster the clogged arteries responsible for angina, your doctor may prescribe a cholesterol-lowering drug. See the entry on clogged arteries for more information.

Over-the-Counter Drugs

If you have angina, your doctor may direct you to take aspirin regularly. Aspirin helps thin the blood so blood clots won't form and block one of your partially obstructed coronary arteries, thus triggering a heart attack. When buying the medication, be sure to get aspirin—not acetaminophen or ibuprofen, which have no blood-thinning effect.

Herbal Remedies

Researchers have found that hawthorn leaf is capable of expanding the blood vessels and enabling more oxygen-rich blood to reach the muscles of the heart. Taken in extract form on a regular basis, it can reduce the tendency to angina, though it won't remedy an acute attack.

Nutritional Support

One of the surest ways to a healthy heart is to keep cholesterol levels under control, and the best way to do that is by eating a low-fat, high fiber diet. For more information, check the entry on clogged arteries.

Alternative Treatments

Although alternative medicine offers no cures for angina, there are several approaches that are said to reduce the risk of heart disease:

Macrobiotic Diet: This Asian-style vegetarian diet is low in fat and high in fiber, qualities that will keep your cholesterol in check. Beware, however, of an overly strict macrobiotic regimen. It can lead to nutritional deficiencies.

Naturopathic Medicine: This style of medicine emphasizes a diet high in fruits, vegetables, and whole grains—all standard recommendations for those facing heart disease.

Orthomolecular Medicine: Orthomolecular practitioners use vitamins as medications to prevent or cure chronic disorders. To lower the risk of heart disease, they recommend 400 IU of vitamin E, 3 milligrams of vitamin B6, and 400 micrograms of folic acid daily.

Vegetarianism: By excluding meat from the menu, vegetarians tend to reduce their intake of fat, cholesterol, and calories. This lowers cholesterol levels, with resulting benefits for the heart.

Stress is especially threatening for those with angina, and alternative medicine offers a variety of methods for fighting it off. If you find yourself under excessive stress, try some of the following:

Alexander Technique: A system of movement and posture training
Aromatherapy: Treatments with concentrated herbal oils
Aston-Patterning: A specialized form of physical training and massage
Guided Imagery: A mind/body therapy involving focused visualization
Hellerwork: A combination of deep massage and movement training
Massage Therapy: Relaxing bodywork to relieve tension
Qigong: Chinese exercises that improve fitness and reduce tension
Reflexology: A specialized foot massage said to relieve stress
Rolfing: A forceful deep-massage technique
Sound Therapy: Use of specially selected music to relieve stress
Yoga: A program of breathing exercises, body postures, and meditation with a proven calming effect

Anorexia

The Basics

Anorexia nervosa—refusal to eat—is not a trivial disorder. At its worst, it can end in life-threatening starvation.

Weight loss is the most visible symptom of anorexia. Stringent dieting leads first to loss of fat, later to loss of muscle tissue. The body begins to look like a skeleton, bones protrude, legs resemble matchsticks, and breasts disappear. Facial muscles tighten because there is no layer of fat beneath the skin to cushion them.

The word anorexia means "loss of appetite," but this name is misleading. Anorexics often have a normal appetite, but refuse to eat because a distorted body image has convinced them that they're obese. Despite an abnormal fear of fatness, they often have an obsessive interest in food. A typical anorexic will read about food, shop for, cook, and constantly think about food—in fact, will do everything with food except eat it.

Many anorexics are also compulsive exercisers, and their typical program is far more strenuous than normal. Women with anorexia often devote a major portion of their waking hours to aerobics, weight training, calisthenics, or running.

How can you tell the difference between a normal concern about weight and destructive anorexia? You should suspect a problem if you:

- Have lost at least 25 percent of your original weight, or weigh only 85 percent of what is considered normal weight for your height
- Still think of yourself as fat
- Fear being overweight and losing control of your eating behavior
- Refuse to eat enough to maintain or return to a normal weight
- Have not had your period for three months in a row
- Feel that all of your energy is going into controlling your weight
- Feel that staying hungry is the only way to keep your weight under control

The malnutrition that accompanies anorexia eventually triggers a variety of physical symptoms. Depriving the body of nutrition interferes with the hormonal cycles that regulate menstruation, bringing it to a halt. Many anorexic women also have glandular disorders leading to low levels of estrogen. Other common consequences of anorexia include:

- Constipation, digestive discomfort, and bloating
- Dehydration, muscle cramps, and tremors
- Growth of fine, downy body hair, especially on the face, back, or arms
- Flattened breasts
- Dull, brittle, thinning hair
- Cracked or dry skin, often with a yellow or gray cast
- Sensitivity to cold and icy hands and feet
- Irregular heartbeat
- Brittle bones (in severe cases)
- Depression and anxiety
- Anemia
- Dental problems
- Insomnia
- Lack of concentration

- Indecisiveness
- Mood swings
- Irritability
- Fatigue and lethargy

Anorexia is considered a behavioral disorder. While the specific cause is unknown, the condition seems to stem from a mixture of psychological, biological, familial, and cultural factors.

Certain personality traits increase the risk of developing anorexia. Anorexic girls are often described as "model children" or perfectionists. Faced with the impossible task of always being perfect, these girls discover that they can take charge of at least one aspect of their lives by exerting control over their eating and their weight.

Family background may also predispose a woman to anorexia. Many anorexics have parents who are themselves fascinated by fitness and appearance. If you have a mother or sister with anorexia, you are more likely to have the problem than someone with no history of the disorder in her family.

For some adolescents, ordinary biology poses a problem. As their bodies mature, many girls discover that they can no longer eat as they used to without gaining weight. Most can cut back as needed; a few lose control. Also, some experts theorize that girls who refuse to eat may be expressing a desire to remain childlike, free of adult bodies.

Anorexia is one of the most stubborn disorders a person can face. It is often complicated by other intractable psychological problems such as obsessive-compulsive behavior, social isolation, anxiety, and a revulsion toward fat and self-indulgence. Often a hidden depression lies at the core. It takes a combination of medical, psychological, and nutritional therapy to overcome this constellation of disorders. Treatment usually involves the patient's family as well, especially in the case of adolescent girls.

If anorexia remains untreated, it can be fatal. Roughly 10 to 20 percent of anorexics die from problems brought on by malnutrition—literally starve themselves to death. Others commit suicide. But treatment substantially improves the odds of survival. The mortality rate among those undergoing therapy is only 5 percent.

An estimated 50 to 70 percent of anorexics in treatment return to their normal or near-normal weight. Reaching this goal takes at least 6 months. About 15 to 20 percent will have an occasional relapse. Fifteen to 20 percent of anorexics need treatment for many years. Group therapy or an informal support group also can make a big difference.

Denial is one of the most consistent features of this disorder, and most anorexics resist treatment. It is usually up to a family member or close friend to recognize the problem and get the patient into treatment.

Call Your Doctor If . . .
■ You suspect that you or someone you know is anorexic.

Seek Care Immediately If . . .
■ You begin to have thoughts of suicide.
■ The situation seems life-threatening.

What You Can Do
Self-help doesn't work for anorexia because most victims are convinced that their attitudes toward food and weight are reasonable. They rarely seek medical care on their own.

If you have even a faint suspicion that you may be anorexic, or are worried about a friend or family member, ask your doctor for an evaluation or call a crisis hotline (listed in the Yellow Pages under Crisis Intervention Service). You may also wish to call the National Association of Anorexia Nervosa and Associated Disorders, an educational and self-help organization with information on this disorder.

Once you have begun treatment, if your doctor prescribes a medication, be sure to take it regularly, exactly as directed. Antidepressants, in particular, may take weeks to begin working. If the medication causes drowsiness, don't use mechanical equipment or drive.

What Your Doctor Can Do
The first step for the doctor will be to restore a normal or near-normal body weight. When an anorexic has lost so much weight that her life is in danger, the priority is to save her from starvation. Treatment may include forced nutrition through intravenous infusions and tube feeding. Hospitalization is usually advised if you weigh less than 70 percent of your recommended body weight, have rapidly progressing weight loss, and have symptoms such as irregular heartbeat, dizziness or fainting, and low potassium levels. Anorexia is probably the only psychiatric illness for which the most effective initial treatment is often a long stay in the hospital.

Stopping dangerous weight-loss tactics can produce some side effects such as temporary weight gain as the body becomes rehydrated. Cramps, abdominal fullness, and constipation may continue for some time during the readjustment period. If you experience any of these symptoms, don't panic and revert to the habits that made you sick.

After stabilizing her weight, the anorexic must relearn normal eating behavior and abandon drastic weight loss strategies. This can't be achieved without coming to grips with the personality and family problems that have helped cause the illness. Individual psychotherapy will help the anorexic face her problem, while family therapy helps those close to her change patterns of behavior that may have contributed to the disorder. In most instances, cases caught at an early stage can be treated in a clinic or doctor's office. You may need 1 to 4 appointments a month.

Prescription Drugs

No medicine can provide a quick cure for anorexia. Tranquilizers can reduce anxiety caused by hospitalization and a forced end to dieting. Certain antidepressant medications have also proved helpful for some patients. Typical choices include Adapin or Sinequan (doxepin), Aventyl or Pamelor (nortriptyline), Prozac (fluoxetine), Surmontil (trimipramine), and the manic-depression drug lithium. To relieve digestive problems that accompany readjustment to a normal diet, the doctor may also prescribe Propulsid (cisapride) or Reglan (metoclopramide). Periactin (cyproheptadine) is sometimes used as an appetite stimulant.

Over-the-Counter Drugs

There are several over-the-counter drugs that claim to suppress appetite, but none that do the opposite.

Herbal Remedies

Dozens of herbs have been found to give the appetite a mild stimulus, but none are likely to help an anorexic.

Nutritional Support

Nutritional counseling can offer practical help in developing a balanced, healthy diet.

Alternative Treatments

There are no holistic therapies aimed specifically at anorexia. To the extent that depression underlies the problem, however, certain forms of alternative therapy may help. The most likely candidates are *biofeedback* (a means of gaining control over involuntary responses and depression), *hypnotherapy* (often effective for depression, addictions, and compulsions), *massage therapy* (a remedy for excessive stress), and *sound therapy* (a mood-modulator).

Anxiety

The Basics

People suffering from anxiety disorders don't just feel "butterflies" in their stomachs—they feel a herd of elephants. It is this marked difference in intensity that distinguishes normal, everyday worrying from a true anxiety disorder. The ability to tolerate anxious feelings varies from person to person. When anxiety occurs at inappropriate times, however, or is so intense and long-lasting that it interferes with normal activities, then it's time to seek treatment.

Anxiety disorders are far from rare. They afflict an estimated 19 million Americans—more than any other emotional disorder, including depression, manic depression, and substance abuse. Potential causes are numerous. Researchers are currently investigating a number of possibilities, including chemical imbalances, enzyme deficiencies, emotional traumas, and the interaction between emotions and brain chemistry.

Diagnosis of an anxiety disorder is based largely on *physical* symptoms, which often include the following:

- Cold/clammy hands
- Diarrhea
- Dizziness
- Dry mouth
- Fast pulse
- Fatigue
- Jitteriness
- Lump in the throat
- Numbness/tingling of hands, feet, or other body parts
- Racing or pounding heart
- Rapid breathing
- Shakiness
- Sweating
- Tension
- Trembling
- Upset stomach

In addition, people plagued by anxiety are likely to harbor other distressing thoughts and feelings, such as impatience, apprehensiveness, irritability, and decreased ability to concentrate. They may also worry, for no particular reason, that something bad is going to happen to themselves or their loved ones. Although sufferers often realize that these thoughts are irrational, they find that they can't control them.

Anxiety disorders are divided into several (sometimes overlapping) categories. The American Psychiatric Association defines them as:

Generalized anxiety disorder: The hallmark of this problem is chronic worry and tension with no apparent cause. Sufferers often worry excessively about health, money, family, or work, while anticipating disaster. Although they are usually aware that their feelings are more intense than the situation warrants, they can't seem to let it go. This disorder often leads to depression.

Panic disorder: This condition is marked by brief episodes of intense fear—accompanied by pronounced physical symptoms, such as chest pains or sweating—that occur repeatedly and unexpectedly without an external threat. Because panic attacks "come out of the blue," people with this disorder grow anxious about the possibility of another attack. They then begin to avoid situations that they fear could trigger an attack.

Phobias: Unlike generalized anxiety disorder and panic disorder, in which symptoms arise without apparent reason, phobias are always focused on a specific threat. People with phobic illness feel terror, dread, or panic when anticipating a confrontation with the feared object, situation, or activity. There are three main types of phobias.

- *Specific phobias* involve fear of a particular object or situation, such as animals, heights, or driving. If the object of dread is easy to avoid, the sufferer may go through life without seeking treatment.
- *Social phobias* are marked by extreme anxiety about being judged by others or an exaggerated fear of public embarrassment. People with social phobias don't just feel uneasy around others—they experience extreme anxiety and avoid situations because of it.
- *Agoraphobia* is the fear of being alone or trapped in a public place. It often accompanies panic disorder if episodes have occurred outside the home.

Obsessive-compulsive disorder: Formally classified as an anxiety disorder, this illness inflicts persistent, unwanted thoughts on its victims, who often feel compelled to perform senseless rituals in an effort to quell their unwelcome feelings. The problem often goes hand-in-hand with depression, other anxiety disorders, and eating disorders. For a complete discussion, see the separate entry for this disorder.

Post-traumatic stress disorder: This condition develops in the aftermath of a severe physical or mental trauma, such as a rape, war, or kidnapping. Unlike other anxiety disorders, where tension or dread is the primary symptom, this condition is distinguished by the reliving of the traumatic event in a number of ways, such as nightmares and flashbacks.

Luckily, great strides have been made in treating anxiety disorders. They are no longer considered character flaws to be defeated by willpower or positive thinking. Treatment usually combines drug therapy—which is useful for short-term relief—with psychotherapy—which promotes longer-lasting behavioral and lifestyle changes.

Call Your Doctor If . . .

■ You have been excessively worried about a number of everyday problems for at least six months, and have at least six of the common anxiety symptoms listed earlier.

■ You have suffered four or more panic attacks and live in constant fear of having another.

■ You have a phobia that causes distress or interferes with your ability to work or socialize.

■ You have experienced or witnessed a recent trauma, such as a car or plane crash, sexual abuse, war, or natural disaster. Be alert for the following symptoms, especially if they last for more than a month:
  • Nightmares and flashbacks
  • Feeling numb or emotionally detached, or losing interest in favorite activities
  • Desire to withdraw from social activities
  • Feeling jumpy or "on guard"
  • Having violent thoughts or feelings
  • Insomnia
  • Problems concentrating
  • Physical distress when a memory arises

Seek Care Immediately If . . .
You are afraid that you will hurt yourself or someone else.

What You Can Do

■ Have a checkup to rule out disorders that can mimic anxiety, such as irregular heartbeat and thyroid disease.

■ Tell your doctor what prescription and over-the-counter drugs you are taking or have taken in the past. Stopping or starting certain medicines—diet pills, for example—can induce anxiety.

■ Seek counseling to remedy the underlying causes of abnormal anxiety.

■ Join a support group to learn how others have dealt with anxiety.

■ Learn breathing exercises and other relaxation techniques to help keep anxiety from escalating. (Check the suggestions under "Alternative Treatments.")

■ Exercise to reduce stress. Talk to your doctor about starting a program, with the goal of exercising for at least 20 minutes, six to seven days a week.

■ Seek help for any coexisting emotional problem—such as depression or substance abuse—in addition to receiving treatment for your anxiety.

What Your Doctor Can Do

The initial step is screening for underlying medical problems and medications that could be causing or contributing to your anxiety. After ruling these out, your doctor will probably take a dual approach, prescribing medication to control your symptoms quickly and recommending psychotherapy to return misdirected thought patterns to normal.

Research shows that two types of psychotherapy—behavioral therapy and cognitive-behavioral therapy—are especially effective treatments for several anxiety disorders. Behavioral therapy focuses on creating specific changes in action and behavior, while cognitive-behavioral therapy focuses on not only how to change behavior but also how to correct faulty thought patterns. This type of approach may be time-consuming, but it's well worth it: Cognitive-behavioral therapy has a low rate of relapse, while treatment with medication alone does not.

Prescription Drugs

In addition to tranquilizers, a number of antidepressant medications are now prescribed for anxiety—particularly panic disorder and obsessive-compulsive disorder. The medications you're most likely to encounter include:

Atarax or Vistaril (hydroxyzine)
Ativan (lorazepam)
BuSpar (buspirone)
Etrafon or Triavil (amitriptyline with perphenazine)
Klonopin (clonazepam)
Librium (chlordiazepoxide)
Limbitrol (amitriptyline with chlordiazepoxide)
Mebaral (mephobarbital)
Miltown (meprobamate)
Paxil (paroxetine)
Phenergan (promethazine)
Serax (oxazepam)
Tranxene (clorazepate)
Valium (diazepam)
Xanax (alprazolam)
Zoloft (sertraline)

Over-the-Counter Drugs

Anxiety disorders can't be treated with over-the-counter drugs.

Herbal Remedies

St. John's wort—traditionally used to treat depression—may also quell anxiety accompanying the depression. Several other herbs are considered remedies for nervousness, including bugleweed, hops, kava, lavender, lemon balm, passion flower, rauwolfia, and valerian.

Nutritional Support

Limit your intake of caffeine and alcohol. In sensitive individuals, the jitteriness precipitated by caffeine can reach panic levels. And even though alcohol is a depressant, both excessive consumption and abrupt withdrawal can lead to anxiety.

Alternative Treatments

Aromatherapy: This approach administers concentrated herbal oils by a variety of means—inhalation, massage, bathing, and compresses—in hope of relieving tension and anxiety. Although aromatherapy has no documented physical effects, it can serve as a comforting, relaxing ritual.

Biofeedback: This specialized technique uses equipment to monitor physiological reactions such as heart rate, blood pressure, brain waves, and muscle tension. You are then taught exercises to help gain control over these reactions. Biofeedback isn't a cure for anxiety disorders, but may help you limit exaggerated symptoms of fear.

Guided Imagery: This mind/body technique uses focused visualization to induce changes in the body, thereby alleviating stress and anxiety. It has no proven benefit in treating anxiety disorders, but it can be used to supplement other stress-reduction methods.

Hypnotherapy: With its ability to enhance the power of suggestion, this mind/body technique has been found effective for problems that hinge on emotions, habits, and even the body's involuntary responses. However, not everyone is susceptible to hypnosis.

Massage Therapy: With systematic manual application of pressure and movement to the soft tissues, massage can help relieve muscle strain, tension, and other symptoms of anxiety.

Meditation: The calming mental exercises of meditation—including the repetition of a phrase and concentration on breathing—are a proven antidote for stress, tension, anxiety, and panic.

Qigong: This ancient Chinese discipline uses visualization, movement, and breathing to improve overall physical fitness, balance, and flexibility. The ability of Qigong to treat any actual disorder remains to be verified, but it can enhance well-being and promote relaxation.

Sound Therapy: Treatment with specially selected music can reduce heart rate, blood pressure, and anxiety. It's often used to induce sleep, counteract fear, and reduce muscle tension.

Therapeutic Touch: This series of hand movements performed just above the body—akin to the "laying on of hands"—is said by its advocates to help relieve stress.

Yoga: This program of breathing exercises, body postures, and meditation has a proven calming effect and is an excellent supplement to mainstream anxiety treatments.

Appendicitis

The Basics

Each year, appendicitis (inflammation of the appendix) strikes about 1 person in 500. It is most common in people 15 to 25 years old.

The appendix is a small pouch hanging from the large intestine. If the entrance to the appendix gets blocked, infection can take hold, causing the appendix to become swollen, reddened, and filled with pus. The most common symptoms are abdominal pain (usually in the right lower side), fever, nausea, constipation, and vomiting. Occasionally there is diarrhea.

Your doctor may have trouble deciding whether the problem is really appendicitis. You probably will need some blood tests, plus an examination called abdominal ultrasound. If the appendix turns out to be infected, you'll need to have it surgically removed as quickly as possible. Left in place, it may burst, spreading dangerous infection throughout the abdomen.

Appendicitis can easily be fatal if left untreated, so be quick to call the doctor if you think it's developing.

Call Your Doctor If . . .

■ You have a high temperature.

■ Your pain gets worse or you start to vomit.

■ You pass out, become dizzy, or have a headache.

■ You notice blood in your stool or vomit.

After surgery, call if . . .

■ Your incision is swollen and red, or you see any pus. These are signs of infection.

■ Your stitches or staples come apart.

■ Your bandage becomes soaked with blood.

■ You develop a high temperature.

■ The pain in your abdomen gets worse.

Seek Care Immediately If . . .

■ You feel dizzy or confused, are urinating less, or have a dry mouth and tongue. These are signs of dehydration.

After surgery, seek emergency care if . . .

■ You suddenly have trouble breathing or start to have chest pain. You could have a blood clot in your lung or an allergy to one of your medicines.

What You Can Do

Before you go to the hospital . . .

■ To keep abdominal pain to a minimum, stay quietly seated in a chair.

■ Check with your doctor before taking painkillers or any of your regular medications.

■ You should not have anything to eat or drink just before surgery. Ask your doctor when to begin fasting.

■ Do not wear contact lenses to the hospital. You may wear your glasses.

After surgery . . .

■ Keep all incisions clean to prevent infection. When you are allowed to bathe or shower, carefully wash the stitches or staples with soap and water. Then put on a clean, new bandage. Change your bandage any time it gets wet or dirty.

■ For pain or swelling, you may put ice in a plastic bag, cover it with a towel, and place it over the incisions for 15 to 20 minutes out of every hour. Do not sleep on the ice pack. Treatment with ice is most effective when started right after the operation and used for 24 to 48 hours.

■ After the first 24 to 48 hours you may use heat for pain or swelling. Apply a heating pad (turned on low) or a hot water bottle, or sit in a warm water bath for 15 to 20 minutes out of every hour as long as you need relief. Do not sleep on the heating pad or hot water bottle. Heat brings blood to the area of the operation and helps it heal faster.

■ Get extra rest while you recuperate. Try to gradually increase your activity each day, resting whenever you feel it's needed. Avoid any heavy lifting until your doctor gives the OK.

What Your Doctor Can Do

Today doctors have two ways of removing the appendix. Both operations take 1 to 2 hours and require hospitalization for a few days after surgery.

■ **Open Appendectomy:** This is the traditional approach, in which the doctor removes the appendix through a large incision in the lower right-hand side of the abdomen.

■ **Laparoscopic Appendectomy:** In this newer type of procedure, the surgeon works through three small incisions in the abdomen instead of a single large one. Watching through a long tube equipped with a tiny lens and light, he maneuvers miniature surgical instruments into the abdomen and over to the appendix, which is then snipped off and pulled out. To give the surgeon an unobstructed view, the abdomen is inflated with carbon dioxide, which may leave you with shoulder pain for the first 2 days after the operation.

Prescription Drugs

While you are hospitalized for appendicitis, you will be treated with a number of prescription medicines:

■ **Antibiotics:** These medicines help prevent bacterial infection. They may be given by IV, as a shot, or by mouth.

■ **Pain Medicine:** To ease pain after the operation, your doctor will probably prescribe medication to be given by IV, as a shot, or by mouth. Tell the doctor or your nurses if the pain won't go away or keeps coming back.

■ **Anti-Nausea Medicine:** This medicine calms your stomach and controls vomiting. Your doctor may suggest you take it at the same time as your pain medicine, which sometimes upsets the stomach.

■ **Stool Softeners:** These medications make bowel movements softer so you won't need to strain.

Over-the-Counter Drugs

If you have constipation with the appendicitis, do not try to treat it with a laxative. This could cause the infected appendix to burst.

After an appendectomy, follow your doctor's directions regarding pain and fever medications.

Herbal Remedies

There are no herbs that will cure—or even relieve—appendicitis.

Nutritional Support

Appendicitis is an immediate medical emergency that diet can't help. To speed healing after the operation, a zinc supplement may help.

Alternative Treatments

There is no alternative to surgery.

Arthritis

The Basics

Afflicting one person in seven, arthritis is one of the most common ailments in America. Although there is still no cure, there are numerous ways to ease its debilitating effects.

Arthritis literally means "inflamed joints," and it lives up to its name by attacking joints and surrounding tissue anywhere in the body. It may amount to nothing more than mild stiffness in the hands or knees or may plague you with several painfully swollen, severely inflamed joints. The three most common types of arthritis are osteoarthritis, rheumatoid arthritis, and gout.

OSTEOARTHRITIS

Osteoarthritis (OA) is the most widespread type of arthritis and the only form directly related to age. Half of all adults over age 65 develop this problem.

Osteoarthritis occurs when the cartilage that normally cushions a joint becomes soft and breaks down. Bone surfaces in the affected joint can then make direct contact during movement, causing pain.

Symptoms of OA include joint stiffness, pain, and—occasionally—swelling. The most notable symptom is a dull aching in the joints at the end of the day. Usually, there is no fever, redness, or heat. The problem generally affects only one or two joints.

Factors linked to OA include heredity, excess weight, previous injuries, and overuse in sports and work-related activities.

RHEUMATOID ARTHRITIS

Rheumatoid arthritis (RA) is one of the more disabling forms of arthritis, though it varies in severity. While the cause is unknown, scientists suspect it may result from a malfunction of the immune system. Some people may have a hereditary tendency to the disease.

Hallmarks of rheumatoid arthritis include stiffness in muscles and joints, swelling in three or more joints, swelling of the hands and wrists, and swelling of the same joints on both sides of the body (such as both knees or wrists). Symptoms are most prominent in the morning. Fever, fatigue, and loss of appetite may accompany the inflammation. Swelling in the joints may lead to deformities and ultimately total immobility.

GOUT

Gout is caused by excess uric acid, a normal human waste product found in blood. When the body produces too much uric acid, crystal-like deposits form in and around the joints, causing agonizing pain.

Gout is marked by sudden swelling and pain, often in the big toe. Swelling may cause the skin to pull tightly around the joint and become very tender. Ankles, knees, elbows, wrists, and hands can also be affected.

Call Your Doctor If . . .

■ You have symptoms of arthritis that last more than two weeks.
■ You have any problems that may be related to the medicine you are taking for arthritis.

Seek Care Immediately If . . .

■ You develop chills, fever, or redness and tenderness of the affected joint.

What You Can Do

You can take a number of steps to ease the discomfort of arthritis and to improve and maintain your mobility.

■ Use appropriate medications. You may use over-the-counter drugs, ointments, and lotions; and your doctor can prescribe a variety of more potent medications.

■ Exercise. Regular exercise will keep your joints from becoming stiff, strengthen muscles around the joints, and maintain bone and cartilage. A daily walk, a swim, or a program that includes range-of-motion (stretching and flexibility) exercises can keep your joints working efficiently.

■ Rest. Exercise should be balanced with rest. Alternate heavy or repetitive tasks with easy ones. Plan rest breaks during walks and other daily activities. Rest is especially important when you have a joint that has become very painful. Resume normal activity when you feel better.

■ Protect joints. You should minimize the stress on affected joints. Use sturdy shoes and insoles to reduce stress on affected hips or knees. Try to position grocery bags, household appliances, tools, and other items to avoid joint stress. A good rule of thumb is to use the largest or strongest joints to support an object. For instance, grocery bags should be braced with forearms or palms instead of fingers.

■ Watch your weight. If you are overweight, lose the extra pounds and stay as close as possible to your recommended weight. Excess weight burdens joints like knees and hips.

■ Apply heat or cold. Heat or cold temporarily relieves pain and stiffness. Put a warm heating pad or warm, moist towels on the painful joint. Use ice compresses or cold packs to numb a joint. Whichever you choose, don't use either treatment for more than 20 minutes at a time.

■ Eat a healthy diet. A well-balanced diet, low in fats and cholesterol contributes to overall health. Arthritis pain can easily interfere with food shopping or cooking. Don't pass up nutritious foods because they tax swollen and aching joints—instead use prepared or frozen versions.

What Your Doctor Can Do

Medications are the first line of defense against the ravages of arthritis. For mild symptoms, the doctor may recommend an over-the-counter painkiller. For more advanced cases, he can select from a wide variety of prescription drugs.

If drug therapy fails to provide sufficient relief, the next step is often surgery to repair or replace the joint. In replacement surgery, the damaged joint is removed and a wear-resistant artificial joint made of metal and plastic is installed in its place. If you opt for the less radical repair procedure, the operation will probably be done through a special instrument called an arthroscope, which allows the surgeon to view the joint and repair any damage through a small incision.

Prescription Drugs

A class of drugs called nonsteroidal anti-inflammatories (NSAIDs) is the first choice for both rheumatoid and osteoarthritis. Drugs in this category include:

Anaprox and Naprosyn (naproxen)	Daypro (oxaprozin)	Nalfon (fenoprofen)
Arthrotec (diclofenac with misoprostol)	Dolobid (diflunisal)	Naprelan (naproxen sodium)
Cataflam and Voltaren (diclofenac)	Ecotrin (aspirin) Feldene (piroxicam) Indocin (indomethacin)	Orudis and Oruvail (ketoprofen)
Clinoril (sulindac)	Lodine (etodolac) Motrin (ibuprofen)	Relafen (nabumetone) Tolectin (tolmetin)

NSAIDs quell pain and inflammation by inhibiting the effect of a natural enzyme called COX-2. Unfortunately, they also interfere with a similar substance, called COX-1, which protects the stomach lining. As a result, they sometimes cause bleeding and ulcers in patients—such as arthritis sufferers—who have to take such medications regularly.

To overcome this problem, researchers recently introduced a new type of NSAID that interferes with COX-2 without defeating the protective effect of COX-1. The first of these drugs, dubbed "COX-2 inhibitors," is a product called Celebrex (celecoxib). It can be taken once or twice a day for osteoarthritis and twice a day for rheumatoid arthritis. If painkillers are giving you serious stomach disorders, another approach is to take the anti-ulcer drug Cytotec (misoprostol).

For severe arthritis, steroids such as Decadron (dexamethasone) and Deltasone (prednisone) can be used to reduce inflammation. These drugs are available in tablet form, or can be injected directly into the joint. For severe symptoms of rheumatoid arthritis, your doctor may turn to potent "second-line" drugs such as gold compounds. These medications come in capsule form—Ridaura (auranofin)—and as an injection—Solganal (aurothioglucose) and Myochrysine (sodium thiomalate). Newer drugs such as Cuprimine and Depen (penicillamine) work like gold salts, but cause fewer side effects.

Drugs that suppress the immune system head the last line of defense against RA. They include azathioprine (Imuran), etanercept (Enbrel), leflunomide (Arava), and methotrexate (Rheumatrex). Certain drugs for other medical conditions have also proved beneficial. These include an antimalarial drug called Plaquenil (hydroxychloroquine); Azulfidine (sulfasalazine), an anti-inflammatory medicine used for chronic bowel disease; anticancer drugs such as Cytoxan (cyclophosphamide) and Leukeran (chlorambucil); and Sandimmune or Neoral (cyclosporine), a drug used to prevent tissue rejection.

Gout, the third major form of arthritis, is treated in a completely different way. The usual prescription is a combination of colchicine and probenecid (ColBenemid), which work together to block joint inflammation and increase the elimination of uric acid. Sulfinpyrazone (Anturane) also is used to increase the elimination of uric acid, and allopurinol (Zyloprim, Lopurin) is used to prevent the formation of uric acid in the body.

Over-the-Counter Drugs

The safest choice for mild arthritis symptoms is plain old acetaminophen (Tylenol and others). Aspirin (Bayer, Bufferin) and ibuprofen (Advil, Nuprin, Motrin) are other frequently recommended remedies. Some ointments also offer short-term relief of minor arthritis pain.

Herbal Remedies

The most popular natural remedies for osteoarthritis are chondroitin and glucosamine. The herb colchicum (source of the prescription drug colchicine) can be used for gout. Products made with the cayenne pepper extract, capsaicin (Capsagel, Capzasin-P, Zostrix), provide temporary relief from rheumatoid arthritis pain. Other herbs considered effective for rheumatism include:

Arnica	Devil's Claw	Pine Oil
Ash	Eucalyptus	Rosemary
Balsam	Guaiac	Stinging Nettle
Boswellia	Larch	White Willow
Cajuput Oil	Mistletoe	Wintergreen
Camphor	Mustard	

Nutritional Support

Diets that attempt to counteract the effects of arthritis include:

■ Elimination diets, which aim to relieve the symptoms of arthritis by avoiding foods thought to aggravate the disease. Leading suspects include corn, wheat, red meat, fruit, and eggs.
■ Supplementation diets, which are based on the belief that high doses of vitamins, minerals, or fish oil will reduce inflammation.

Despite the popularity of these diets, experts have never been able to agree on their effectiveness. What works for one patient often fails for another. Most doctors simply recommend a healthy, balanced diet rich in all vitamins and minerals.

Still, if you suspect that something in your diet may be aggravating your arthritis, keep a diary of everything you eat, noting any change in your arthritis symptoms. Once you suspect a certain food is the culprit, stop eating it for at least five days; then add that food back into your diet to see what happens.

Research has shown that diets high in purines (organ meats, fish eggs, sardines, anchovies, beer, and wine) definitely *can* aggravate gout in people who have trouble dealing with uric acid. Alcohol also can trigger a gout attack. Eliminating these foods may help reduce chances of an attack, but won't cure the underlying disease.

Alternative Treatments

■ *Acupuncture* is often effective for short-term pain relief. It requires the insertion of tiny needles at specific "acupoints" on the skin. Scientists suspect that the needles trigger the release of natural painkillers within the body. The ancient Chinese believed that they enhanced the flow of vital energy.
■ *Alexander Technique,* a form of muscular reeducation, seeks to relieve arthritis by improving overall strength and mobility.
■ *Aromatherapy* uses highly concentrated essential oils extracted from herbs as a comforting ritual. Although some people say it eases the

pain of arthritis, medical science can find no physical reason for this effect.

■ *Biofeedback* captures information about your body's involuntary response to chronic pain, then relays it back to you so you can learn to modify counterproductive reactions.

■ *Energy Medicine* preys on desperate patients with a variety of unproven devices. However, there is one technique—transcutaneous electrical nerve stimulation (TENS)—that has been found effective in at least a few trials. It is thought to work by "drowning out" pain signals. It seems most effective against moderate, localized pain.

■ *Hydrotherapy* combines systematic application of hot and cold wet towels with administration of mild electrical stimulation in order to detoxify and balance the system.

■ *Magnetic Field Therapy* seeks to relieve joint pain with magnetic disks taped to the body. Some say the magnets change the electrical charges in the nervous system. Others think they pull on the charged particles in bodily fluids, thus improving circulation.

■ *Reconstructive Therapy* calls for a series of injections into damaged joints in order to speed healing of the damaged area. The injected solution is said to dilate blood vessels and trigger the migration of healing cells into the damaged tissue. Although reconstructive therapy has been validated in several clinical trials, qualified practitioners are still very hard to find in the U.S. Check with the American Association of Orthopedic Medicine for further details.

Asthma

The Basics

During an asthma attack, the airways in the lungs grow swollen and constricted, making it difficult to breathe. Symptoms include wheezing, coughing, and a tight feeling in the chest. Asthma cannot be cured, but it can be relieved with medicine. Repeat attacks are common.

A variety of irritants can trigger an asthma attack. Leading culprits include pollen, dust, animals, molds, some foods, sinus or lung infections, hormonal changes, smoke, exercise, high amounts of air pollution, changes in temperature or humidity, and stress. About 5 percent of those with asthma react badly to sulfite-containing foods, suffering mild to severe breathing difficulties and symptoms such as flushing, faintness, weakness, cough, and a bluish tinge to the skin. Severe sulfite reactions can end in loss of consciousness and death.

An estimated 10 million Americans have asthma. One-third of them are under 10 years of age.

Call Your Doctor If . . .
- Your symptoms get worse despite your regular medicine.
- You develop a high temperature.
- You have muscle aches or chest pain.
- Your sputum turns yellow, green, gray, or bloody, or becomes too thick to cough up.
- You have any problems that may be caused by your medicine (such as a rash, itching, swelling, or trouble breathing).

Seek Care Immediately If . . .
- You find that you can't say more than a few words without pausing for breath.
- You develop rapid, shallow breathing.
- Your heart rate speeds up and you begin to sweat.
- Your lips and nail beds turn pale or blue.
- You begin to feel tired and weak.

These are symptoms of a severe attack that may require emergency treatment. **Call 911 or 0 (operator)** to get help immediately. **Do not drive yourself!**

What You Can Do
There are a variety of prescription drugs that—if taken regularly—will keep asthma attacks to a minimum. Be sure to take the medication faithfully, exactly as prescribed. Do not quit taking it on your own; if you feel it is not helping, check with your doctor.

To reduce the chance of an asthma attack:
- Try to avoid pollen, dust, animals, molds, smoke, and anything else that could cause an attack.
- Keep the amount of dust in your home at a minimum. If necessary, hire a company to clean out the air ducts and vents in your house.
- Replace your pillows or mattress with materials that don't cause allergies. Look for bedding that is made of urethane or foam rubber and is labeled nonallergenic.

- Remember to drink 8 to 10 large glasses of water each day. This helps thin the sputum so it can be coughed up more easily.
- If animals are the cause of your asthma, you may need to find another home for your pets.
- If you smoke, make a determined effort to quit. Ask your doctor about quit-smoking aids such as the prescription drug Zyban and nicotine patches, inhalers, and gum.
- Do not use aspirin, which is known to trigger attacks in many asthma sufferers. Also be cautious with other nonsteroidal anti-inflammatory drugs, such as Naprosyn and Motrin.

If you have an asthma attack:
- Use your inhaler. If this does not help, repeat the inhaler one more time after waiting the number of minutes recommended by your doctor. If the second try doesn't work, check to see whether there's any medication left in it. The inhaler is empty if it floats in a bowl of water.
- You may find it easier to breathe if you straddle a chair backwards, placing your elbows up on the back of the chair.

If you do not know what causes your attacks:
- Make a note of the time of each attack and what your surroundings were at the time.
- Consider allergy testing if you have not already had it done.

What Your Doctor Can Do

Doctors often prescribe one medication to prevent or reduce the number of attacks, and another to relieve attacks once they're under way. For a really acute attack, you may need oxygen, breathing treatments, and airway-opening medications given by IV injection in the hospital. If a bacterial infection is complicating your condition, the doctor may prescribe an antibiotic.

Prescription Drugs

Treatment of asthma usually includes administration of medicines that reduce inflammation and open the air passages. For patients with daily symptoms, inhaled steroids such as Azmacort, Beclovent, Vanceril, and AeroBid are frequently prescribed, as are cromolyn sodium (Intal), nedocromil sodium (Tilade), theophylline (Theo-Dur, Uniphyl), and albuterol (Proventil, Ventolin). For prevention of attacks, the choices include zafirlukast (Accolate), montelukast (Singulair), salmeterol (Serevent), and zileuton (Zyflo).

Over-the-Counter Drugs

Primatene Mist (epinephrine) or Primatene tablets (ephedrine and guaifenesin) can provide temporary relief from the shortness of breath, chest tightness, and wheezing that mark an asthma attack. They work by reducing spasms in the muscles of the bronchial passages. Primatene tablets also include an ingredient that loosens phlegm to keep the passageways clear.

Do not use these medications without your doctor's approval if you have heart disease, high blood pressure, thyroid disease, diabetes, an enlarged prostate gland, chronic cough, or cough with excessive phlegm. Also check with your doctor before using them if you have ever been hospitalized for asthma.

Herbal Remedies

There are no herbs deemed effective specifically for asthma. However, you might want to experiment with those recommended for bronchitis (inflammation of the airways)—including ephedra, the original source of ephedrine.

Nutritional Support

A study reported in the *British Medical Journal* has linked high salt consumption with deaths from asthma in men and children. Although the results of the small-scale study were by no means conclusive, they did demonstrate a relationship between high-sodium diets and asthma that should not be overlooked by parents of asthmatic children.

Alternative Treatments

Acupuncture: Some research suggests that acupuncture may be useful—along with other more conventional therapies—in the treatment of asthma. Acupuncture relies on the insertion of fine needles at special "acupoints" on the skin to work beneficial changes inside the body.

Biofeedback: For asthmatics, biofeedback offers the possibility of controlling bronchial spasms and reducing the severity of attacks. Biofeedback training enables patients to alter specific, measurable physiological functions that are ordinarily beyond conscious control.

Hypnotherapy: This approach doesn't work for everybody, but for those who are susceptible, it has successfully alleviated an amazing range of symptoms, including those of asthma. Hypnosis often provides symptomatic relief, but it can't cure any physical disorders, and should never be used as a replacement for conventional therapy. Seek standard medical care first and use hypnosis as an adjunct.

Trager Integration: This light, gentle form of massage therapy has been advocated as a treatment for asthma. By rhythmically stretching tense muscles and rocking stiff joints, Trager therapists attempt to release deeply ingrained tensions, promoting a sense of relaxation and freedom.

Attention Deficit Disorder

The Basics

Kids will be kids—full of energy and hard to control—but you're likely to know it when a child is afflicted with a full-blown case of attention deficit disorder. Kids with this problem are unusually impulsive and easily distracted. Although hyperactivity is *not* always an issue, victims typically seem exceptionally fidgety or jittery. Tip-offs of this condition include some or all of the following:

- Constant talking or motion
- Trouble following directions
- Inattention to what people are saying
- Inability to focus on a single activity for long
- Moving from task to task without completing the job
- Difficulty staying seated in school
- Squirming and fidgeting while seated
- Difficulty playing quietly
- Failure to wait their turn
- A tendency to lose things and to be disorganized
- Doing and saying things without thinking
- Lack of control over their actions, sometimes resulting in damage or injury
- Failure to consider the consequences of an action. For example, running into the street without checking for traffic.

The problem is not uncommon; it affects an estimated 5 to 10 percent of school-aged children. It's 10 times more likely among boys than girls.

The disorder usually starts before age 4, and invariably before age 7. It's almost certain to interfere with schoolwork, and often disrupts relations with friends and family. Many children never fully grow out of the problem, carrying impulsivity, restlessness, and attitude problems along into adulthood.

Scientists have yet to find a cause, although an imbalance in the brain's chemical messengers seems a likely culprit. The problem seems to run in families. Psychoactive medications are the standard remedy.

Call Your Doctor If . . .
■ The child can't sleep or sleeps too much.
■ The child is hurting himself or others.
■ You feel you can no longer cope with the situation.
■ You fear you're going to lose patience and hurt the child.

Seek Care Immediately If . . .
This condition does not constitute an emergency.

What You Can Do
■ Make sure the child takes his prescribed medicine regularly, exactly as directed.
■ Take advantage of family counseling services. They can give you valuable advice for dealing with the situation.
■ Sessions with the doctor can also help. They give both you and the child a chance to discuss the problem away from your usual routine.
■ Make lists and use a calendar to help the child remember obligations. Be sure to praise him for doing well.
■ Establish well-defined limits on conduct and apply them consistently.
■ Call a time-out when the child acts up at home. After he calms down, discuss what happened.
■ Make sure that the people in the child's life are familiar with the disorder. Work with his teachers to help solve classroom problems.
■ Each month have meetings at home where family members can ventilate their feelings about the way things are going.
■ Provide plenty of opportunities for exercise and active play.
■ Regular sleep is very important for a child with this problem. If your child can't sleep, let your doctor know.

What Your Doctor Can Do

Doctors have found that several stimulant drugs tend to have a paradoxical calming effect on children with this disorder. The doctor may also recommend various forms of non-drug therapy, such as role-playing and self-monitoring of behavior.

Prescription Drugs

Methylphenidate (Ritalin), a mild central nervous system stimulant, is the usual remedy for attention deficit disorder. The antidepressant drug imipramine (Tofranil) is sometimes prescribed instead. Other possibilities include the amphetamine product Adderall, dextroamphetamine (Dexedrine, DextroStat), methamphetamine (Desoxyn), and pemoline (Cylert).

Ritalin, Cylert, and the various amphetamine products all have abuse potential and must be taken exactly as directed. Potential side effects include insomnia, loss of appetite, and weight loss.

Over-the-Counter Drugs

Nothing available over the counter relieves this disorder.

Herbal Remedies

There are no herbs known to affect this problem.

Nutritional Support

If your child is hyperactive or prone to temper tantrums, food may be one of the problems. Some children are sensitive to salicylates (a group of compounds related to aspirin), certain food additives, monosodium glutamate (MSG), other food enhancers, and sugary foods. You may wish to discuss with your pediatrician the Feingold diet, for example, which is completely additive- and salicylate-free, and therefore highly restrictive and difficult to follow. Studies of this diet have been contradictory and inconclusive. One found that roughly one-third of a group who faithfully followed the diet enjoyed a dramatic improvement in behavior. Another found no beneficial effect at all.

Even if you do not choose to follow a diet, per se, it is still wise to avoid chocolate, cola, and anything else containing caffeine if your child is jittery or hyperactive. Although most experts agree that sugar has been overrated as a cause of hyperactivity, some children do react to specific sugars such as cane or beet sugar. You may wish to avoid foods with excessive amounts of processed sugars and see if any difference in behavior results. Natural sugars, such as those found in fruits, are usually not a problem.

Alternative Treatments

Biofeedback: This specialized training allows people to gain control over physiologic reactions that are ordinarily unconscious and automatic. It has successfully reduced the symptoms of attention deficit disorder in some patients.

Sound Therapy: Proponents of certain auditory feedback treatments report positive results for attention deficit disorder and various learning difficulties. Possibilities to investigate include the *Tomatis Method,* the *Berard Method,* and *SAMONAS (Spectral Activated Music of Optimal Natural Structure).* However, studies of the effectiveness of these treatments have so far been inconclusive.

Back Pain

The Basics

Back pain is almost universal. An estimated 80 percent of Americans suffer from back problems at one time or another. Failure to find the cause is also quite common. As many as 85 percent of patients can't get a definitive diagnosis from their doctors. But here's the good news: Even with no treatment at all, nine out of ten patients will recover in a month.

Potential causes are numerous. Problems often result from a combination of bad habits, heredity, and normal wear and tear on the body. Lack of movement and slouching may cause pain in people who sit or stand for long periods. Conversely, muscle strain from repetitive motion and bad posture while bending, lifting, or twisting can affect those who are more active.

Other potential troublemakers include:
- Being overweight by more than 20 pounds
- Wearing high-heeled shoes
- Carrying heavy tote bags, purses, or briefcases
- Childbirth
- Osteoporosis ("brittle bone" disease)
- Arthritis of the spine
- An infection or tumor

■ A ruptured disk or nerve damage
■ Hardening and stiffening of the spinal cord

Back pain usually stems from an injury in one of three areas: (1) the soft tissues attached to your spine—the muscles, ligaments, and tendons, (2) the joints between the vertebrae that make up the spine, and (3) the disks between the vertebrae. The disks are the spine's shock absorbers and, when injured, can become ruptured or herniated (sometimes referred to, inaccurately, as a slipped disk). A ruptured disk in the lower back can put pressure on the sciatic nerve, causing sciatica—sharp, shooting pain that runs from the buttock and down the back of the leg to the foot.

Sometimes back pain is caused by problems in organs unrelated to the back's machinery. Trouble in the kidneys, liver, ovaries, or pancreas is occasionally signaled by pain in the back. Less serious ailments—menstrual cramps, for example—can also take the form of backaches.

Back pain doesn't always require a doctor visit. You can try treating it yourself with over-the-counter painkillers, rest, ice packs, and warm, moist compresses or a heating pad. Physical manipulation, such as chiropractic therapy, can be used to relieve pain when self-treatment fails to help. However, if your pain lingers or worsens, or if you remain unable to perform everyday activities, see a doctor immediately.

Call Your Doctor If . . .
■ You have any of the following symptoms:
  • Sudden severe pain
  • Pain limited to the spine
  • Shooting pains in your buttocks, groin, or legs
  • Unsteadiness or falling when walking
  • Pain associated with a recent fall or traumatic experience
  • Pain accompanied by fever or weight loss
  • Pain that does not lessen over time

Seek Care Immediately If . . .
■ You have trouble urinating or lose control of your bladder or bowels.
■ You develop numbness or weakness in your legs or feet.

What You Can Do

To ease the pain:

■ A short stay in bed—up to 24 hours—is okay if it hurts too much to move. Walk a little every few hours to keep the blood flowing and the muscles toned.

■ For the first day or two, apply ice to the injury for 10 to 20 minutes each hour. Put the ice in a plastic bag and place a towel between the bag and your skin.

■ After 2 days, you may apply heat to the injury to help relieve pain. Use a warm heating pad, whirlpool bath, or warm, moist towels for 10 to 20 minutes every hour for 48 hours.

■ Resume light activities such as walking as soon as possible.

To prevent an encore:

■ When picking things up, never bend from the waist. Instead, bend at the hips and knees.

■ Wear low-heeled shoes.

■ When sleeping:
  • Use a firm mattress, or put a ½- to 1-inch piece of plywood between the mattress and box springs.
  • Do not use a waterbed; it will not support your back correctly.
  • Choose a position that supports your back. You can either (1) sleep on your back with a pillow under your knees, or (2) sleep on your side with your knees bent and a pillow between them.

■ The right kind of exercises will strengthen your back and reduce the chances of another strain. However, some types can cause further injury. Check with your doctor before undertaking any exercise program.

What Your Doctor Can Do

Your doctor will probably ask a series of questions meant to rule out disk problems and other disorders, then conduct a hands-on examination of the spine and its movement. You'll also be asked to report any changes in the type or degree of pain you feel as you perform a variety of movements.

Be aware that unless there are signs of other trouble—such as a possible fracture, damaged nerve, or infection—costly scans and x-rays usually aren't needed. The reason? When spine abnormalities appear on such tests, they may be purely coincidental. Many people with normal scans have back pain, and others with abnormal scans have no pain at all.

For most types of back pain, treatment with medication, chiropractic, or physical therapy is all that's recommended. Most experts believe that people with typical back pain—that is, pain that does *not* radiate down a leg—do not need surgical treatment. Surgery should be performed only in the rarest of emergencies and never before other treatments have been given a fair chance.

Prescription Drugs

If over-the-counter painkillers have not been helpful, your doctor may prescribe a stronger medication such as oxaprozin (Daypro), or muscle relaxers such as methocarbamol (Robaxin) or diazepam (Valium). The doctor may also offer an injection of an anesthetic such as procaine (Novocain) to relieve a muscle spasm. Rarely, the doctor may inject a steroid such as cortisone to reduce inflammation in a joint or relieve the pressure of a disk on a nerve.

Over-the-Counter Drugs

Nonprescription painkillers are not only permissible but actually recommended for most cases of back pain. You can choose from a broad array of products:

Actron	Doan's	Nuprin
Advil	Ecotrin	Orudis
Aleve	Excedrin	Pamprin
Ascriptin	Excedrin, Aspirin	Panadol
Backache Caplets	Free	St. Joseph
Bayer	Goody's	Tylenol
BC Powder	Midol	Vanquish
Bufferin	Motrin	YSP

Herbal Remedies

While no herbal remedy can cure a back problem, a few can provide pain relief. Applied externally as a cream, capsaicin (an ingredient of cayenne pepper) helps relieve painful muscle spasms in the spine. Japanese mint oil rubbed on the skin can relieve muscle and nerve pain. And white willow, an aspirin-like compound taken internally, is considered a remedy for all types of pain.

Nutritional Support

No dietary measures seem to help this problem.

Alternative Treatments

Acupuncture: This ancient Chinese therapeutic technique calls for insertion of tiny needles at specific points on the skin in an effort to redirect the flow of vital energy along hypothetical channels within the body. Surprisingly, it affords significant relief to many back-pain sufferers.

Chiropractic: Spinal adjustments—manual pressure on the joints of the spine—can relax muscles, break up adhesions or scar tissue, and move displaced vertebrae back into place. Mounting evidence shows that this form of manipulation can provide genuine relief for sudden low back pain.

Energy Medicine: A wide variety of electrical devices promise to relieve pain, but few if any have been proven effective. *Transcutaneous Electrical Nerve Stimulation (TENS)* appears to show the most promise.

Hydrotherapy: The application of hot and cold water or water-soaked compresses has long been a standard remedy for pain.

Hypnotherapy: This mind/body technique, which relieves symptoms through the power of suggestion, is capable of relieving virtually any type of pain—provided you're susceptible.

Massage Therapy: With systematic manual application of pressure and movement to the soft tissues, massage can relieve the muscle strain that underlies many attacks of back pain.

Myotherapy: This specialized form of deep-muscle massage focuses on "trigger points"—damaged, tender spots in the muscles.

Osteopathic Medicine: This branch of medicine supplements standard care with physical manipulation—ranging from light pressure on soft tissue to high-velocity thrusts on the joints. Osteopathic manipulation is considered particularly effective for musculoskeletal disorders such as back pain.

Reconstructive Therapy: With a series of injections made directly into damaged joints, this form of therapy aims to jump-start the healing process. Low back pain is one of its primary targets.

Rolfing: A type of vigorous, deep-tissue massage, this technique seeks to loosen and relax the fascia—the membranes that surround the muscles.

Trager Integration: This form of therapy attacks back pain with light, gentle massage, then follows up with special exercises done between sessions.

Several other alternative forms of treatment address the poor balance, posture, and coordination that often foster back problems. Options to consider include:

Alexander Technique: A system of movement training that focuses on the relationship of the head, neck, and torso

Aston-Patterning: A specialized form of physical training and massage

Feldenkrais Method: A system that combines movement training with gentle manipulation of muscles and joints

Hellerwork: An offshoot of Rolfing that combines deep-tissue massage with movement training

Breast Cancer

The Basics

Breast cancer is frighteningly common: It strikes 1 out of every 8 American women. There are 175,000 new cases each year, and before age 55, more women die of breast cancer than any other cause. Yet the news is not all bad. When the disease is discovered early enough, over 95 percent of the victims are cured.

How worried should *you* be? We know that some women are more likely to get breast cancer than others. For example, if your mother or sister (or both) have had breast cancer, your estimated risk is 10 to 15 times higher than that of a woman whose close female relatives are breast cancer-free. Risk also increases with age. If your periods started before age 12 or continued after age 55, you're at higher risk. And women who have their first baby after age 35 are twice as likely to develop breast cancer as those who give birth in their teens.

Breast cancer is most common among Caucasian women and least common among Asians. It occurs more frequently in women who are overweight, who live in big cities, who earn high incomes, and in those who have been exposed to radiation. Some researchers used to blame birth control pills for an increased risk of breast cancer, but modern contraceptives seem to be free of any danger. There's also a theory that failure to breastfeed increases your risk, but the jury remains out on the validity of this idea.

For most women, the first sign of breast cancer is a mass or lump in a breast. (Remember, however, that 3 out of every 4 lumps discovered are *not* cancerous.) The second most common sign is a clear, bloody, or colored discharge from a nipple. (But, again, a discharge can be perfectly normal, even in women who are not breastfeeding.) Other signs include a change in shape or size of the breast or swelling of the skin that covers it. Breast tissue may feel thicker, or you may notice pain or redness of the skin.

Call Your Doctor If . . .

■ You notice any lumps or changes in your breasts.
■ You have breast pain or a discharge from your nipples.

Remember: Your best protection against the disease is an early diagnosis. Don't let fear prevent you from investigating signs or changes.

Seek Care Immediately If . . .

Discovery of a lump is not an immediate emergency. But don't put off making an appointment to check it out.

What You Can Do

One of the most important things a woman can do is *monthly breast self-examinations (BSEs).* Getting to know your breasts and being able to notice the slightest changes in them are your best protection.

The best time to check your breasts is about 1 week after your period ends, when the breasts are usually not swollen, lumpy, or tender. If your periods have stopped due to pregnancy or menopause, pick a regular day each month to do the exam. If you've had a hysterectomy, your doctor can tell you which day to choose. Even if you have breast implants, you should do an exam each month.

Use the following procedure to check your breasts:

■ Stand in front of a mirror with your arms at your sides. Look at each breast and nipple to check for swelling, lumps, dimpling, scaly skin, or other skin changes.
■ Join your hands behind your head, then push them forward while looking at your breasts in the mirror. Next, press your hands firmly on your hips and bow slightly towards the mirror, pulling your shoulders and elbows forward. Inspect the breasts again.
■ Lie down and put a pillow or towel under your left shoulder. Put your left hand over your head, then begin to gently press into the skin of your left breast using the pads of the first 3 fingers of your

right hand. Start at the outer part of the breast and slowly move around it in a clockwise direction. Vary the pressure at each spot from light to heavy. Squeeze your nipple to check for liquid coming from it. Check your right breast the same way.

■ Finally, check the lymph nodes near each breast. Raise your left arm and, using the pads of the first 3 fingers of your right hand, feel in and around your armpit. Do the same thing with the other armpit.

Your breasts can also be checked while you are bathing. Lumps can be felt more easily when your skin is wet.

In addition, be sure to have a physician or other health care professional examine your breasts once a year from age 20 onward. Start getting mammograms (breast x-rays) when you reach age 40. Between ages 40 and 49, you should get one every one or two years. Starting at age 50, they should be conducted annually. They are important because they can spot lumps that are too small to feel during a breast examination.

What Your Doctor Can Do

If you notice a lump or anything else that seems suspicious, the next step will be an examination, followed by a mammogram and perhaps a *biopsy*. Remember, most lumps are not cancerous. One type of biopsy, known as a *fine needle aspiration*, can be performed quickly in your doctor's office under a local anesthetic. But if this procedure does not provide the answers the doctor is looking for, you may need a *core needle biopsy*. This alternative, which also can be performed with a local anesthetic, uses a larger needle to take a sample of the mass.

If neither procedure provides definitive answers, your doctor will probably recommend a *surgical biopsy* in order to obtain a sample of the tumor and surrounding tissue for microscopic examination. Surgical biopsies are usually performed on an outpatient basis at a hospital or clinic.

Sometimes *ultrasound*—which forms a picture by bouncing sound waves off the mass—is useful for locating lumps in younger women, whose breast tissue is typically more dense and harder to penetrate with x-rays. Ultrasound is also used for evaluating masses that lie deep within the breast and cannot be felt or reached with a needle.

If cancer is diagnosed, the doctor will discuss treatment options with you. The goal of therapy is always to prevent the spread of cancer if the disease is confined to the breast and to minimize the possibility of a recurrence of cancer in the future.

Often the leading option is some form of *mastectomy*—surgical removal of part or all of the breast. The extent of mastectomy is determined mostly by the extent of disease. Another surgical option is a *lumpectomy*—removal of only the tumor and possibly a few lymph nodes located around the breast and armpit. Removal of lymph nodes is sometimes necessary to prevent the cancer cells from spreading to other parts of the body. Various forms of *breast reconstruction* are possible after a mastectomy is performed.

Your doctor may also recommend *radiation*. Radiation therapy involves beaming x-rays at the site of the tumor to kill the growing cancer cells. It is a promising option during the early stages of cancer. In fact, some studies show it to be just as effective as a mastectomy. It is also often used after a lumpectomy to make sure no cancer cells remain. And doctors sometimes employ it to shrink especially large tumors prior to surgery or to slow the growth of inoperable tumors. Some women who undergo radiation develop red, peeling, or itchy skin similar to a sunburn, but find it disappears as soon as treatment ceases.

Prescription Drugs

Chemotherapy is a follow-up to surgery or radiation. It typically calls for a combination of potent drugs that will destroy cancer cells no matter where they may remain in the body. This anticancer "cocktail" is usually administered intravenously (though some drugs may be swallowed or injected into the muscle) every 3 to 4 weeks for anywhere from 4 to 24 months. Though these drugs are highly effective against cancer cells, they also tend to destroy healthy cells, often causing debilitating side effects such as nausea, vomiting, fatigue, and hair loss. They also make the body less able to fight infections and other diseases.

Hormone therapy, a relatively new addition to the therapeutic arsenal for breast cancer, is aimed at preventing a return of the cancer. Some cancer cells have hormone receptors for estrogen and won't grow—or won't grow as fast—if they are deprived of estrogen. The most drastic way to eliminate estrogen is to remove the ovaries, which produce virtually all of the body's supply. A much more common approach is use of the drug called Nolvadex (tamoxifen), which works by attaching itself to the estrogen receptors and blocking the estrogen from doing its cancer-promoting work. The drug is taken twice a day for up to 5 years. A related drug, Evista (raloxifene), has not been studied for the treatment of breast cancer, but may have a preventive effect when taken before cancer develops.

Over-the-Counter Drugs

Nothing available over the counter can help against cancer.

Herbal Remedies

There are no herbs known to be capable of curing cancer.

Nutritional Support

To *prevent* breast cancer, one of the most important things you can do is to eat a low-fat, high-fiber diet. Make sure that no more than 30 percent of your daily calories come from fat, and that no more than 10 percent derive from saturated fat. At the same time, boost your intake of fiber to between 20 and 30 grams a day (roughly twice the amount in the average American diet). You can do this by eating more fruits, vegetables, and whole grains.

Also be sure to get an adequate supply of *antioxidant* vitamins. These include vitamins E and C and beta carotene. Boost your intake of other *carotenoids* as well. Lycopene (in tomatoes) and lutein and zeaxanthin (in broccoli) appear to be especially potent cancer fighters.

An assortment of other *phytochemicals* (naturally occurring compounds in plants) may also help to protect against breast cancer. Foods especially rich in these chemicals include garlic, broccoli, cauliflower, cabbage, brussels sprouts, parsley, carrots, citrus fruits, berries, cucumbers, peppers, squash, yams, tomatoes, eggplant, and soy products.

Alternative Treatments

Hyperthermia: Some cutting-edge physicians are experimenting with a procedure called diathermy—a form of heat treatment that uses electricity, ultrasonic waves, or microwaves to boost the temperature of diseased tissue. Some studies indicate that the technique may make cancer cells more vulnerable to other forms of treatment.

Broken Bones

The Basics

Some very minor fractures (the medical term for a break) may cause only passing discomfort, but most broken bones are a source of considerable pain, swelling, bruising, and possibly even bleeding. An affected limb may feel weak or numb, or may tingle. It may look injured or out of alignment. You may have difficulty moving it, or may not be able to move it at all.

If a broken bone isn't set properly, it may become permanently disfigured, fail to regain normal function, or turn into a source of chronic pain. To keep the bone from moving out of alignment while it heals, the doctor will probably need to put a cast or a splint on it. A serious fracture may need surgery. Healing time depends on the location and nature of the fracture, and can take from weeks to months.

Call Your Doctor If . . .
■ The cast gets damaged or breaks.
■ Your pain gets worse instead of better.
■ You have more swelling than you did before the cast was put on.
■ The skin or the nails below the cast turn blue or gray.
■ The skin below the cast feels cold or numb.
■ There is a bad smell from the cast.
■ There are new stains coming from under the cast.
■ The fracture needed surgery and
  • Your incision is swollen and red, or you see any pus. These are signs of infection.
  • Your stitches or staples come apart.
  • Your bandage or cast becomes soaked with blood.
  • You are running a high temperature.

What You Can Do
Always see a doctor if you suspect a broken bone. Don't try to ignore it or set it yourself. Once the bone is properly set, follow these guidelines to reduce pain and prevent complications.

■ To relieve swelling, keep an injured arm or leg elevated above your heart.
■ Apply ice to the injury for 15 to 20 minutes each hour for the first 1 to 2 days. Put the ice in a plastic bag and place a thin towel between the bag of ice and your cast.
■ If you have a plaster or fiberglass cast:
  • Do not try to scratch the skin under the cast by pushing a sharp or pointed object down the cast.
  • Check the skin around the cast every day. You may put lotion on any red or sore areas.

• If your fiberglass cast gets a little wet, it can be dried with a hair dryer.

■ If you have a plaster splint:

• Wear the splint for as long as directed or until your follow-up examination.

• You may loosen the elastic around the splint if your toes or fingers become numb or begin to tingle.

■ Do not push, lean, or put pressure on any part of the cast or splint; it may break.

■ Keep the cast or splint dry. During bathing, protect it with a plastic bag. Do not lower it into water.

■ If your doctor prescribes pain medication, take no more than directed. If the medication makes you drowsy, don't drive. You may also use over-the-counter painkillers.

■ If you've had a leg injury, you'll need to use crutches, a cane, or a walker while the fracture heals. Ask your doctor or nurse for instructions. A sling may be necessary to support a cast on an elbow, arm, wrist, or hand.

What Your Doctor Can Do

Most fractures can be treated by putting a cast around the break. The cast can be made of plaster or fiberglass. Plaster looks and feels smooth, while fiberglass looks like woven cloth and feels rough on the outside. Fiberglass also comes in many different colors. The cast will feel hard within 10 to 15 minutes after it is applied. However, it takes 24 hours to dry completely, so be careful with it for the first day, while it still can easily crack.

If you suffer a severe fracture in one of the bones of an arm or leg, the doctor may need to realign the pieces through a surgical incision, then apply metal screws or plates to hold them together while they heal. The surgical realignment is called an open reduction. Application of the screws and plates is known as internal fixation. In addition to the internal fixation, you may need to wear a cast or a splint after the operation. You could be in the hospital 1 to 3 days, or might be allowed to go home the same day.

During the operation, the doctor may have to take x-rays to make sure the pins and plates are positioned correctly. Drills and other devices may come into play. Surgeons sometimes use a microscope to help them see small bones and nerves. After the operation, the incision will be closed with thread or staples. The surgery may last 1 to 3 hours.

There are always risks with surgery. Even after the operation, the bone may not heal correctly. If the nerves or blood vessels that lead to the bone were injured when it was broken, the bone could die. There's also a slight danger of developing a body-wide infection. However, if you have a bad fracture, the chances of the bone returning to normal without surgery are very slim.

After surgery, the incision will be bandaged to keep the area clean and prevent infection. You'll need to stay in bed until the doctor says it's safe to get up. You may need to take several medicines, including: antibiotics to prevent infection, pain medicine, anti-nausea medicine to control vomiting, stool softeners to prevent constipation, and blood thinners to prevent blood clots from forming.

Prescription Drugs

While the pain remains severe, the doctor can prescribe a variety of pain-killing pills. Typical medications include:

DHCplus (acetaminophen with dihydrocodone)
Dilaudid (hydromorphone)
Hydrocet, Lorcet, Lortab, Vicodin, or Zydone (acetaminophen with hydrocodone)
Kadian, MS Contin, or MSIR (morphine)
Levo-Dromoran (levorphanol)
OxyContin, OxyIR, or Roxicodone (oxycodone)
Percocet or Tylox (acetaminophen with oxycodone)
Percodan (aspirin with oxycodone)
Talwin Nx (naloxone)
Toradol (ketorolac)
Tylenol with Codeine (acetaminophen with codeine)
Ultram (tramadol)
Vicoprofen (hydrocodone)

Over-the-Counter Drugs

Once the pain has subsided, it can be controlled with standard non-prescription painkillers such as aspirin, acetaminophen, or ibuprofen.

Herbal Remedies

Two herbs also offer relief from mild pain: Japanese mint and white willow.

Nutritional Support

While the bone is healing, it's especially important to maintain a diet rich in amino acids and such building blocks of bone as calcium and phosphorus.

Alternative Therapies

A form of magnetic field therapy is sometimes prescribed to speed the healing of severe fractures. Don't, however, bother experimenting with the small magnetic disks occasionally advocated for pain. Only a large magnetic field generator has any chance of making a difference.

Broken Hip

The Basics

The threat of a fractured hip looms especially large for people with bone cancer or osteoporosis (the brittle-bone disease that strikes some older women). When they suffer a fracture, the doctor will probably have to realign the fragments through a surgical incision, then apply metal screws or plates to hold them together while they heal. The surgical realignment is called an open reduction. Application of the screws and plates is known as internal fixation.

There are always risks with surgery. Even after the operation, the hip may not heal correctly. If the nerves or blood vessels that lead to the bone were injured when it was broken, the bone could die. The long period of bed rest required after the surgery also poses a danger. It can promote clot formation in the blood vessels, and if one of these clots breaks free and travels to the lungs, a dangerous condition called pulmonary embolism can be the result. However, without the operation, the hip is unlikely to heal properly.

If your hip has undergone extensive damage, you may need total hip replacement, also called hip joint replacement. In this operation, the damaged hip joint is replaced with a new joint made of metal or a mixture of metal and plastic. Total hip replacement is often recommended when nothing else will relieve the symptoms of really bad osteoarthritis or rheumatoid arthritis of the hip. Most hip replacements are totally successful, but it takes most patients at least 3 to 5 months to get back their strength and energy.

Call Your Doctor If . . .

After your operation, you develop any of the following problems:

■ The incision becomes swollen and red, or you see any pus. These are signs of infection.
■ Your stitches or staples come apart.

■ Your bandage becomes soaked with blood.

■ You start to run a high temperature.

■ The pain in your hip doesn't go away or becomes worse.

Seek Care Immediately If . . .

■ You fall and injure your hip.

■ You suddenly have trouble breathing.

■ The leg or toes on the side of the surgery feel numb and tingly or cool to the touch, or turn blue or pale.

What You Can Do

■ You'll probably need to stop taking aspirin and ibuprofen before the operation. The doctor will tell you when. If you're taking aspirin for your heart, don't stop without asking the doctor first. Also ask whether you can take any other over-the-counter medicines.

■ You may need traction to pull the bones into place before surgery. If so, a pin will be placed in the bone and hooked to ropes and a pulley. Sandbags attached to the ends of the ropes will provide the force needed to keep the bones in place.

■ Just before surgery, you should not eat or drink anything (even water). Your doctor will tell you when to begin fasting. Check with your doctor before taking insulin, diabetes pills, blood pressure medicine, heart pills, or any other medication on the day of surgery.

During Recovery:

■ To ease pain and swelling after surgery, you may put ice in a plastic bag, cover it with a towel, and place it over the incision for 15 to 20 minutes out of every hour as long as necessary. Do not sleep on the ice pack. Treatment with ice is most effective when started right after the operation and used for 24 to 48 hours.

■ After the first 24 to 48 hours, heat is a better remedy for pain and swelling. Apply a heating pad (turned on low) or a hot water bottle for 15 to 20 minutes out of every hour as long as you need relief. Do not sleep on the heating pad or hot water bottle. Heat brings blood to the area of the operation and helps it heal faster.

■ When you are allowed to bathe or shower, carefully wash the stitches or staples with soap and water. Then put on a clean, new bandage. Change the bandage any time it gets wet or dirty.

■ For the first 3 months after the operation, you must take the following precautions when using your legs:

• Do not cross your legs when you are sitting, lying, or standing.

• Keep the affected leg facing front at all times, even in bed. Do not turn your hip or knee in or out.

• Keep a pillow between your legs when lying on your side.

• Do not bend at the hips to reach into cupboards or drawers or to pick things up from the ground.

• Do not sit on low chairs, stools, or toilet seats, and avoid reclining chairs. When sitting, you should always have your knees lower than your hips. You may need to use a firm cushion to raise chair seats. Consider renting or buying a raised toilet seat.

• Sit only in chairs that have arms. When you need to get up from the chair, move to the front edge, place the affected leg in front of your stronger leg, and push up with the stronger one only. Push on the chair arms with your hands to finish bringing yourself upright.

■ Slowly start to do more each day, resting as needed. Once the hip is stronger, your doctor may prescribe physical therapy and a regular exercise program. Do check with your doctor first, however, before starting any exercise; and don't lift anything heavy until your doctor says it's OK.

■ Until you can spend time walking, you may need to wear support hose to reduce swelling in the legs.

■ Once the hip is better, you'll probably be able to swim, play golf, walk, and bicycle. Do not play tennis, jog, or do other exercises that jar the hip joint.

What Your Doctor Can Do

Hip surgery usually lasts 2 to 4 hours. It requires an incision over the hip bone that will be closed with thread or staples after the operation. To reduce the risk of dangerous blood clots developing during recovery, you'll be encouraged to get out of bed as soon—and as much—as possible.

Prescription Drugs

To reduce the risk of infection, the doctor may prescribe an antibiotic. He's also likely to prescribe a medication such as Zofran (ondansetron) and Tigan (trimethobenzamide) to help quell nausea after the surgery. To prevent clotting in the veins, he may order a blood-thinning drug such as Coumadin (warfarin), Lovenox (enoxaparin), Orgaran (danaparoid), or heparin. And to relieve post-op pain, you're likely to be given prescription painkillers, first by injection, later in the form of pills. Typical medications include:

DHCplus (acetaminophen with dihydrocodone)
Dilaudid (hydromorphone)
Hydrocet, Lorcet, Lortab, Vicodin, or Zydone
(acetaminophen with hydrocodone)
Kadian, MS Contin, or MSIR (morphine)
Levo-Dromoran (levorphanol)
OxyContin, OxyIR, or Roxicodone (oxycodone)
Percocet or Tylox (acetaminophen with oxycodone)
Percodan (aspirin with oxycodone)
Talwin Nx (naloxone)
Toradol (ketorolac)
Tylenol with Codeine (acetaminophen with codeine)
Ultram (tramadol)
Vicoprofen (hydrocodone)

Over-the-Counter Drugs

To ease bowel movements after the operation, the doctor may recommend a stool softener so you won't need to strain. Options include Colace, Correctol Stool Softener, Dialose, and Ex-Lax Stool Softener Caplets.

Once post-op pain has subsided, you'll be able to switch to a standard over-the-counter painkiller. The leading choices are:

Actron	Bufferin	Orudis KT
Advil	Excedrin	Panadol
Aleve	Excedrin, Aspirin-	St. Joseph
Alka-Seltzer	Free	Tylenol
Ascriptin	Goody's	Unisom with Pain
Ascriptin, Enteric	Motrin IB	Relief
Bayer	Nuprin	Vanquish
BC Powder		

Herbal Remedies

Two herbs—Japanese mint and white willow—are generally judged effective for relief of mild pain.

Nutritional Support

While the bone is healing, it's especially important to maintain a diet rich in amino acids and such building blocks of bone as calcium and phosphorus. Your doctor may want you to take calcium supplements and eat foods high in calcium, such as milk, cheese, ice cream, fish, and dark green vegetables, like spinach. The doctor probably will also tell you to drink 6 to 8 large glasses of water each day. Keep a record of exactly how much liquid you drink. Limit your intake of beverages that contain caffeine such as coffee, tea, and soda.

Alternative Treatments

A form of magnetic field therapy is sometimes prescribed to speed the healing of severe fractures. Don't, however, bother experimenting with the small magnetic disks occasionally advocated for pain. Only a large magnetic field generator has any chance of making a difference.

Bronchiolitis

The Basics

Confined almost entirely to children less than 18 months of age, bronchiolitis is a viral infection of the airways in the lungs. The disease breaks out in epidemics, particularly during winter and early spring. About one child in ten gets it during the first year of life.

Bronchiolitis usually begins like a common cold, with sneezing and a runny nose. The virus then spreads into the smaller passageways of the lungs, causing them to swell and interfere with breathing. Typical symptoms include increased heart rate, rapid breathing, and a hacking cough. The child may begin to wheeze, and is likely to develop a fever. He may seem more tired than usual.

The condition usually clears up on its own in 3 to 5 days, and can be treated at home. However, if the child begins to suffer from oxygen deprivation, fatigue, or dehydration, a short stay in the hospital may be necessary. Children have been known to die from bronchiolitis, but with proper treatment, the danger is very small.

Call Your Doctor If . . .

■ The child is sleepier than usual, urinates less, has a dry mouth and cracked lips, cries without tears, or seems dizzy. These are signs of dehydration.

■ The child develops a high temperature.

■ The child begins tugging his ears or shows other signs of an ear infection.

Seek Care Immediately If . . .

■ You notice any of the following signs: the skin between the child's ribs is being sucked in with each breath, the lips or fingernails are turning blue or white, or the child shows trouble breathing or swallowing. These are warnings of oxygen deprivation. **Call 911 or 0 (operator)** for help.

What You Can Do

■ Run a cool-mist humidifier in the child's room, out of reach of the bed. Direct the mist stream towards the child's face. This will help to loosen the sputum in the child's throat, making it easier to breathe.

■ Hang wrung-out wet towels or sheets in the child's room to add moisture to the air.

■ Raise the child's head with extra pillows. This will make it easier to breathe.

■ Keep the child warm and give plenty of room-temperature clear liquids (water, apple juice, lemonade, tea, or ginger ale). Fluids keep the sputum thin and prevent dehydration.

■ Use a rubber-bulb suction device to keep the child's nose as free of mucus as possible.

■ Try to keep the child calm and rested. Crying will make breathing and coughing worse.

■ Do not let anyone smoke near the child.

What Your Doctor Can Do

Home care is usually all that's needed. For a severe case, however, hospitalization may be best. There, the child can be given oxygen and intravenous fluids—as well as aerosol doses of the antiviral drug ribavarin—until the infection subsides.

Prescription Drugs

There is nothing you can give at home that will hasten recovery. Antibiotics are useless against this viral infection. Steroid medications, sometimes prescribed for other types of lung inflammation, are also ineffective. Drugs that open the airways in other ailments such as asthma usually have little effect on bronchiolitis—and could harm a young infant.

Over-the-Counter Drugs

It's important for the child to get rid of as much sputum as possible, so over-the-counter cough medicine may not be advisable. Check with your doctor before you proceed.

If the child develops a fever, give acetaminophen, not aspirin. When given to children with viral infections, aspirin sometimes helps to trigger a dangerous condition called Reye's syndrome.

Herbal Remedies

A number of herbs have been said to help with coughs, colds, and breathing problems, but check with your doctor before giving any to a child with bronchiolitis.

Nutritional Support

Your most important objective is to keep the child well hydrated by supplying as many room-temperature clear liquids as possible. This includes water, apple or white grape juice, lemonade, ginger ale, and tea. You may also wish to try a commercial hydration solution such as Pedialyte.

Alternative Treatments

A number of alternative treatments that center on the concept of relaxation (Alexander Technique, Hellerwork, Meditation, Yoga) have been suggested to help ease breathing difficulties, but none are appropriate for children in this very young age group.

Bronchitis

The Basics

Bronchitis is the medical term for any inflammation of the windpipe and the airways in the lungs. There are two forms, acute and chronic.

Acute bronchitis occurs most often in the winter and usually starts as a cold. The cold then spreads from the nose and throat to the windpipe and airways. Acute bronchitis is usually caused by germs (virus or bacteria) spread through the air or by direct contact with someone who is infected. It can also result from an allergy or from breathing air that contains chemical fumes, dust, or smoke. Your chances of getting bronchitis increase if you have lung disease, smoke, go out in cold or humid weather, have a poor diet, or become run down from another illness.

The most common symptom is a dry cough. Later in the illness the cough may bring up sputum. Other complaints may include a low fever, burning chest pain or pressure behind the breastbone, noisy breathing (wheezing), and trouble breathing. Most people can be treated at home, but if you don't follow the doctor's instructions, your illness can get worse and turn into pneumonia, in which case you may need to be hospitalized.

Chronic bronchitis is a much more serious problem. This debilitating condition comes under the heading of *chronic obstructive pulmonary disease* and affects about 13.8 million people in the U.S. In chronic bronchitis, the airways are constantly inflamed and filled with mucus. Victims have difficulty coughing up the mucus because of damage to the hairlike structures called cilia that ordinarily sweep mucus out of the air tubes. This damage is usually the result of substances in tobacco. (About 80 to 90 percent of cases of chronic bronchitis are linked to cigarette smoking.) Other causes include exposure to dust and air pollutants and frequent colds and flu, which can irritate the airways.

Chronic bronchitis is marked by a very specific set of symptoms: People who cough up mucus on most days for at least 3 months of the year for 2 consecutive years are said to have this condition.

Call Your Doctor If . . .
- You develop a cough that lasts more than a few days.
- You cough up green, gray, or bloody sputum.

Seek Care Immediately If . . .
- You have chills, increasing chest pain, trouble breathing while resting, or vomiting.
- Your lips or nail beds turn blue or pale.
- You can't stop coughing, or your constant coughing makes you feel light-headed.

What You Can Do
- If you are taking antibiotics, use up the entire prescription, even if you begin to feel better. If you stop too soon, some germs in your lungs may survive and eventually cause a relapse.
- Some medications for bronchitis occasionally cause drowsiness. Do not drive or use heavy equipment until you know how a drug affects you.
- When recovering from acute bronchitis, rest until you feel better. You can return to work or school when your temperature is normal.

■ If you're a smoker and develop chronic bronchitis, quitting is the most important thing you can do.

■ Avoid dairy foods if they seem to make your sputum thicker.

■ Drink 8 to 10 large glasses of water each day. This helps thin sputum so it can be coughed up more easily.

■ To help keep your lungs free of infection, stop to take 2 or 3 deep breaths and then cough. Do this often during the day.

■ Use a humidifier to help keep the air moist and your sputum thin, but be sure to clean it every day.

■ Stay inside on days that are very hot or cold or on days when the air pollution is high.

What Your Doctor Can Do

If you have acute bronchitis, your doctor can prescribe medicines that will quiet your cough and make breathing easier. He may also prescribe antibiotics if you have an infection.

An especially severe case of bronchitis may require hospitalization. There you will receive oxygen to help you breathe easier and perhaps medicines that you inhale to help open your breathing passages. You can also expect a number of diagnostic procedures, including a chest x-ray, tests to measure the level of oxygen in your blood, and an electrocardiograph (ECG) to monitor your heartbeat.

If you complain of cough, shortness of breath, or wheezing, are older than 50, and smoke, the first test the doctor is likely to perform is spirometry, a test that measures how long it takes to exhale and how much air is expelled in the first second. The less air expelled, the more likely one has chronic bronchitis.

Prescription Drugs

If you have an infection in the lungs, you'll be given *antibiotics* to help clear it up. To help open your airways, you may be given a *bronchodilator*, such as albuterol (Proventil, Ventolin), metaproterenol (Alupent, Metaprel), ipratropium (Atrovent), terbutaline (Brethine, Bricanyl) or theophylline (Slo-bid, Theo-Dur). To decrease the swelling and inflammation of the tissue in your lungs, the doctor may also prescribe a *steroid*, such as beclomethasone (Beclovent, Vanceril), triamcinolone (Azmacort), or flunisolide (AeroBid).

Your doctor may also prescribe a *cough suppressant* to help quiet your cough or an *expectorant* to make it easier for you to cough up sputum. Those with chronic bronchitis may have to inhale pure oxygen for a certain number of hours each day to keep enough oxygen in their blood.

Over-the-Counter Drugs

There are no nonprescription drugs specifically for bronchitis. However, you may find over-the-counter cough suppressants and expectorants helpful. Over-the-counter decongestants can help relieve cold symptoms, swelling, and congestion. Aspirin, acetaminophen (Tylenol), or ibuprofen (Advil, Motrin) may be useful for relieving general aches and reducing fever. For more information, see the entry on colds and flu.

Herbal Remedies

An immense number of herbs have been found to provide at least some relief from bronchitis. Candidates include:

Adonis	Ephedra	Mustard
Anise	(Ma Huang)	Nasturtium
Balsam	Eucalyptus	Niauli
Balsam of Peru	Fennel	Onion
Blue Mallow	Galangal	Peppermint
Brewer's Yeast	Garlic	Pimpinella
Camphor	Gumweed	Pine Oil
Caraway	Hemp Nettle	Primrose
Cardamom	Horehound	Radish
Chamomile	Horseradish	Red Clover
Chinese	Iceland Moss	Sandalwood
Cinnamon	Japanese Mint	Sanicle
Cinnamon	Khella	Seneca Snakeroot
Cloves	Knotweed	Soapwort
Couch Grass	Larch	Star Anise
Dill	Licorice	Sundew
Echinacea	Linden	Thyme
Elder	Lungwort	Watercress
English Ivy	Marshmallow	White Nettle
English Oak	Meadowsweet	Wild Cherry
English Plantain	Mullein	Wild Thyme

Nutritional Support

The most effective measure you can take is to drink 8 to 10 glasses of water or other clear liquids daily. This will help to keep mucus thin, making it easier to bring up.

Alternative Treatments

Several alternative therapies are considered especially helpful for all types of breathing disorders:

Alexander Technique: A specialized movement training program, the Alexander Technique encourages people to shed ingrained and inappropriate muscular reactions, allowing healthy natural reflexes to take over.

Hellerwork: A combination of deep tissue massage and movement reeducation, this form of therapy is also advocated for breathing disorders.

Meditation: The calming mental exercises of meditation are said to help everything from stress, tension, and anxiety to high blood pressure, chronic pain, respiratory ailments, and headaches.

Yoga: This age-old discipline, which entails breathing exercises, body postures, and meditation, offers a significant variety of proven health benefits.

Burns

The Basics

Heat, electricity, chemicals, and radiation all can cause burns. Healing usually takes 1 to 3 weeks. There are three degrees of severity:

■ *First-degree* burns are mild and injure only the outer layer of skin. The skin becomes red, but will turn white when touched. The area may also be painful to the touch.

■ *Second-degree* burns are deeper, more severe, and very painful. Blisters may form on the burned area. This type of burn takes about 2 weeks to heal.

■ *Third-degree* burns are the deepest and most serious kind. The skin becomes white and leathery, but does not feel very tender when touched.

There may be swelling in the burned area. Serious burns may be accompanied by headache, fever, and dizziness.

Electrical burns are especially worrisome. They occur when current jumps from an electrical outlet, cord, or appliance and passes through your body. The electricity can burn the skin—sometimes very deeply—and may also cause internal damage.

When treating minor burns, the goal is to promote healing and prevent infection. How quickly you heal depends on the severity of the burns and injuries. Your doctor may prescribe an antibiotic ointment. Use it as directed, and follow the first-aid steps outlined below. If the burn is severe, you may need to be hospitalized to avoid infection and receive special care.

Call Your Doctor If . . .

■ You have increasing pain and redness in the burned area or bad-smelling drainage from the burn. These are signs of infection.

■ You develop a high temperature.

■ You've suffered any sort of electrical burn.

Seek Care Immediately If . . .

■ The burn covers a large surface area.

■ You've received a serious electrical shock. (Do not drive yourself to the hospital.)

■ You develop swelling, numbness, or tingling below a burn on your arm or leg.

■ A child with a burn has trouble swallowing or breathing.

What You Can Do

■ Soak the burned area in cold water for 10 minutes.

■ Gently wash the burn with warm, soapy water. Pat it dry with a clean towel, and cover it with a clean, dry bandage.

■ Clean the burn and put on new bandages several times a day. Be sure that everything that touches the burn is clean. If your doctor has prescribed a medication, use only this prescription. When changing bandages:

•Wash your hands well with soap and water. Dry them with a clean towel.

•Remove the old bandage by cutting it off with a pair of scissors. Do not pull off a bandage if it is sticking to the burn. Instead, soak it in warm water for a few minutes and then remove it slowly.

•Gently wash the burn with warm, soapy water. Use a clean, soft washcloth to help remove any old cream, blood, and loose skin. Do not break blisters. This may increase the pain.

•Rinse the burn with clear warm water. Pat dry with a clean towel.

•With a clean tongue depressor, apply antibiotic cream (or other recommended burn medication) to a gauze pad in a thin layer. Throw the tongue depressor away when you're done. Do NOT put it back in the container of medication.

• Cover the burn with the gauze. Be careful not to touch the gauze that comes in contact with the burn. Carefully rewrap the burn with a clean bandage.

■ Keep the bandage clean and dry. Change it if it gets wet.

■ If the burn is on your arm or leg, keep it raised or propped up for the first 24 hours to help reduce swelling.

■ You may use aspirin, acetaminophen, or ibuprofen for pain.

■ Do not bump or overuse the burned area.

■ Drink plenty of water or juice to prevent dehydration.

■ For mouth burns (often suffered by children):

• Feed the child bland, soft, cold foods such as baby foods, soft cooked eggs, cooked cereal, ice cream, and yogurt. Give lots of liquids such as water, milk, and fruit juices.

• Brush the child's teeth 3 or 4 times a day. Use a soft toothbrush, with or without toothpaste.

• If the child is given a special device called a microstoma to help prevent scarring, use it exactly as directed.

■ To prevent burns from heat:

• Teach your children not to play with matches or touch the stove (even when it is not on).

• Test bathwater before getting into a bathtub or putting your child in one.

• Do not set your hot water heater too high. Usually the dial should be set in the middle between hot and cold.

• Do not smoke in bed.

■ To prevent electrical burns:

• Never stick foreign objects into an electrical plug. Cover unused electrical outlets with childproof plug covers, available in hardware stores and the baby section of department stores.

• Do not use electrical appliances near standing or running water.

• Do NOT stick forks or knives into toasters or other appliances when they are plugged in.

• Repair or replace any frayed or worn electrical cords. Teach children to NEVER suck or chew on these cords.

What Your Doctor Can Do

Your doctor may need to clean up the tissue surrounding the burn. If you have not had a recent tetanus booster, he may give you a tetanus shot. If the burn becomes infected, you may be prescribed antibiotics to be taken by mouth. In severe cases, hospitalization may be required.

Prescription Drugs
Silvadene Cream 1% (silver sulfadiazine)
Sulfamylon Cream (mafenide acetate)

Over-the-Counter Drugs
A+D Ointment
Aquaphor Healing
  Ointment
Barri-Care Antimicrobial
  Ointment

Betadine
Desitin
Mycitracin
Polysporin

Herbal Remedies
The following herbal remedies are considered useful for the treatment of wounds and burns:

Balsam of Peru
Chamomile
English Plantain
Horsetail

Marigold
Poplar
Shepherd's Purse

Slippery Elm
St. John's Wort
Witch Hazel

Nutritional Support
There are no special dietary recommendations specifically for burns. Be sure to get plenty of protein, which the body needs to build new cells and promote healing. Maintain ample fluid intake, especially if the burns are severe.

Alternative Treatments
Hydrotherapy: The application of hot and cold water or water-soaked compresses to manage the pain and swelling of soft tissue injuries and burns is standard practice. It has been proven effective in a variety of well-controlled clinical trials.

Oxygen Therapy: Hyperbaric oxygen therapy is a procedure in which patients go into an airtight chamber and inhale 100 percent oxygen under pressures of up to 2 atmospheres. It is sometimes used as an additional treatment for burns. Oxygen plays a key role in every cellular process; it supports the immune system, destroys toxic substances, fuels metabolism, and promotes new cell growth.

Bursitis

The Basics

Although people tend to think of bursitis as a disorder of the shoulder, this painful ailment can strike in a number of areas, including the knee, hip, elbow, and big toe. The problem stems from swelling and inflammation of a bursa—one of the fluid-filled sacs that act as shock absorbers between the bones and nearby tendons and muscles. These sacs serve to minimize friction and encourage normal movement. With more than 78 of them on each side of the body, it's not surprising that bursitis is common.

Injury and overuse of a joint are the usual causes of bursitis. It can occur after a single incident—such as a fall or a blow—but it usually develops after long-term stress. Bursitis often strikes people who are active in sports that require repetitive motions, such as running, dance, or tennis. The problem can also stem from your job. Carpet layers, for example, and other people who work on their knees are prone to bursitis of the knee joint. Other causes of bursitis include infection, arthritis, or gout (a painful joint inflammation).

The hallmark of bursitis is a sudden burning pain in the joint. The area may also swell and be tender to the touch. Depending on the location, movement is often limited. For example, it's usually painful to raise your arm if you have bursitis in the shoulder. Or you might feel pain while climbing stairs if the problem is in your knee. Symptoms are sometimes accompanied by fever.

Acute bursitis happens suddenly. The inflamed joint is painful when moved or touched. If the problem is caused by an infection or gout, the affected area is likely to be red and warm to the touch.

Chronic bursitis takes hold after repeated injuries or previous bouts of acute bursitis. An already damaged bursa is susceptible to additional inflammation from excessive exercise or strain. Long-standing pain that limits movement can cause surrounding muscles to weaken or even shrink. Attacks of chronic bursitis may last a few days to several weeks, and they frequently recur.

Call Your Doctor If . . .

■ Your pain increases during treatment.

■ You develop a high temperature.

Seek Care Immediately If . . .

Bursitis usually doesn't require emergency care.

What You Can Do

■ Take an over-the-counter nonsteroidal anti-inflammatory drug such as ibuprofen or naproxen. This type of medication is one of the best remedies for bursitis pain.

■ Apply ice to the injury for 10 to 20 minutes each hour for the first 1 to 2 days. Put the ice in a plastic bag and place a towel between the bag of ice and your skin.

■ After the first day or two, you may apply heat to the joint to help relieve pain. Use a warm heating pad, whirlpool bath, or warm, moist towel for 10 to 20 minutes every hour for 48 hours.

■ If the bursitis is sports- or job-related, refrain from the offending activity, if possible, until the inflammation goes away.

■ Rest the injured joint as much as possible. When the pain decreases, begin normal, slow movements.

■ Ask your doctor if carefully stretching the tendons in your muscles might help. You can also ask about specific exercises to increase the joint's range of motion.

What Your Doctor Can Do

If the bursa is noticeably swollen, your doctor may use a needle to remove a sample of fluid from the sac. The fluid can be tested for causes of the inflammation, such as an infection or gout. X-rays are usually not helpful. Infected bursas must be drained and then treated with the appropriate antibiotics.

If infection is not the cause, acute bursitis is usually treated by rest and temporary immobilization of the joint. Your doctor may advise you to take an over-the-counter nonsteroidal anti-inflammatory drug or may order a stronger, prescription version of one of these drugs. If this doesn't work, your doctor can reduce the inflammation by injecting a mixture of a local anesthetic and a steroid directly into the bursa. The injection may have to be repeated. People with severe bursitis can also take steroids by mouth for a few days.

Chronic bursitis is treated in a similar way. However, rest and immobilization are less likely to help. Disabling bursitis may be eased by several injections of steroids and intensive physical therapy to restore the joint's function. The exercises will help strengthen weak muscles and improve the joint's range of motion.

Prescription Drugs

Prescription nonsteroidal anti-inflammatory drugs recommended for bursitis include the following:

Anaprox or Naprelan
  (naproxen sodium)
Clinoril (sulindac)
Indocin (indomethacin)

Naprosyn (naproxen)
Trilisate (choline magnesium
  trisalicylate)

The doctor can also use one of the following steroid medications:

Celestone (betamethasone)
Cortone (cortisone)
Decadron (dexamethasone)
Hydrocortone (hydrocortisone)

Pediapred or Prelone
  (prednisolone)
Solu-Medrol
  (methylprednisolone)

Over-the-Counter Drugs

Anti-inflammatory painkillers available over the counter include:

Actron
Advil
Aleve
Ascriptin
Bayer
BC Powder

Bufferin
Ecotrin
Excedrin
Goody's
Motrin

Nuprin
Orudis
St. Joseph
Vanquish
YSP

Herbal Remedies

Applied externally as a cream, cayenne helps relieve pain. Researchers have found that capsaicin, the active ingredient in cayenne, depletes the chemical messengers that send signals through the pain-sensing peripheral nerves. This deadens the sensation of pain even when its cause remains present.

Nutritional Support

It's a good idea to watch your weight since extra pounds can burden inflamed joints. If your bursitis is due to gout, it's important to decrease your intake of foods high in purines, which can aggravate gout. The foods to avoid include liver, kidney, mussels, anchovies, peas, and beans.

Alternative Treatments

Reconstructive Therapy: Although not widely used in the United States, this form of therapy has been scientifically validated as a possible treatment for bursitis. It's performed by making a series of injections directly into the damaged area. The injected solution is made up of natural irritants aimed at mobilizing the healing process in the damaged joint.

Carpal Tunnel Syndrome

The Basics

As the signature ailment of the computer age, carpal tunnel syndrome has been gaining considerable notoriety lately. Often fostered by repeated flexing of the wrist, it occurs when the median nerve leading from the arm to the hand gets pinched as it passes through the carpal tunnel, a narrow, hollow area in the wrist. One or both hands can be affected.

Pressure on the nerve is usually the result of irritation and swelling of the tissues within the tunnel. Although repetitive tasks such as typing or working with power tools are considered leading culprits, carpal tunnel syndrome can also be caused by a wrist injury, arthritis, diabetes, or water retention during pregnancy and menopause.

The defining symptoms of the ailment are loss of feeling in part of the hand—usually the thumb, index, and middle fingers—accompanied by pain that shoots from the wrist up the arm, especially at night. Other symptoms include stiffness of the wrist in the morning, cramping of the hands, inability to make a fist, weakness in the thumb, a feeling of burning in the fingers, and a tendency to drop things.

Call Your Doctor If . . .

■ There is no improvement after two weeks of care.
■ You develop new unexplained symptoms.

Seek Care Immediately If . . .

This problem doesn't require emergency treatment.

What You Can Do

■ If your doctor recommends a splint to keep your wrist from bending, be sure to leave it on at night. Wear it as long as you have pain and numbness in your hand—from 1 to 2 months.

- If you are troubled by pain at night, it may help to rub or shake your hand, or hang it over the side of the bed.
- To speed healing, you must give the wrist a rest and stop the activity that caused the problem. If your symptoms are work-related, you may need to ask your employer about changing to a job that doesn't require as much wrist action.

What Your Doctor Can Do

If nonsteroidal anti-inflammatory medications, splinting, and rest fail to relieve the problem, your doctor can give you a steroid injection to combat inflammation and temporarily ease the pain. If all else fails, you'll need surgery to release the pressure on the nerve.

Prescription Drugs

Nonsteroidal anti-inflammatory drugs such as Motrin, Naprosyn, and Orudis often prove helpful. See the entry on arthritis for a complete list. Injectable steroids the doctor can use include the following:

Celestone (betamethasone)
Cortone (cortisone)
Decadron (dexamethasone)
Hydrocortone (hydrocortisone)

Pediapred or Prelone
(prednisolone)
Solu-Medrol
(methylprednisolone)

Over-the-Counter Drugs

Over-the-counter painkillers such as aspirin, acetaminophen (Tylenol), and ibuprofen (Advil, Motrin) can all provide at least some relief.

Herbal Remedies

White willow, the original source of aspirin, is said to be useful for all types of pain.

Nutritional Support

There are no dietary measures that seem to help this problem.

Alternative Treatments

Acupuncture: This traditional Chinese therapy often proves effective for all types of pain. The treatments require insertion of tiny needles at points located along an invisible system of energy channels called meridians.

Energy Medicine: Of all the electrical therapies currently available, transcutaneous electrical nerve stimulation is the closest to adoption by the mainstream. It is used for any type of localized pain.

Hypnotherapy: With its ability to enhance the power of suggestion, hypnosis has been found effective for a variety of problems that hinge on emotions, habits, and even the body's involuntary responses. Some people have found it helpful for carpal tunnel syndrome.

Magnetic Field Therapy: This hotly debated form of therapy uses magnets to quell pain.

Myotherapy: A specialized form of deep muscle massage, this therapy is said to relieve virtually any sort of muscle-related pain, including the pain of repetitive stress injuries such as carpal tunnel syndrome.

Reconstructive Therapy: With a series of injections into the joints, this therapy endeavors to speed healing of torn, damaged, injured, pulled, or weak joints, ligaments, tendons, and cartilage. It may successfully reduce the swelling that underlies carpal tunnel syndrome.

Cervicitis

The Basics

Cervicitis is probably the most common of all female disorders, affecting half of all women at some point in their lives. Any inflammation of the cervix (the lower end of the uterus) is technically a case of cervicitis, but the problem is usually the result of a sexually transmitted infection.

The three most common causes are chlamydia, gonorrhea, and trichomonas. An IUD (intrauterine device) or a forgotten tampon is sometimes at fault. Chemicals in douches may also be responsible.

The first sign of cervicitis is often a yellow discharge from the vagina. The discharge typically becomes more pronounced just after your menstrual period, and may or may not have a bad odor. Other symptoms include bleeding, itching, pain during sex, or a burning feeling when you urinate. You may have abdominal or lower back pain. If the infection spreads, you may experience nausea and vomiting.

Call Your Doctor If . . .

■ You notice a vaginal discharge or any kind of lower abdominal pain.

■ Your discomfort lasts longer than a few days.

■ Your symptoms get worse.

■ During or after treatment, you have vaginal bleeding between periods.

Seek Care Immediately If . . .

You experience severe abdominal pain.

What You Can Do

■ If you have an infection:
- Be sure to take the prescribed medication for as long as directed. If the germs aren't completely eliminated, the infection may spread up into the pelvic area, causing damage that may make it hard to get pregnant.
- To prevent the infection from being passed back and forth, your sexual partner must be examined and treated as well.
- It is best to avoid having sex while you are being treated. If you do have sex, your partner should use condoms.
- During treatment, use sanitary pads instead of tampons.
- Do not use a douche during treatment.

■ If you have had a biopsy, avoid intercourse, douching, and the use of tampons for a week.

■ To prevent cervicitis:
- Limit your sexual contacts, know the history of your partner, and make condoms a routine part of sex.
- See your doctor immediately if your partner has been diagnosed with urethritis or has symptoms of the condition such as pain or burning during urination or a thin discharge from the penis.
- Avoid chemical irritants in deodorized tampons, douches, or sprays.

What Your Doctor Can Do

During the examination, your doctor may take a "smear" to be tested for infection. He may also perform a colposcopy, in which he examines the cervix with a binocular-like instrument called a colposcope. If necessary, he may take a photograph of the cervix and send it to an expert for interpretation (a procedure called "cervicography").

If the cervix appears abnormal, a biopsy may be needed. In this procedure, the doctor removes a small piece of tissue for examination under the microscope. It is usually done in the office without anesthesia and causes only minor discomfort.

If an infection proves to be the cause, you'll be prescribed a medication to eliminate the germs.

Prescription Drugs

A chlamydial infection calls for treatment with an antibiotic. Typical choices include:

Doryx or Vibramycin   Floxin (ofloxacin)
(doxycycline)   Zithromax (azithromycin)
E.E.S., EryPed, Ery-Tab or PCE
(erythromycin)

Gonorrhea is usually attacked with one of the following antibiotics:

Cefizox (ceftizoxime)   Penetrex (enoxacin)
Cipro (ciprofloxacin)   Rocephin (ceftriaxone)
Floxin (ofloxacin)   Vantin (cefpodoxime)
Noroxin (norfloxacin)

Trichomonas infections are treated with the antibacterial drugs Flagyl or Protostat (metronidazole).

Over-the-Counter Drugs

There are no nonprescription remedies for this kind of infection. Products such as Gyne-Lotrimin and Monistat will cure a yeast infection, but have no value here.

Herbal Remedies

Herbs are generally useless against infections, and cervicitis is no exception.

Nutritional Support

There are no dietary measures that can rid you of this type of infection.

Alternative Treatments

There is no better alternative than standard antibacterial drugs.

Chickenpox

The Basics

Still one of the most common childhood diseases, chickenpox is most likely to strike between the ages of 3 to 9 years. It is caused by the varicella-zoster virus, which in adults is also responsible for the painful skin condition known as shingles. A shot to prevent the disease is now available.

Chickenpox is highly contagious from the moment the first symptoms appear until the last blisters have crusted over. It is spread by close contact with an infected individual. After exposure, some 2 to 3 weeks pass before the child begins to get sick.

Fever, mild headache, and an uneasy feeling are often the first signs. Within 24 to 36 hours, these symptoms are followed by an eruption of small red bumps, usually starting on the torso. After a few hours, these bumps turn into itchy blisters that break and crust over. New crops of blisters keep forming for 3 or 4 days, spreading over most of the body. It usually takes a week for the blisters to subside, and 2 weeks for all the scabs to fall off.

There is no cure for chickenpox. Antibiotics will not help; the disease must simply run its course. The illness is usually mild, but can be dangerous in children with serious health problems such as leukemia, and in adults who contract the disease. Once a child has chickenpox, he or she will not get it again. However, the infection may re-emerge as shingles later in life.

Call Your Doctor If . . .

■ The child has sores in the eyes.
■ The skin blisters get bigger or have pus in them.
■ The child's fever does not go away in 3 or 4 days, or exceeds 102 degrees.

Seek Care Immediately If . . .

■ The child starts vomiting, acts confused or sleepy, or has seizures.
■ The child has trouble breathing or starts breathing very fast.

What You Can Do

■ Make sure the child gets plenty of rest and liquids.
■ DO NOT GIVE ASPIRIN to a child with chickenpox who is under 18 years of age. This could lead to a condition called Reye's syndrome, which causes brain and liver damage. Instead, give acetaminophen for fever. Carefully check for aspirin on the label of any over-the-counter medicines.
■ To control itching:
  • Apply wet compresses to the blisters.

- Your doctor can prescribe medicine for itching. You also may use an over-the-counter antihistamine product.
- You may use calamine lotion on the blisters. Follow the directions on the label. Do not use on sores in the mouth.
- Give the child baths in lukewarm water for the first few days. Add ½ cup of baking soda to the water. Let the child soak for about 30 minutes, several times a day. You may also use an oatmeal bath product purchased from the drugstore.

■ Try to keep the child from scratching the rash or picking off the scabs; this can lead to infection and may cause scars. Keep the child's fingernails cut short. Put socks on the child's hands at night. Use a soap that kills germs for hand washing.

■ If your child has painful sores in the mouth, make tea twice as strong as usual, add a little sugar, and use as a mouthwash or gargle.

■ Keep the child quiet and cool. Heat and sweating makes the itching worse. Keep the child out of the sun.

■ The child should stay home from school or day care for about 1 week. Be especially careful to keep him or her away from babies and pregnant women.

What Your Doctor Can Do

Your doctor may be able to diagnose the problem over the telephone, especially if you know the child has recently been exposed to others with the illness. If the doctor wants to see you, he will examine the blisters to rule out other diseases that cause fever and rash.

Although there is no cure for this disease, the doctor can prescribe medications to make the child more comfortable and to remedy any complications that develop.

Prescription Drugs

The prescription drug Atarax or Vistaril (hydroxyzine) can help relieve itching, as can antihistamine pills such as Benadryl (diphenhydramine). In severe cases, the anti-viral medication Zovirax (acyclovir) may be needed. Antibiotics will be prescribed only if the blisters get infected.

Over-the-Counter Drugs

For fever, give NON-ASPIRIN products such as Advil, Motrin IB, Panadol, and Tylenol. It's safe to use calamine lotion on the blisters, but check with your doctor before using other lotions, ointments, or creams.

Herbal Remedies
No herbs seem to relieve the itching and blistering that characterize this disease.

Nutritional Support
Your child should drink plenty of fluids, such as water, milk, and apple juice. Avoid salty foods and orange juice.

Alternative Therapies
There are no alternative therapies that have any significant effect on this—or any other—viral infection.

Chronic Fatigue Syndrome

The Basics
People plagued with this frustrating illness say that it feels like a terrible case of the flu that never gets better. Although most victims are in their 20s and 30s, the problem can develop at any age. It attacks both genders, but favors women two to one. Doctors are not sure what causes it, and they have no cure.

While debilitating fatigue is the hallmark of chronic fatigue syndrome (CFS), a feeling of exhaustion is not, by itself, a sure sign of the illness. CFS produces a very specific kind of fatigue—a persistent weariness that cuts your activity in half, doesn't improve with bed rest, and can't be explained by any other form of illness. A true case of the disease is also marked by at least four of the following symptoms:

■ Sore throat
■ Painful lymph nodes
■ General muscle pain
■ Prolonged fatigue after physical activity
■ Generalized headaches
■ Pain that moves from one joint to another without swelling or redness
■ Forgetfulness, excessive irritability, confusion, or inability to concentrate
■ Sleep disturbance

CFS often begins with a flu-like illness that never completely clears up. The symptoms may come and go, vary in intensity from mild to incapacitating, and last for months or years. Exercise often makes the problem worse.

Debate over the cause of CFS is reflected in its many names. Among experts who believe the condition stems from problems with the immune system, it's known as *chronic fatigue immune dysfunction syndrome*. The disease has also been blamed on a variety of viral infections, and is sometimes called chronic *Epstein-Barr* by those who believe this stubborn virus is at fault. Speculation that the condition results from a nerve inflammation has led to the title *myalgic encephalomyelitis*. And recent studies have linked the problem with neurally mediated *hypotension,* a condition marked by a dramatic drop in blood pressure each time the victim stands up for more than a few minutes.

Call Your Doctor If . . .
■ You can't seem to shake an infection and feel constantly wrung out.

Seek Care Immediately If . . .
CFS does not constitute an emergency.

What You Can Do
■ Eat a balanced diet, get adequate rest, and exercise as much as your condition allows—walking is most frequently recommended.
■ Set limits and pace yourself; stress can often make the symptoms worse.
■ Changes in lifestyle may be necessary, such as taking a job closer to home or switching to a less stressful occupation. Few people can work full-time throughout the course of the illness.
■ Consider specialized treatment. For example, pain management programs may help with severe muscle pain or headache, while sleep disorders can often be treated at a specialized sleep disorder center; relaxation training may help reduce stress. Support groups and counseling may also be useful.

What Your Doctor Can Do
Chronic fatigue syndrome shares symptoms with conditions such as lupus, multiple sclerosis, Lyme disease, and depression, so your doctor's first task will be to rule out a look-alike illness. If the problem does turn out to be CFS, the doctor can prescribe medication to relieve some of the symptoms.

Prescription Drugs

Drug treatment for CFS has met with mixed results, and the doctor may have to try a variety of medications before you find one that helps. Successes have occasionally been reported for antiviral drugs, certain antidepressants (tricyclics), blood pressure medications, and drugs that boost the immune system, but few drugs have gone through formal clinical testing for CFS, and none have shown clear benefits. Recent tests of antiviral agents such as acyclovir (Zovirax), and immunoglobulin (Gamimune, Gammagard, others) have been inconclusive, working no better than dummy pills in some tests.

Over-the-Counter Drugs

For relief of the aches and pain that accompany this illness, some doctors recommend nonsteroidal anti-inflammatory drugs such as ibuprofen (Advil, Motrin, Nuprin), ketoprofen (Orudis KT), and aspirin.

Herbal Remedies

There are no herbs that have been found effective specifically for chronic fatigue syndrome, but a wide variety appear to boost the immune system and might be worth trying. They include:

Anise	Cinnamon	Japanese Mint
Balsam	Cloves	Larch
Balsam of Peru	Couch Grass	Mustard
Barberry	Dill	Onion
Brewer's Yeast	Echinacea	Peppermint
Caraway	English Oak	Pine Oil
Cardamom	English Plantain	Radish
Cat's Claw	Galangal	Sandalwood
Chamomile	Garlic	Siberian Ginseng
Chinese Cinnamon	Iceland Moss	Yellow Dock

Nutritional Support

Some doctors recommend vitamin B_{12}, and magnesium for relief of general symptoms.

Alternative Treatments

Alexander Technique: This specialized form of movement training aims to bring the body's muscles into natural harmony. It may be helpful in relieving the muscle pain often associated with CFS.

Biofeedback: This technique uses a variety of sensors to alert people to changes within the body, enabling them to gain control over physiological reactions that are ordinarily unconscious and automatic. It has helped many people overcome chronic fatigue.

Other treatments, such as *acupuncture, chiropractic, massage,* and *yoga,* have also proved helpful for some patients.

Clogged Arteries

The Basics

Clogged arteries are largely the result of high cholesterol levels in the blood. While it's true that diabetes, high blood pressure, smoking, obesity, and lack of exercise all contribute to the problem, cholesterol stands out as the major culprit. For example, the majority of heart attacks occur in people whose total blood cholesterol levels are between 180 and 240 and who have at least one other risk factor. The good news is that for every 1 percent decrease in cholesterol, the heart attack rate goes down 2 percent, and often nothing more than a healthy, low-fat diet and regular exercise are required to accomplish the reduction.

Cholesterol is not intrinsically bad. In fact, this waxy, fat-like substance is a necessary part of our body chemistry. Dietary cholesterol is a problem only because the human liver normally produces all that we need. When there's an excess, it finds its way into the blood vessels, where it is deposited as a thick, fatty gunk called plaque. A build-up of plaque eventually narrows the arteries and stiffens their walls, slowing down the flow of oxygen-rich blood. If this condition, known medically as atherosclerosis, develops in an artery in the head or neck, it can lead to a stroke. If it happens in the arteries serving the heart muscle, it can cause the intense pain known as angina pectoris and, left untreated, can lead to a heart attack.

Low-density lipoprotein (LDL) cholesterol, the "bad cholesterol," contributes to the buildup of plaque. High-density lipoprotein (HDL) cholesterol, commonly referred to as the "good cholesterol," works to keep the arteries clear. Therefore, the lower your total and LDL cholesterol levels and the higher your HDL cholesterol level, the better. According to the National Cholesterol Education Program, adults should have:

■ A total blood cholesterol level less than 200 milligrams per deciliter of blood

■ An LDL level less than 130 milligrams per deciliter

■ An HDL level greater than 35 milligrams per deciliter

Triglycerides (blood fat) may also contribute to clogged arteries. Ideally, your triglyceride levels should be less than 200 milligrams per deciliter. Dietary and lifestyle changes that reduce total cholesterol and LDL levels should also have a positive impact on triglycerides.

Call Your Doctor If . . .

■ You are experiencing chest pain that:
- Is more painful each time you have it, or is returning more frequently.
- Lasts longer than 10 to 15 minutes even after you rest.
- Wakes you from sleep.
- Occurs during exercise and doesn't go away with rest.

Seek Care Immediately If . . .

■ You develop the following warning signs of a heart attack:
- Uncomfortable pressure, fullness, squeezing, or pain in the center of the chest that lasts more than a few minutes, or goes away and comes back.
- Pain that spreads to your shoulders, neck, or arms.
- Discomfort in your chest associated with light-headedness, fainting, sweating, nausea, or shortness of breath.

■ You develop the following warning signs of stroke:
- Sudden weakness or numbness of the face, arm, or leg on one side of the body.
- Sudden dimness or loss of vision, especially in only one eye.
- Loss of speech, difficulty talking, or difficulty understanding speech.
- Unexplained dizziness.

What You Can Do

■ To prevent clogged arteries and ward off heart disease, one of the most important things you can do is stick to a low-fat diet. Most Americans eat much more fat than they need.

■ Exercise regularly. This raises "good" HDL levels while reducing total cholesterol. It also improves blood circulation and strengthens the heart.

■ Take other measures to improve overall heart health. If you smoke, quit. If you're overweight, shed some pounds. Keep stress to a minimum. And seek treatment for conditions, such as high blood pressure and diabetes, that increase the danger of heart disease.

What Your Doctor Can Do

Your doctor can make specific recommendations for dietary and lifestyle changes that will keep your cholesterol levels in check. When diet and exercise fail to do an adequate job, he can prescribe cholesterol-lowering medications that have a proven track record for reducing the risk of heart attack.

If your coronary arteries are severely clogged, the doctor may recommend a procedure called *percutaneous transluminal coronary angioplasty (PTCA)*, or *"angioplasty"* for short. The technique involves threading a catheter (a long, thin tube with an inflatable balloon-like tip) through an artery in the arm or groin until it reaches the area of blockage. The balloon is then inflated, flattening the fatty plaque and widening the arterial passage. *Angioplasty* is typically performed under local anesthesia and, although invasive, does not involve traditional open heart surgery or the use of a heart-lung machine.

Another surgical option for hopelessly clogged coronary arteries is a *coronary artery bypass graft*, more commonly known as a bypass operation. In this procedure, the narrowed coronary artery is bypassed with a vessel taken from a less critical part of the body. The new vessel reestablishes an adequate blood supply to the heart muscle.

If the problem is a severely clogged artery serving the brain, the doctors may recommend a surgical procedure called *carotid endarterectomy*. In this operation, plaque buildup in the carotid artery is cut out and removed.

Prescription Drugs

Cholesterol-lowering medications work by preventing the body from manufacturing cholesterol, reducing absorption of dietary cholesterol, or combining with cholesterol to facilitate its removal from the bloodstream. The most common of these drugs are niacin (Nicolar, Nicobid), lovastatin (Mevacor), pravastatin (Pravachol), simvastatin (Zocor), cholestyramine (Questran), gemfibrozil (Lopid), colestipol (Colestid), and fluvastatin (Lescol). Some of the "statin" drugs, such as Mevacor and Pravachol, have now been conclusively proven to reduce the chances of a heart attack in people with high cholesterol.

For additional protection against heart attack and stroke, the doctor can also prescribe a drug called Plavix (clopidogrel) that keeps blood platelets slippery and discourages the formation of clots in already narrowed arteries. For people at greatest risk, doctors often prescribe anticoagulant medications such as heparin or warfarin (Coumadin).

Over-the-Counter Drugs

If you have significantly clogged arteries, aspirin can be one of the most important safety measures available. Like the prescription drug Plavix, aspirin thins the blood, helping to prevent the formation of blood clots that can block constricted arteries and cause a heart attack. Be sure, however, to use only aspirin (Bayer, Ecotrin, Empirin), and not other painkillers such as acetaminophen (Tylenol) or ibuprofen (Advil, Motrin). The other products do not have the same blood-thinning effect.

Herbal Remedies

Herbs considered helpful for clogged arteries include onion, garlic, fo-ti, and kudzu. In addition, psyllium, soy lecithin, and wild yam have been shown to combat high cholesterol.

Garlic seems to work in at least three ways to protect against heart disease. It helps lower total cholesterol and raise HDL, lowers blood pressure, and keeps blood platelets slippery, helping to prevent clots. Onions have been found to have similar beneficial effects.

In addition to using fresh garlic in cooking, you can take garlic in the form of various pills, powders, and capsules. The exact amount to take is unknown, but if you regularly use aspirin or another anticoagulant drug, consult your doctor before adding large amounts of garlic to your diet.

Nutritional Support

One of the best ways to maintain plaque-free arteries is to keep cholesterol levels under control, and the best way to do that is by eating a low-fat, high fiber diet.

Most experts feel that healthy individuals should derive no more than 30 percent of their daily calories from fat, and that those with signs or symptoms of heart disease should try to keep it down to 20 percent. If you are typical, however, over 35 percent of the calories in your diet probably come from fat.

Some fats are more harmful than others. Saturated fats represent the biggest threat because they raise your cholesterol levels. Butter, whole milk, cheese, ice cream, egg yolks, and fatty cuts of beef, pork, and lamb are all particularly high in these potentially dangerous fats. Experts say they should account for only 7 to 10 percent of your total daily calories.

Substituting unsaturated fats (both mono- and polyunsaturated) for the saturated kind will lower your blood cholesterol level and stave off hardening of the arteries. Monounsaturated fats—found in olive, peanut, canola, avocado, and certain fish oils—should account for 10 to 13 percent of your daily caloric intake.

Polyunsaturated fats—found in corn, soybean, safflower, sunflower, and sesame seed oils, as well as tuna and salmon—should make up 10 percent of your total calories.

In addition to keeping your intake of fats to a minimum, eat more unprocessed whole grains, fruits, vegetables, and beans. These filling foods not only serve as stand-ins for richer meat and dairy products, but also deliver powerful arterial plaque fighters: carotene, vitamins C and E, selenium, and soluble fiber.

Alternative Treatments

Macrobiotic Diet: This Asian-style vegetarian diet is low in fat and high in fiber, qualities that will keep your cholesterol in check. Beware, however, of an overly strict macrobiotic regimen. It can lead to nutritional deficiencies.

Naturopathic Medicine: This style of medicine emphasizes a diet high in fruits, vegetables, and whole grains—all standard recommendations for those with clogged arteries.

Orthomolecular Medicine: Orthomolecular practitioners use vitamins as medications to prevent or cure chronic disorders. To lower the risk of clogged arteries, they recommend 400 IU of vitamin E, 3 milligrams of vitamin B_6, and 400 micrograms of folic acid daily.

Vegetarianism: By excluding meat from the menu, vegetarians tend to reduce their intake of fat, cholesterol, and calories, thus benefiting their cholesterol levels and reducing their chances of developing atherosclerosis.

Cluster Headaches

The Basics

Named for their tendency to strike in "clusters" or waves, recurring day after day at the same hour, these headaches are typically sudden and severe, and may be accompanied by watery eyes, sweating, restlessness, nausea, or a runny nose. The pain is usually one-sided, starting near the eye and shooting up to the temple and top of the head. The headaches often start at night and last from 15 minutes to 2 hours. They're more likely to develop in the spring and fall, when they may come and go for several days, weeks, or months at a time. They occur mainly in men.

The underlying cause is still a mystery, but we do know some of the leading triggers. They include:

■ Smoking or drinking alcohol
■ Napping in the daytime
■ Inhaling solvents, gasoline, or oil-based paints for long periods of time
■ Air travel or trips to high-altitude areas (above 5,000 feet)

Call Your Doctor If . . .
■ You have a series of headaches that fit the "cluster" profile. Prescription medication from the doctor is the most effective remedy.

Seek Care Immediately If . . .
■ You have a headache that gets worse or lasts more than 2 hours despite medication.
■ You develop a high temperature.
■ You faint or develop weakness, numbness, double vision, difficulty with talking, or neck pain or stiffness.

What You Can Do
■ Try to avoid the triggers that seem to set off the headaches for you.
■ Before an airplane trip, take a preventive dose of the headache medication your doctor has prescribed. Using oxygen during the flight can also be a help.
■ When you have a headache, avoid bright lights, alcohol, and stressful situations that cause you to become angry or excited; they can worsen the pain.
■ During headaches, try applying a cold pack to your head. For many people, this eases the pain.
■ Supervised exercise often helps prevent cluster headaches. Be sure to talk to your doctor, however, before starting an exercise program.

What Your Doctor Can Do

There is no permanent cure for this problem, but the doctor can make sure that the headaches are not a warning sign of a more dangerous disorder, and can prescribe medications to relieve them when they occur.

Prescription Drugs

Some of the drugs used for migraine headaches are also prescribed for the cluster variety. Included among these medications are:

Ergomar (ergotamine)
Imitrex Injection (sumatriptan)
Sansert (methysergide)

Indocin (indomethacin)
Wigraine (ergotamine and
  caffeine)

Over-the-Counter Drugs

You can try over-the-counter pain relievers such as ibuprofen (Advil, Motrin), aspirin, acetaminophen (Tylenol), and others, but many people find they don't do much good for cluster headache pain.

Herbal Remedies

Small doses of feverfew taken daily have a preventive effect against migraine headaches. Although there's no documentation of a similar action against cluster headaches, you might want to give it a try. White willow, the original source of aspirin, also has some pain-relieving properties.

Nutritional Support

Avoid alcohol and caffeine. They can help bring on or worsen a cluster headache.

Alternative Treatments

Acupressure: Often called acupuncture without needles, this therapy seeks to remedy illness through the application of deep finger pressure at points located along an invisible system of energy channels called meridians. Some doctors consider it a reasonably effective remedy for headache pain.

Acupuncture: This traditional Chinese therapy often proves effective for all types of pain, including headache. The treatments require insertion of fine needles at certain very specific "acupoints" on the skin.

Biofeedback: This specialized type of training allows people to gain control over physiologic reactions that are ordinarily unconscious and automatic. For some people, it helps to reduce the pain associated with headaches.

Chiropractic: This therapy focuses on hands-on joint manipulation as a means to relieving pain. Particularly effective for back pain, it is also said to relieve headache pain.

Environmental Medicine: Certain toxins are known to trigger cluster headaches. Environmental medicine aims to remedy the effects of such toxins, and its advocates recommend it for all types of chronic disorders.

Feldenkrais Method: Not a therapy or cure, this is a type of supportive therapy that can help in any situation where improved movement patterns (and awareness of those patterns) can help with recovery from illness or injury. Its practitioners have found it helpful for chronic headaches.

Hypnotherapy: With its ability to enhance the power of suggestion, hypnosis has been found effective for a variety of problems that hinge on emotions, habits, and even the body's involuntary responses.

Magnetic Field Therapy: This hotly debated form of therapy is sometimes advocated for headache. It relies on small magnetic disks taped over areas of the body that radiate pain (known as trigger points).

Massage Therapy: While massage isn't capable of curing anything, it can provide welcome relief from all kinds of pain.

Meditation: The calming mental exercises of meditation are a proven antidote to stress, tension, anxiety, and panic. Some people find it helpful for headaches as well.

Myotherapy: This specialized form of deep muscle massage is said to quickly relieve virtually any sort of muscle-related pain, including that associated with some types of headaches.

Osteopathic Medicine: Born over a century ago from the belief that displaced bones, nerves, and muscles are at the root of most ailments, osteopathy has long since merged into the medical mainstream. Many modern osteopaths still offer manipulative treatments, but they can also prescribe the most effective new medications.

Qigong: The exercises typical of this well-known Chinese discipline can reduce stress and anxiety, while improving overall physical fitness, balance, and flexibility. By alleviating tension, they may also combat insomnia and relieve certain types of headache, although their effectiveness for cluster headaches remains unverified.

Reflexology: Reflexologists say the foot is a microcosm of the entire body and press on various "reflex points" along the foot to relieve symptoms elsewhere in the body. Such treatments, they insist, can ease the pain of headaches.

Colds and Flu

The Basics

Colds (known medically as upper respiratory infections) affect the air passages in the head, neck, and chest. The nose, throat, sinuses, ears, windpipe (trachea), and airways of the lung (bronchi) all can be involved. Without treatment, a cold will improve in a week or two.

Colds are caused by viruses. They can spread easily, especially during the first 3 or 4 days of illness. You can catch a cold simply by touching someone who has one, or by being nearby when an infected person coughs or sneezes. You are most likely to get a cold in the winter, and are most susceptible if you are tired, under stress, or plagued with allergies (especially hay fever).

Typical symptoms include sneezing, runny nose, stuffy nose, headache, cough, sore throat, trouble breathing, fatigue, muscle aches, and red, watery eyes. Most cold sufferers do not run a fever.

Colds are the most common illness among children. Although youngsters often feel better within 3 or 4 days of developing the infection, they may continue coughing for 2 to 3 weeks. Many children have 6 colds a year.

There is still no cure for the common cold. Antibiotics will not kill cold viruses. The symptoms can, however, be relieved by a variety of prescription drugs, over-the-counter medicines, and herbal remedies.

Flu, like the common cold, is an infection of the nose, throat, windpipe, and airways in the lung. Unlike a cold, it usually starts with chills and fever, and is likely to be accompanied by headache, body aches, and fatigue. Other symptoms include sore throat, cough, and red, watery eyes. Children may also develop earaches, vomiting, and diarrhea. The disease is worst during the first 1 to 2 days. Cough and tiredness may last another week or more.

Known medically as influenza, flu is caused by a wide variety of influenza viruses. Infected individuals quickly spread the germs through coughing and sneezing. An annual flu shot can protect you from some—but not all—of the most common influenza viruses. Even with the shot you may still get the flu, but it may not last as long as it would otherwise.

Antibiotics are no help against the flu. There are a couple of prescription medicines that will weaken the virus, but they won't provide a cure. Symptoms such as congestion, sore throat, and cough can be relieved with an assortment of prescription medicines, over-the-counter drugs, and herbal remedies. Still, your best strategy is plenty of rest, lots of liquids, and acetaminophen or ibuprofen for pain and fever.

Call Your Doctor If . . .

■ Your fever lasts more than 3 or 4 days or you have a high temperature.
■ You have a sore throat that gets worse, or you see white or yellow spots in your throat.
■ Your cough gets worse or lasts more than 10 days.
■ You develop a rash.
■ You feel large and tender lumps in your neck.
■ You develop an earache or a bad headache.
■ You cough up thick yellow, green, gray, or bloody mucus (a sign of bacterial infection).
■ You have nausea, vomiting, or diarrhea.
■ Your child's eyes get red and become coated with a yellow discharge.

Seek Care Immediately If . . .

■ You get really bad neck pain or stiffness.
■ You feel confused, start acting strangely, or have a seizure.
■ You have trouble breathing or develop chest pain.
■ Your skin or nails look gray or blue.
■ A youngster with a cold seems sleepier than usual, urinates less than normal, has a dry mouth and cracked lips, cries without tears, or seems dizzy. These are signs of dehydration.

What You Can Do

■ Use prescription and over-the-counter medicines exactly as directed. Extra doses can lead to side effects.
■ Use a cool-mist humidifier to increase air moisture. This will make it easier for you to breathe and will help relieve your cough.
■ Gargling may help relieve your sore throat. Use warm salt water (1 teaspoon of salt in a cup of water) or warm or cold double-strength tea.
■ Wash your hands often to avoid spreading germs. This is especially important after blowing your nose and before touching food. Cover your mouth and nose when you cough or sneeze.
■ Rest until your temperature is normal (98.6° F or 37° C). This usually takes 3 to 4 days. Get plenty of sleep.
■ You may want to get a flu shot in the fall to reduce your odds of

catching the disease, particularly if you are over 65 or have a chronic heart or lung disease.

■ DO NOT GIVE ASPIRIN if a child with influenza is under 18 years of age. This could lead to brain and liver damage (Reye's syndrome). Carefully check for aspirin on the label on any over-the-counter medicines. Acetaminophen will help relieve fever and body aches.

■ To keep a young child's nose free from mucus, soak a cotton ball with warm water and put 3 drops into each nostril. Wait about 1 minute, then have the youngster blow his or her nose. If the child is too young for this, use a soft rubber suction bulb: Close one nostril, squeeze the bulb, insert it into the open nostril, and release the bulb so that it sucks up the mucus.

What Your Doctor Can Do

If you have a cold or the flu, there is little your doctor can do other than to prescribe medications to relieve the worst of the symptoms. (If you want to spare yourself a visit to the doctor, you can find over-the-counter remedies that contain most of the prescription products' ingredients.) Antibiotics are useless unless the doctor finds that you also have a bacterial infection in the lungs.

Prescription Drugs

Two prescription drugs—Flumadine and Symmetrel—attack and weaken the flu virus itself. There are also a variety of prescription drugs that offer symptomatic relief of problems such as congestion, runny nose, and cough. Among the available medicines are:

Atrohist products	Duravent products	Nucofed products
Bromfed-DM	Entex PSE	Ornade
Codimal-L.A.	Exgest LA	Phenergan products
Congess	Extendryl	Rynatan products
D.A. II	Fedahist	Trinalin
Duratuss products	Kronofed-A	Tussionex

Over-the-Counter Drugs

Over-the-counter painkillers such as acetaminophen or ibuprofen can relieve headache, pains, and fever. Decongestants can clear a stuffy nose. Cough suppressants and expectorants are also helpful. However, taking antihistamines for a runny nose is useless unless you have a nasal allergy. Among the many cough and cold remedies available without a prescription are:

Actifed products	Cheracol products	Ryna products
Actron	Comtrex products	Sinarest
Advil products	Contac products	Sine-Aid
Aleve	Coricidin products	Sine-Off
Alka-Seltzer Plus	Delsym	Singlet
products	Dimetapp products	Sinulin
Allerest No	Drixoral products	Sinutab products
Drowsiness	Goody's	St. Joseph
Ascriptin	Halls Cough Drops	Sucrets
Bayer	Motrin IB	Sudafed products
BC Powder	N'Ice Lozenges	Theraflu products
products	Novahistine	Triaminic products
Benadryl products	Nuprin	Triaminicin
Benylin products	Orudis KT	Tylenol products
Bufferin	Panadol	Vicks 44M
Cepacol products	Pertussin DM	Vicks DayQuil
Cepastat Lozenges	Robitussin products	Vicks NyQuil
Cerose DM		

For a child with a cold or the flu, you can select from a variety of special pediatric formulations:

Advil, Children's	Halls Juniors	Robitussin Pediatric
Bayer, Children's	Motrin children's	Cough Suppressant
Chewable	products	Tylenol children's
Benylin Pediatric	Panadol Children's	products
Cough Suppressant	Pediacare	Vicks 44 E,
Dimetapp children's	Pertussin CS	Pediatric
products		

Herbal Remedies

You can also choose among an extensive assortment of herbs for relief of the problems that typically accompany a cold or the flu. Listed below are the natural remedies judged effective for each type of problem:

COLD SYMPTOMS IN GENERAL

Anise	Brewer's Yeast	Chinese Cinnamon
Ash	Caraway	Cloves
Balsam	Cardamom	Couch Grass
Balsam of Peru	Chamomile	Dill

Echinacea
English Oak
English Plantain
Galangal
Garlic

Iceland Moss
Japanese Mint
Larch
Mustard
Onion

Peppermint
Pine Oil
Radish
Sandalwood

COUGH

Anise
Balsam
Balsam of Peru
Blue Mallow
Brewer's Yeast
Camphor
Caraway
Cardamom
Chamomile
Chinese Cinnamon
Cinnamon
Cloves
Couch Grass
Dill
Echinacea
Elder
English Ivy
English Oak
English Plantain
Ephedra
  (Ma Huang)

Eucalyptus
Fennel
Galangal
Garlic
Gumweed
Hemp Nettle
Horehound
Horseradish
Iceland Moss
Japanese Mint
Khella
Knotweed
Larch
Licorice
Linden
Lungwort
Marshmallow
Meadowsweet
Mullein
Mustard

Nasturtium
Niauli
Onion
Peppermint
Pimpinella
Pine Oil
Primrose
Radish
Red Clover
Sandalwood
Sanicle
Seneca Snakeroot
Soapwort
Star Anise
Sundew
Thyme
Watercress
White Nettle
Wild Cherry
Wild Thyme

FEVER

Anise
Ash
Balsam
Balsam of Peru
Caraway
Cardamom
Chamomile
Chinese Cinnamon
Cinnamon

Cloves
Couch Grass
Dill
Echinacea
English Oak
English Plantain
Galangal
Garlic
Iceland Moss

Japanese Mint
Larch
Mustard
Onion
Peppermint
Pine Oil
Radish
Sandalwood

SORE THROAT

Agrimony
Anise
Balsam
Balsam of Peru
Bilberry
Blackberry
Blackthorn
Brewer's Yeast
Caraway
Cardamom
Chamomile
Chinese Cinnamon
Cinnamon
Cloves
Coffee Charcoal

Couch Grass
Dill
Echinacea
English Oak
English Plantain
Galangal
Garlic
Iceland Moss
Jambolan
Japanese Mint
Knotweed
Larch
Marigold
Mustard
Myrrh

Onion
Peppermint
Pine Oil
Potentilla
Radish
Rhatany
Rose Flower
Sage
Sandalwood
Slippery Elm
Tormentil
Usnea
White Nettle
Witch Hazel

Nutritional Support

Drink plenty of fluids (8 to 10 glasses daily). Liquids such as juice, water, broth, gelatin, and lemonade are all appropriate. If a sick child won't eat, don't worry about giving solid food until the illness passes.

Alternative Treatments

Environmental Medicine: According to practitioners of this approach to medicine, pollution is responsible for common ailments such as nasal congestion, sneezing, and sinus headaches. Environmental therapists aim to relieve such symptoms through four types of treatment:

■ Nutritional therapies, such as vitamins and minerals
■ Detoxification therapies to remove harmful metals and chemicals from the body
■ Immunotherapy to strengthen the immune system
■ Desensitization to train the immune system to ignore allergic triggers

Colic

The Basics

Colic is the term used to describe a pattern of symptoms in newborn infants. A colicky infant cries for hours for no known reason. The cry often takes the form of a fussy screaming. Colic frequently follows the "Rule of Threes": It begins in the first three months of life, the crying lasts for 3 hours a day, and the colicky symptoms occur at least 3 days a week.

The exact cause of colic is unknown. Tiredness, food allergy, overly warm milk, hunger, and overfeeding may play a part. Stress in the home, loneliness, and pain may also have a role. A colicky infant may simply want to be held or to go to sleep. Many doctors blame the problem on intestinal gas.

Symptoms often seem to run in cycles. The infant may cry once or twice a day for several hours. Between these crying spells, the baby may seem fine. Crying often starts in the late afternoon or early evening and tends to stop when you hold the child. The crying does no harm, but can be very stressful for the parents.

It is hard to treat colic since its cause is unknown. Holding, cuddling, and rocking the baby usually works best. The over-the-counter medication simethicone has also proven helpful for many colicky babies.

Call Your Doctor If . . .

■ The baby seems to be in pain or acts sick.
■ The baby has been crying constantly for more than 3 hours.
■ The baby develops a high temperature.

Seek Care Immediately If . . .

You are afraid that you will hurt the baby.

What You Can Do

■ Burp the infant after each ounce of formula. If you are breastfeeding, burp the baby every 5 minutes. Always hold the child while feeding, and allow at least 20 minutes for each session.
■ Do not give a feeding every time the baby cries. Wait at least 2 hours between feedings. Check to see if the baby is in a cramped position, is too hot or cold, has a soiled diaper or an open diaper pin, or needs to be cuddled.

■ When trying to comfort a crying infant, use soothing, gentle motions. Use a rocking chair or cradle, put the baby in a wind-up swing, or carry the child in a front-pack. If the crying continues after more than 20 minutes of gentle motion, let the baby cry himself to sleep.

■ When the baby is having an attack of gas, hold him or her securely and gently massage the lower part of the stomach. You may also apply a heating pad set on *low* (or a warm water bottle) to the stomach. Be very careful not to burn the baby. Do not lay the infant on the heating pad.

■ Try not to let the baby sleep more than 3 hours at a time during the day.

■ The baby's constant crying can be very aggravating. Try to be patient and stay calm. Ask someone to care for the infant so you can get out for an hour or two. Don't blame yourself. Remember that you're not the cause of the baby's colic.

What Your Doctor Can Do

Your doctor will examine the baby to rule out other causes of pain. He may recommend trying a milk substitute formula to make sure the problem is not the result of milk intolerance. If you are breastfeeding your baby, he may suggest changing your diet.

The doctor may recommend simethicone drops for your baby to help break up gas bubbles. Ask your doctor how much to give and how often to administer it. A prescription drug called hyoscyamine is sometimes used to control intestinal spasms.

Prescription Drugs

Levsin (hyoscyamine sulfate)
Cystospaz (hyoscyamine)

Over-the-Counter Drugs

Infants' Mylicon Drops
Phazyme Infant Drops

Herbal Remedies

Angelica root is considered a remedy for gas.

Nutritional Support

If your infant is formula-fed, it may be helpful to try a different type of infant formula. Ask your doctor for suggestions.

If you are breastfeeding your baby, you may want to eliminate gas-producing foods from your diet. Beans, broccoli, cabbage, garlic, onions, prunes, turnips, and large amounts of fruit may make your breast milk difficult on the baby's digestive system. If you suspect any food is making the infant uncomfortable, try eliminating it from your diet for several weeks to see if the symptoms improve.

Alternative Treatments
Infant massage may help calm a crying, uncomfortable baby.

Colitis

The Basics
Stubborn, troubling, and—in the most severe cases—life-threatening, colitis is an inflammation of the large intestine that upsets the movement of waste through the bowel. The exact cause of colitis is still a mystery. Until recently, it was believed to be triggered by certain foods and medicines, infections, and stress. However, researchers now know that an overzealous and misdirected immune system plays a major role in destroying intestinal tissue. Colitis appears to run in families and most often affects young adults.

The most prominent symptom of colitis is profuse diarrhea brought on by the diseased bowel's failure to absorb enough water. The diarrhea is usually combined with blood and pus from the many tiny ulcers that develop in the intestine as a result of the disease.

Colitis also causes cramping, abdominal pain, fever, chills, nausea, weight loss, anemia, and tiredness. Constipation may also occur, either due to obstructions in the intestines or because nerves damaged by chronic inflammation fail to produce an urge. Symptoms outside the digestive system can include eye problems, such as pinkeye (conjunctivitis) and inflammation of the iris, canker sores, skin rashes and sores, and joint pain. Symptoms typically come and go from day to day.

There are different kinds of colitis, named according to the extent of the inflammation or the specific areas affected. Universal colitis involves the entire colon (large intestine), while sigmoid colitis extends only a short distance beyond the rectum. The mildest form of colitis, proctitis, affects only the rectum.

Call Your Doctor If . . .

■ You go for several days without a bowel movement.

Seek Care Immediately If . . .

■ You have a high temperature.

■ Your stool is black or has blood in it.

■ You have severe pain in your abdomen.

■ You develop a skin rash.

What You Can Do

■ Rest often. When you feel better, you can begin normal activities.

■ Avoid raw vegetables and fruit, spicy foods, alcohol, chocolate, nuts, and drinks that have caffeine in them (coffee, tea, cola). Milk, cheese, and ice cream may also upset the colon.

■ Drink 8 to 10 large glasses of water each day. You need plenty of water to replace the liquid lost in watery stools.

■ For pain relief, take acetaminophen. Do not take aspirin or ibuprofen; they may irritate the colon.

■ A cool towel or heating pad (set on low) on the abdomen may also ease pain.

■ If your rectal area is sore from loose stools and rough toilet paper, ask your doctor to recommend an ointment.

What Your Doctor Can Do

Your doctor will diagnose the disorder by analyzing your symptoms, conducting a physical exam, and studying the appearance of the inflamed areas. The doctor will run tests on your blood and stools and have x-rays taken. A new blood test, ANCA, can detect the presence of a liver and bile duct abnormality known as PSC (primary sclerosing cholangitis) that accompanies colitis.

At times, endoscopy is used to diagnose colitis. This technique employs fiberoptic technology to transmit an image of the inside of the intestines. There are two types of endoscopy: flexible sigmoidoscopy and colonoscopy.

Flexible sigmoidoscopy can be performed during an office visit and without sedation. During this procedure, a soft, lighted tube about 2 feet long is inserted through the rectum and maneuvered up the sigmoid colon and the descending colon (up the left side). The procedure is quick (usually about 5 minutes) and usually painless. If there is pain, it is usually due to the difficulty of passing the probe through the curvy sigmoid colon ("sigmoid" means S-shaped). Virtually all cases of colitis can be diagnosed through this procedure.

Colonoscopy also uses a soft, lighted tube, but the device is longer in order to allow your doctor to see further into the colon, and sedation is often required. The procedure is more time-consuming than sigmoidoscopy (average time is about 18 minutes) and more painful. It can be useful, however, in gathering tissue samples from various sites along the gut wall and in looking for signs of cancer—important because people with long-standing colitis have a higher risk of colorectal cancer.

Short of surgery, there is no definitive cure that will end colitis once and for all. However, four out of five colitis patients find sufficient relief from drug therapy.

Prescription Drugs

A drug called mesalamine (also known as 5-ASA) is now the mainstay of therapy for inflammatory bowel disease. Brands include Asacol, Pentasa, and Rowasa. This drug is used to control first attacks and relapses, and to maintain recovery. A related drug, olsalazine sodium (Dipentum) is used for cases involving the large intestine. An older drug, sulfasalazine (Azulfidine), has lost popularity due to potential side effects.

If these drugs fail to do the job, steroids are the next line of defense. Steroid products approved for this purpose include betamethasone (Celestone), cortisone (Cortone), dexamethasone (Decadron), hydrocortisone (Hydrocortone), prednisolone (Pediapred, Prelone), and methylprednisolone (Medrol).

For mild cases of colitis, doctors often prescribe the anti-diarrhea medication diphenoxylate, found in Lomotil.

Over-the-Counter Drugs

Over-the-counter medications can relieve diarrhea during mild attacks. Your options include Donnagel, Imodium, Pepto-Bismol, and Rheaban. Check with your doctor, however, before using any anti-diarrhea medication during a severe attack. It could trigger a dangerous ballooning of the lower intestine.

Herbal Remedies

A number of herbs can help control mild diarrhea. They include:

Agrimony	English Oak	Potentilla
Bilberry	Green Tea	Psyllium
Blackberry	Jambolan	Tormentil
Coffee Charcoal	Lady's Mantle	Uzara

Nutritional Support

Proper diet is important. Foods with high residue tend to aggravate the symptoms of colitis. Your doctor may prescribe a diet of low-residue, easily absorbed foods such as meat, fish, rice, white bread, pasta, gelatin, and hard-boiled eggs. You should avoid high-residue foods such as apples, oranges, celery, cabbage, tomatoes, and berries. Some people find that a dairy-free diet is also helpful.

Regular servings of yogurt could also provide relief. A number of inflammatory bowel disease patients participated in a clinical trial of live-culture yogurt as a remedy for their symptoms. Participants ate 8 ounces of yogurt in the morning and another 8 ounces at bedtime. Overall, most of those who participated in the trial reported at least a 50 percent improvement in such symptoms as pain, diarrhea, and bloody stools.

Antioxidant vitamins, such as beta carotene, vitamins C and E, selenium, and methionine also have been shown to help keep inflammatory bowel disease in remission. One small study of people with mild to moderate colitis showed that treatment with omega-3 fatty acids could improve symptoms.

Folic acid, a B vitamin that can be depleted by bowel disease, is being studied for its protective effect against colon cancer. Researchers suggest that people with colitis take 1 milligram of folic acid a day to diminish colon cancer risk. Check with your doctor, though, before starting this type of regimen.

Alternative Treatments

Colitis is one of the many serious disorders that refuse to yield to any form of alternative therapy. However, if your problem is not colitis but actually irritable bowel syndrome (a noninflammatory condition with which colitis is often confused) there are several therapeutic possibilities. *Biofeedback,* which trains people to control involuntary reactions such as spasms in the colon, might prove helpful. *Hypnotherapy* also claims some success, and you may find *meditation* beneficial.

Conjunctivitis

The Basics

Sometimes called "pinkeye," this annoying and often painful ailment results from irritation of the inner eyelid and the surface of the white part of the eye. Infections and allergies are the most common causes.

If an infection is the culprit, you'll typically have painful red eyes, puffy eyelids, or a gritty feeling when you blink. There may be a clear, yellow, or green-colored discharge that forms crusts and cause the eyelids to stick together, especially in the morning. A copious discharge usually signifies a bacterial infection; viral infections cause less. The disease spreads easily from person to person through hands, towels, and handkerchiefs.

If an allergy is at fault, the eyes tend to get red, itchy, and watery, but don't exude pus. The problem develops when pollen, spores, dust, or other pollutants blow into the eyes.

Whatever the cause, the problem should begin to clear up within a few days after starting treatment.

Call Your Doctor If . . .

■ The eye is still pink 3 days after starting treatment.
■ Pain in the eye increases, the redness spreads, or your vision becomes blurred.
■ You develop a high temperature.

Seek Care Immediately If . . .

Symptoms of pinkeye rarely demand emergency treatment.

What You Can Do

■ To ease discomfort, apply a clean, warm or cool washcloth to your eye several times a day for 10 to 20 minutes.
■ Do not touch or rub your eyes with your hands.
■ Gently wipe away any discharge from the eyes with tissues.
■ To keep from spreading the infection, wash your hands often with soap and dry them with paper towels. Do not share towels or washcloths. Keep children with pinkeye home from school or day care until the condition clears up.
■ Sunglasses may be helpful if light bothers your eyes.
■ Until the irritation subsides, do not use eye makeup or wear contact lenses.

■ If a medication blurs your vision, do not attempt to drive.

■ If the problem is due to allergies, do your best to avoid the cause.

What Your Doctor Can Do

The doctor will probably test the discharge for the presence of bacteria or viruses. If a bacterial infection is the culprit, the doctor may prescribe antibiotic medication.

Prescription Drugs

For bacterial eye infections, a variety of antibiotic drops and ointments are available. The more commonly prescribed products include:

Garamycin Ophthalmic (gentamicin sulfate)
Neosporin (polymyxin B, neomycin, and bacitracin)
Polysporin (polymyxin B and bacitracin)
Sodium Sulamyd or Bleph-10 (sulfacetamide sodium)

If there is no evidence of infection, the doctor may prescribe a steroid ointment or drops to reduce the inflammation. Leading choices include:

Decadron or Maxidex (dexamethasone)
FML or Flarex (fluorometholone)
Inflamase or Pred Forte (prednisolone)

It's also possible to prevent expected allergic symptoms with cromolyn sodium eyedrops (Crolom, Opticrom).

Over-the-Counter Drugs

To relieve allergic symptoms, you can buy antihistamine eyedrops over the counter at any drugstore. The most common choices are:

Naphcon A or OcuHist (pheniramine with naphazoline)
Vasocon-A (antazoline with naphazoline)

Antihistamine tablets also can help.

Herbal Remedies

No herbs are considered effective for this problem.

Nutritional Support

There are no nutritional measures that can provide relief.

Alternative Treatments

Because an infection may be involved, your best course is to see a conventional physician.

Constipation

The Basics

Constipation (infrequent and difficult bowel movements) strikes an estimated 10 percent of the population in Western countries. Older adults are five times more likely to suffer the problem than the young.

The normal frequency of bowel movements ranges from daily to every third day, with perfectly healthy people falling outside both ends of this range. However, if you don't have a bowel movement at least every 3 days, the intestinal contents may harden, making elimination difficult or even painful.

Resulting complications include hemorrhoids or fissures (painful cracks near the anus). Bleeding can occur for either of these reasons, signaled by bright red streaks on the surface of the stool. Fecal impaction is also a possibility, particularly in older adults. This problem may be accompanied by a loss of control, with liquid flowing around the hard-packed stool. Rectal prolapse, in which a small amount of intestinal lining is pushed through the rectal opening during straining, is another potential side effect.

Constipation is usually the result of a shortage of fiber in the diet or a failure to drink enough liquids daily. Plentiful in fruits, vegetables, bran, and whole-grain cereals, fiber absorbs water in the intestines, making the stool softer and easier to pass. It also adds more weight to the stool, and the heavier the stool, the more easily it moves through the gut. Fiber also encourages the growth of gas-producing bacteria in the colon, which serves to add forward pressure on the intestinal contents.

There are a variety of other problems that occasionally lead to constipation. Potential culprits include:

- Irritable bowel syndrome
- Poor bowel habits
- Lack of exercise

■ Laxative abuse
■ Travel, with its inevitable changes in diet, activity, and schedule
■ Hormonal disturbances
■ Pregnancy
■ Fissures and hemorrhoids
■ Neurological or muscular disorders, such as lupus and multiple sclerosis
■ Depression
■ Loss of body salts
■ Spinal cord damage
■ Medications, including pain medications, antihistamines, diuretics, antacids containing aluminum, antispasmodic drugs, antiparkinsonism medications, antidepressants, tranquilizers, iron supplements, anticonvulsants, and antibiotics.

Like adults, children vary greatly in the frequency of their bowel movements, and constipation is rarely serious. However, you should suspect the problem if the child grunts, strains, draws up his legs, and becomes red in the face when having a bowel movement. Leading causes of constipation in the very young include chocolate; eating or drinking too many milk products; medicines such as iron; waiting too long to go to the bathroom; stress during toilet training; and diaper rash that causes pain during a bowel movement.

Call Your Doctor If . . .
■ Constipation lasts longer than 3 weeks.
■ The problem is accompanied by fever and abdominal pain.
■ There is bright red blood or pus in the stool.
■ The symptoms are severe and disabling.
■ The rectal area has tears that fail to heal.
■ A child has not had a bowel movement in several days.
■ A child's bowel movements are very hard or painful.

Seek Care Immediately If . . .
■ A child suffers constant, severe abdominal pain for more than 2 hours.

What You Can Do
■ You can use over-the-counter laxatives for relief of occasional constipation; but try to avoid relying on them. If you need them for more than a week, you should check with your doctor.

■ Maintain good bowel habits. Set aside a time for an undisturbed visit to the bathroom and don't ignore the urge to have a bowel movement. Bending forward so your chest touches your thighs helps move the stool out.

■ Be sure to include plenty of fiber in your diet, and drink lots of fluids. (See the Nutritional Support section for more information.)

■ Exercise regularly. Walking is a good choice.

For a constipated child:

■ If your baby is less than 4 months of age, give fruit juices twice a day. Apple, grape, or prune juices are especially recommended. Babies also need water every day. Ask your doctor how much you should give.

■ For a baby over 4 months old, give strained fruits, vegetables, and cereal, including apricots, peaches, plums, pears, prunes, beans, peas, or spinach.

■ If the child is 1 year or older, make sure that he or she eats fruits and vegetables 3 times daily. Avoid food that can't be chewed easily.

■ Limit the amount of milk, ice cream, cheese, white rice, bananas, cooked carrots, and applesauce in the child's diet.

■ To help a baby have a bowel movement, gently hold his knees against his chest.

■ Put the child in a warm water tub several times a day. This may relax the rectal area and make it easier to pass a bowel movement.

■ If your child becomes constipated while toilet training, stop for a while and go back to using diapers.

■ Be sure to remedy diaper rash, which can cause constipation. See the entry on Rash for details.

■ Tell the child not to wait too long to go to the bathroom when he feels the urge.

■ Encourage the child to be more physically active.

■ If the child develops small tears near the rectum, let him sit in warm salt water three times daily (your doctor will tell you how much salt to add to the tub water). After the bath, rub ½ percent hydrocortisone cream on the area.

■ Check with your doctor before giving laxatives.

What Your Doctor Can Do

Although minor constipation doesn't require medical care, you may want to see your doctor if the problem becomes chronic. To rule out an underlying disease such as irritable bowel syndrome or cancer, the doctor may conduct a physical exam, including an examination of the rectum, a barium enema, x-rays, and possibly a sigmoidoscopy to exclude rectal disease.

Prescription Drugs

For chronic constipation, the doctor can prescribe a lactulose preparation such as Chronulac Syrup or Duphalac. All other remedies are available over-the-counter.

Over-the-Counter Drugs

For occasional constipation, the following preparations can be used by adults:

Bisacodyl (Correctol, Dulcolax)
Calcium polycarbophil (Fibercon)
Docusate sodium (Colace, Correctol Stool Softener,
  Dialose, Ex-Lax Stool Softener Caplets)
Docusate sodium/casanthranol (Fleet Sof-Lax
  Overnight, Peri-Colace)
Docusate sodium/phenolphthalein (Dialose Plus,
  Phillips' Gelcaps)
Magnesium hydroxide (Phillips' Milk of Magnesia)
Malt soup extract (Maltsupex)
Methylcellulose (Citrucel)
Mineral oil (Kondremul)
Psyllium (Perdiem Fiber)
Senna (Correctol Herbal Tea, Ex-Lax Gentle
  Nature Pills, Senokot)
Sennosides (Ex-Lax)
Sennosides/psyllium (Perdiem)

Children can take senna (Fletcher's Castoria, Senokot Children's Syrup) for an occasional bout of constipation.

For chronic constipation, adults can take calcium polycarbophil (Konsyl Fiber Tablets), casanthranol docusate (Peri-Colace), senna (Senokot), docusate sodium/senna (Senokot-S), methylcellulose (Citrucel), and psyllium (Konsyl Powder, Metamucil). For children there is a senna product (Senokot Children's Syrup).

Avoid using enemas repeatedly; this practice will eventually lead to the loss of bowel function. Likewise, excessive use of laxatives can alter the bowel muscles' ability to advance intestinal contents and thus cause chronic constipation. Overuse of mineral oil also can reduce the body's ability to absorb vitamins A, D, E, and K. Do not combine mineral oil and stool softeners (Colace, Dialose, Fleet Sof-Lax). And if you're pregnant, check with your doctor before using any laxative.

Herbal Remedies

Herbal remedies for constipation include:

Aloe	European Buckthorn	Mountain Flax
Black Root	Fo-Ti	Psyllium
Buckthorn	Gamboge	Rhubarb
Cascara	Linseed	Senna
Castor Oil	Manna	Yellow Dock

Nutritional Support

Dietary improvements are the best long-term solution to this problem. Eat less of those foods that increase the chance of constipation: meat, dairy products, eggs, and refined sugars. Most important, eat more of the foods known to reduce the chances of constipation: vegetables, fruits, and whole grains. Prunes and figs are especially good because they contain naturally occurring substances that stimulate the bowels. People with dental problems can rely on softer fiber-rich foods such as oatmeal, stewed or canned fruits, beans, steamed vegetables, and brown rice. You also can add unprocessed bran to your food. Start with half a cup daily, then increase your intake over the course of several weeks until you reach two cups daily.

Alternative Treatments

Biofeedback: This training technique is designed to put you in control of otherwise involuntary bodily functions. It's under study as a potential remedy for chronic constipation.

Crabs

The Basics

Shaped like its namesake from the sea, the crab louse is a tiny light-brown wingless insect that makes its home in the hairy parts of the body. The lice cling to the hair and feed on blood. The female of the species lays about 50 eggs, called nits, which become so firmly attached to the base of the hair strands that they cannot be removed with normal washing. The average life span is 25 to 30 days.

There has recently been a resurgence of pubic lice, which are often spread during sex. You can also catch them by sharing combs, hats, clothing, or bed linens. They spread easily from person to person, which means that your risk increases if you or your partner have multiple or casual sexual partners. It's easier to get lice than any other sexually transmitted disease. In fact, from just one sexual encounter with an infested person, you have a 95 percent chance of picking them up.

The first symptom is usually itching in the hairy areas of your body, such as the genital area, scalp, or eyebrows. You may see red marks and bumps (called hives) where the insects have bitten your skin. You may even see the lice themselves on your hair. With treatment, however, the lice should be gone in about 5 days.

Call Your Doctor If . . .

■ The bites become pus-filled or crusty, and your hair becomes matted or foul-smelling. These are signs of infection.

■ Itching or red, swollen bite marks return after treatment.

■ You have any problems related to the medicine you are using.

Seek Care Immediately If . . .

Crabs are annoying, but never constitute an emergency.

What You Can Do

■ Apply medication—whether prescribed or over-the-counter—for exactly the recommended amount of time.

■ Lice-killing medicine does not always destroy all the nits. You must remove them from your hair with a fine-toothed comb. A special comb may come with the medicine. If not, you can buy one at a drugstore. Comb the lice-infected hair completely, from the skin outward, once a day until the treatment is complete. You do not have to shave or cut the hair in the affected area.

■ Avoid close contact with anyone until your doctor tells you the lice are all gone.

■ Machine wash all the clothes, towels, sheets, and blankets you used during treatment and the 3 days prior to treatment. Use hot water, then dry them for at least 20 minutes in a hot dryer. If you do not have a washer and dryer, iron the items, seal them up in a plastic bag for 10 days, then have them dry-cleaned or hang them outside for 2 days.

■ Tell all sexual partners you've had during the past month so that they can be checked for lice and treated.

What Your Doctor Can Do

Your doctor can prescribe a lice-killing medication, usually in the form of a shampoo or lotion. If the lice fail to disappear after a week, get another examination. It is normal to still feel itchy for a few days after treatment.

Prescription Drugs

Cure is rapid with either a 1 percent lindane shampoo (Kwell) applied for 4 minutes and then washed off, or a 1 percent permethrin cream rinse (Rid), which is washed off after 10 minutes. Application may be repeated in 10 days to destroy any surviving nits, but prolonged use is not recommended because these products may cause irritation. To avoid a recurrence, be sure to follow all instructions carefully.

Over-the-Counter Drugs

You can buy other pesticide treatments, containing pyrethrin with piperonyl butoxide (A-200, Rid), without a prescription. They are applied for 10 minutes and then washed off. If you are allergic to ragweed, you should avoid these products. There are also products for inanimate objects such as furniture. These should not be used on humans or animals.

Herbal Remedies

No herbal preparations have been tested for this purpose.

Nutritional Support

There are no dietary measures capable of eliminating this problem.

Alternative Treatments

There are no worthwhile alternatives to the standard anti-lice preparations described above.

Croup

The Basics

Croup, known medically as laryngotracheobronchitis, is an inflammation of the voice box (larynx), windpipe (trachea), and airways (bronchi). It is a common illness in infants and children from 6 months to 3 years of age. Croup usually occurs during late fall, winter, and early spring. It can be caused by a wide variety of viruses, and children can develop it more than once.

Croup is usually preceded by a cold. Typically, the child develops a barky cough, noisy breathing, and a hoarse voice. Other signs are fast breathing, problems swallowing, and restlessness. Croup attacks usually occur during the evening or night. The attacks are worst during the first 2 to 3 days.

A severe case of croup can make breathing so difficult that the child requires hospitalization. Milder cases can be cared for at home.

Call Your Doctor If . . .

■ The child is sleepier than usual, is urinating less, has a dry mouth and cracked lips, cries without tears, or seems dizzy. These are signs of dehydration.
■ The child has a high temperature.
■ The child's breathing does not get better after 10 to 15 minutes in a steamy bathroom.
■ The child cannot rest because the coughing won't stop.
■ The cough lasts more than a few days.

Seek Care Immediately If . . .

Call 911 or go to the emergency room if the child shows any of the following signs:

■ Trouble breathing or swallowing.
■ The skin between the ribs is being sucked in with each breath.
■ The lips or fingernails are turning blue or white.
■ The child is leaning over and drooling.

What You Can Do

Most cases of croup can be treated at home as long as breathing problems and coughing don't increase. It typically takes 3 or 4 days before the child feels better.

■ You can help the child's breathing by sitting with him or her in a steamy bathroom. Turn on the hot water in the sink, shower, or bathtub and close the windows and bathroom door. When the room is steamed up, bring the child into the room and sit with him or her on your lap for at least 15 minutes. Do not leave the child alone.

■ Call your doctor if the steam does not improve the child's breathing within 10 to 15 minutes.

■ If it is cool outside, taking the clothed child outside in the cool air for 5 minutes may help make breathing easier.

■ If you have a cold-steam vaporizer or humidifier, place it out of reach by the child's bed. Fill it with cool water. Direct the mist stream toward the child's face. The humidifier will loosen the mucus in the child's throat, making it easier to breathe.

■ Keep the child warm and give clear liquids (water, apple juice, lemonade, tea, or ginger ale) once breathing has improved. The liquids should be room temperature. It's important to make sure the child gets plenty of fluid so the mucus will stay thin.

■ Do not let anyone smoke around the child. The smoke can make breathing difficult and aggravate the child's cough.

■ Do **not** give the child aspirin. Give acetaminophen for fever and discomfort. Ask your doctor before giving ibuprofen.

■ If the child begins to have trouble breathing, call for emergency help. Never try to open your child's airway with your finger.

■ You should try to stay calm and see that the child gets as much rest as possible. His or her breathing and coughing will become worse if the child is afraid and crying.

What Your Doctor Can Do

If the child has trouble breathing, a stay in the hospital may be needed. There, the level of oxygen in the child's blood will be measured with a device called a pulse oximeter, which is placed on an ear, finger, or toe. The nurse may also take a blood sample from an artery to test for oxygen.

Nurses may place an IV tube in one of the child's veins for giving medicine or liquids. To ease breathing, the child will be given moist cool air from a mask, tent, or high-humidity room. The doctor may also use a machine to help the child inhale medicines to keep the airways open. At first, these treatments may be needed quite often. Later, they'll be given less frequently. If breathing gets worse, the doctor may need to put a tube into the child's windpipe to provide enough air.

Prescription Drugs

Antibiotics are useless against croup, and are prescribed only if a bacterial infection sets in. If the child needs to be hospitalized, he or she may be given epinephrine to open the airways and steroid medications such as prednisone to reduce inflammation.

Over-the-Counter Drugs

Several children's remedies are available to relieve the cough that accompanies croup:

Benylin Pediatric	Robitussin Pediatric
Cough Suppressant	Cough Suppressant
Halls Juniors	Vicks 44E, Pediatric
Pertussin CS	

For fever, several brands of children's acetaminophen and ibuprofen are available. Do not give aspirin.

Advil, Children's	Panadol, Children's
Motrin (Junior Strength	Tylenol, Children's and Infants'
and Children's)	

Herbal Remedies

A broad assortment of herbs is considered effective against cough. They include:

Anise	Elder	Khella
Balsam	English Ivy	Knotweed
Balsam of Peru	English Oak	Larch
Blue Mallow	English Plantain	Licorice
Brewer's Yeast	Ephedra (Ma Huang)	Linden
Camphor	Eucalyptus	Lungwort
Caraway	Fennel	Marshmallow
Cardamom	Galangal	Meadowsweet
Chamomile	Garlic	Mullein
Chinese Cinnamon	Gumweed	Mustard
Cinnamon	Hemp Nettle	Nasturtium
Cloves	Horehound	Niauli
Couch Grass	Horseradish	Onion
Dill	Iceland Moss	Peppermint
Echinacea	Japanese Mint	Pimpinella

Pine Oil	Sanicle	Thyme
Primrose	Seneca Snakeroot	Watercress
Radish	Soapwort	White Nettle
Red Clover	Star Anise	Wild Cherry
Sandalwood	Sundew	Wild Thyme

Nutritional Support

Make sure the child gets plenty of liquid. No other special nutritional measures are recommended.

Alternative Treatments

There are no alternative forms of therapy that promise to relieve croup.

Dehydration

The Basics

Dehydration is not a trivial problem. Excessive loss of water and other important body salts can become very dangerous if you allow it to go uncorrected. The condition is especially serious in newborns and infants. Without treatment, it can produce a disastrous drop in blood pressure, leading to shock and even death.

Prolonged vomiting, diarrhea, or high fever can deplete the body's fluids. Even excessive sweating in the sun or heat can produce a dangerous deficit. An overdose of medicines that cause you to lose water and salt, such as diuretics or "water pills," can also cause the problem.

Typical symptoms include a dry tongue and mouth, excessive thirst, and reduced urination. As the condition worsens, additional symptoms may include sunken eyes, wrinkled skin, dizziness, confusion, and a fast heartbeat and breathing. A dehydrated child may be sleepier than usual, urinate less, have a dry mouth and cracked lips, cry without tears, or seem dizzy. In babies less than one year old, the soft spot on top of the head may become sunken.

To correct dehydration, the lost liquids must be replaced. In severe cases, hospitalization may be required.

Call Your Doctor If . . .

■ You develop a high temperature.

■ A child under 3 months old has a temperature above 100 degrees F (37 degrees C).

■ A child over 3 months old has a temperature above 102 degrees F (39.4 degrees C).

■ You do not feel better after drinking liquids for several hours.

■ You are having trouble keeping liquids down.

Seek Care Immediately If . . .

■ You pass very little urine or none at all after a few hours of treatment.

■ You feel dizzy or faint.

■ You have a fast heartbeat.

■ Your skin looks wrinkled or your mouth feels very dry.

■ You lose several pounds in a few days.

■ Your child has signs of worsening dehydration, including listlessness, excessive thirst, little or no urination in more than 6 hours, no tears, wrinkled skin, dizziness, irritability, and weight loss.

What You Can Do

ADULTS

■ If you think you are becoming dehydrated, you should weigh yourself daily and write down the number. If vomiting or diarrhea is the cause, keep track of how much and how often it occurs. Get lots of rest.

■ Be sure to drink plenty of liquids to replace the water your body has lost. Take a small amount of fluid every 30 to 60 minutes. Large amounts may upset your stomach.

■ Drink clear liquids for the first 24 hours.

• You can buy a special ready-made liquid called a rehydration or electrolyte solution at a drug or grocery store. It has the exact amounts of water, salts, and sugar your body needs to replace what you've lost. Follow the directions on the label.

• You also can make your own fluid replacement mixture. Be sure to measure carefully. Add 1 level teaspoon of sugar and ½ level teaspoon of salt to 1 pint (2 cups) of water.

• Do not use liquids such as apple juice, soft drinks, tea, chicken broth, or sports drinks. They have the wrong amounts of water, salts, and sugar.

■ If you have been vomiting and can't keep liquids down, suck on ice chips or flavored ice until you stop throwing up. Drink more liquids as your condition improves.

■ Keep drinking liquids until your urine is pale yellow. You may need to drink 8 to 12 large glasses of liquid a day to bring your water level back to normal.

■ You may slowly return to your normal diet over the next 2 to 3 days.

CHILDREN
■ For the first 24 hours give the child only clear fluids. Use an electrolyte solution from the grocery store or give gelatin water (a 3-ounce package in a quart of water) or a mixture made by adding ¼ teaspoon of salt and 1 tablespoon of sugar to 1 pint of water.
  • If the child is vomiting, give fluid very slowly, starting with 1 or 2 teaspoons every 10 minutes.
  • If there is no vomiting and the child is less than 1 year old, you may give 1 tablespoon every 20 minutes.
  • If there is no vomiting and the child is over 1 year old, give 2 tablespoons every 30 minutes.
■ If there is no vomiting, you may gradually return the child to a normal diet over the next 2 or 3 days.
  • If a baby is taking only formula, dilute it to half strength for the next 24 hours.
  • If you are breastfeeding, give the baby clear liquids for 2 feedings, then start breastfeeding again.
  • If the child is taking solid food, begin with bland foods such as applesauce or bananas and add other foods as tolerated. If the child is over 1 year old, do not include milk, ice cream, butter, or cheese in the diet for the next 3 days.
■ Keep a record of how often you change your baby's diaper and how wet it is each time.

What Your Doctor Can Do
You can treat dehydration yourself, but to remedy the vomiting, diarrhea, or fever that's causing the problem, a trip to the doctor is your best bet. For severe dehydration you may need a short stay in the hospital, where you can be given fluids intravenously.

Prescription Drugs
None of the common rehydration products require a prescription.

Over-the-Counter Drugs
KaoLectrolyte
Rehydralyte
Pedialyte

Herbal Remedies
Only fluids and salts are needed. Herbs won't help.

Nutritional Support

Your only immediate concern is to restore the body's normal fluid and mineral balance.

Alternative Treatments

Alternative treatments are unnecessary.

Depression

The Basics

If you find yourself overcome by uncontrollable feelings of sadness, guilt, and low self-esteem that you can't shake off—even after 2 weeks or more—you're probably suffering from major depression. This illness afflicts more than 15 percent of Americans at some point in their lives. Fortunately, there's no need to be resigned to the problem. A variety of medications are available to bring your mood back to normal and let you get on with your life.

Ordinary bouts of depression come and go, but a major, unshakable depression seems to be the result of a change in brain or body chemistry. It can start spontaneously, or be triggered by a devastating event such as loss of a loved one, loss of a job, an assault, or a rape. Your odds of developing major depression are higher if:

■ You're a woman.
■ Someone else in your family has had a mood disorder.
■ You are between the ages of 25 and 44 years.
■ You abuse drugs or alcohol.

Depression can start very slowly, and become noticeable to other people before you recognize it yourself. It's often accompanied by irritability and anxiety. The chief symptoms are:

■ Constant fidgeting or a slowdown in movement
■ Depressed mood most of the day, every day
■ Difficulty thinking and concentrating
■ Disturbed sleep
■ Fatigue, loss of energy
■ Feelings of guilt, worthlessness, hopelessness
■ Inability to make decisions

■ Loss of interest in pleasurable activities
■ Recurrent thoughts of suicide
■ Significant weight loss or gain

If you have at least 5 of these symptoms every day for 2 weeks, you may have major depression. If you have fewer than 5, or if the symptoms are mild and do not interfere with your daily life, the condition is called mild depression.

Depression is sometimes the result of another illness, such as a thyroid disorder. It can also be caused by certain medications, such as birth control pills and some of the drugs used for high blood pressure. In such cases, correcting the source of the problem will provide relief.

For most people, however, the standard treatment is a prescription for one of the many antidepressant medications currently on the market. Psychotherapy may also be warranted to help you improve your self-esteem, change patterns of negative behavior, and cope with problems arising from depression. If these measures fail to help—or you begin to feel suicidal—a hospital stay may be necessary.

Call Your Doctor If . . .
■ You feel your mood getting worse.
■ You're unable to sleep well or find that you are sleeping more than usual.
■ You have a change in appetite.
■ Your medicine makes you drowsy, dizzy, or sick to your stomach.

Seek Care Immediately If . . .
■ You begin to have thoughts of suicide or violence.
■ Your medicine causes an allergic reaction (swelling or trouble breathing).

What You Can Do
■ Be sure to take your prescribed medication regularly, even if it seems to have no effect at the start. It takes as long as 4 to 6 weeks for some medications to become effective. Since some antidepressants can make you drowsy, be cautious when using machinery or driving until you know how the drug affects you. Check with your doctor before taking any other drugs, either prescription or over-the-counter.
■ Avoid alcohol and recreational drugs while taking an antidepressant. They may interact with it badly.

■ Since it's hard to avoid stress, learn to control it with such techniques as deep breathing, relaxation exercises, meditation, or biofeedback. Try not to bottle up your feelings; talk to your doctors, family, or friends and let them help you. You may also want to join a support group.

■ Encourage those close to you to talk to your doctor. He can give them tips on how to deal with your illness.

What Your Doctor Can Do

Your doctor will begin by looking for an outside cause. He may order blood tests, an x-ray, EKG, or a CT scan to rule out other illnesses. If he finds that you have a standard case of major depression, you will probably need to visit a clinic or doctor's office 1 to 4 times a month.

To relieve the problem, there are several types of antidepressant medication available, including selective serotonin reuptake inhibitors, serotonin/norepinephrine reuptake inhibitors, tricyclic antidepressants, and monoamine oxidase inhibitors. These drugs affect the balance of brain chemicals in slightly different ways. For any given individual, one type may work well, while another has little effect. There is no way to predict which type is best for a specific patient, so don't be surprised if your doctor has to try several different prescriptions before finding the medication that works best for you. Once drug therapy is underway, you'll need additional blood tests to monitor the effects of the drug and guard against side effects.

Treatment for severe depression can require full-time hospitalization, or a partial care program in which you are able to return home after each day's therapy. If medication and psychotherapy doesn't work for you—or isn't fast enough—the doctor may recommend electroconvulsive therapy. Also known as ECT or shock therapy, this form of treatment applies a mild electric current to the brain. Although the shock temporarily disrupts the memory, full recall typically returns within two weeks.

Prescription Drugs

Asendin (amoxapine)
Aventyl (nortriptyline)
Celexa (citalopram)
Desyrel (trazodone)
Effexor (venlafaxine)

Elavil (amitriptyline)
Etrafon (amitriptyline with
  perphenazine)
Limbitrol (amitriptyline with
  chlordiazepoxide)

Ludiomil (maprotiline)
Marplan (isocarboxazid)
Nardil (phenelzine)
Norpramin (desipramine)
Pamelor (nortriptyline)
Parnate (tranylcypromine)
Paxil (paroxetine)
Prozac (fluoxetine)
Remeron (mirtazapine)
Serzone (nefazodone)
Sinequan (doxepin)
Surmontil (trimipramine)
Tofranil (imipramine)
Triavil (amitriptyline with
  perphenazine)
Vivactil (protriptyline)
Wellbutrin (bupropion)
Zoloft (sertraline)

Over-the-Counter Drugs
All antidepressant medications require a prescription.

Herbal Remedies
Only one herb—St. John's wort—has genuine mood-lifting effects. It seems to share some of the properties of serotonin-boosting drugs and monoamine oxidase inhibitors.

Nutritional Support
The amino acid tryptophan is the raw material for serotonin, one of the chemicals in the brain that seems to prevent depression. Tryptophan supplements were briefly outlawed in the U.S. after a contaminated batch caused an outbreak of illness, but they are now available again. If you still prefer to increase your tryptophan intake through diet rather than supplements, the best sources include bananas, dried dates, milk, cottage cheese, turkey, and peanuts.

Alternative Treatments
Biofeedback: This technique enables patients to control otherwise involuntary reactions. After applying sensors to various parts of your body and hooking them up to a computer, a biofeedback therapist will teach you mental and physical exercises that serve to control your body's responses. The therapy has been deemed helpful for depression and similar problems such as seasonal-affective disorder.

Hypnotherapy: After putting you into a "trance-like" state, a hypnotist can help you change the way you perceive stressful problems and help you discover new ways of responding to them. Scientists aren't sure how hypnotherapy works, but it's considered especially helpful for anxiety, phobias, compulsions, and depression.

Massage Therapy: A relaxing massage won't cure depression, but it may help alleviate some of the symptoms you may be experiencing. In one medical study conducted in a group of teenage mothers, massage therapy helped relieve anxiety and depression.

Sound Therapy: Listening to certain types of music can have therapeutic benefits for individuals with a wide variety of ailments, including depression. Employing auditory feedback in a broad range of frequencies, a therapy known as the Tomatis Method, may be especially helpful.

Diabetes

The Basics

Over the years, diabetes—or excess sugar in the blood—can work severe damage on the heart, kidneys, eyes, blood vessels, and nerves. There's no cure for this disease, but fortunately, we do know how to keep it under control.

Diabetes results either from the body's failure to produce enough insulin or from an inability to make use of it efficiently. Insulin is the hormone that helps us convert the starches and sugar we eat into the energy needed for daily life. Without its benefit, sugar builds up in the blood, eventually triggering the problems for which diabetes is feared.

Doctors have divided diabetes into two major categories. In people with "Type 1" diabetes—which usually appears in childhood—the pancreas makes too little insulin or none at all. In those with "Type 2" diabetes—which typically develops in adults—the pancreas continues to manufacture insulin, but the body fails to make use of it. People with Type 1 diabetes usually need regular injections of insulin. Type 2 diabetes can often be controlled with a special diet, exercise, and oral medicines, though temporary insulin injections may be necessary during periods of stress and times of illness.

The onset of diabetes is signaled by a distinctive set of symptoms that includes fatigue, frequent urination, great thirst, weight loss, and increased vulnerability to infection. Wounds may heal slowly. You may also feel as though you are eating more than usual. If the condition isn't brought under control, a variety of complications are likely to follow.

Among the most dangerous possibilities is ketoacidosis. This problem develops when the body, unable to get enough energy from blood sugar, begins to burn fat. As a by-product of this process, chemicals called ketones flood the bloodstream. Together with excess sugar, the extra ketones can build up to dangerous, even life-threatening levels that require immediate, emergency treatment.

Early signs of ketoacidosis include excessive thirst, frequent urination, headache, nausea, and vomiting. Your breath may take on a fruity odor, you may find yourself panting, and you may become unusually sleepy and fatigued. Other symptoms include weight loss and a feeling of fullness or pain in the stomach. Call your doctor as soon as these signs begin to appear. If the condition is left untreated, it could lead to coma and death.

The insulin taken to control diabetes can also cause complications. Although its whole purpose is to reduce the amount of sugar in your blood, it can push the level *too* low, causing the condition known as hypoglycemia. Early warning signs of this problem include headache, hunger, sweating, nervousness, and weakness. As the sugar supply drops further, these symptoms are joined by palpitations, memory loss, double vision, trouble walking, and numbness around the mouth. Ultimately, twitching, fainting, and seizures set in.

You can drive down your blood sugar too far by missing a meal, eating too little, eating late, or exercising more vigorously than usual without eating extra food. Hypoglycemia can also be triggered by an infection, excessive doses of insulin, alcohol, and certain medicines. The remedy for mild hypoglycemia is simple: eat a hard candy or drink a glass of fruit juice. For a severe attack, seek emergency treatment.

Long-standing diabetes can also interfere with the blood supply to your legs and feet. As a result, your skin may become thinner, break more easily, heal more slowly, and become more vulnerable to infection. Since nerve damage, with reduced feeling in the feet, is another complication of diabetes, there's a constant danger of unnoticed infections. To prevent serious damage, it's therefore wise to pay special attention to your feet.

Call Your Doctor If . . .

■ Your medications and treatment plan fail to improve your symptoms.

■ An injury refuses to heal, or you notice redness, numbness, burning, or tingling.

■ You develop pain or cramps in your legs and feet, or they always feel cold.

Seek Care Immediately If . . .

■ You notice the warning signs of ketoacidosis listed above.

■ You have symptoms of low blood sugar, feel you are going to pass out, and can't get something to eat. THIS IS AN EMERGENCY!

- You develop vomiting or diarrhea.
- You feel chest pain.
- You have signs of dehydration, such as decreased urination, increased thirst, or a light-headed feeling.
- Your blood or urine glucose measurement remains higher than the level judged safe by your doctor even when you take 2 extra doses of insulin per 24 hours.

What You Can Do

- Be sure to test your urine or blood for sugar (glucose) as often as your doctor directs, and take your prescribed medications faithfully. The more carefully you keep your sugar level under control, the less your danger of complications.
- Make a point of exercising regularly and bring your weight down to normal. Losing as little as 10 to 15 pounds can improve your blood sugar levels.
- Take orange or apple juice, sugar, or candies if you have any symptoms of low blood sugar. If you have time, check your blood sugar first. Keep sugar (such as candies) and a product called glucagon in your car and at home. Avoid alcohol, which can lower your blood sugar.
- Do not go barefoot, and check your feet daily for blisters, cuts, and redness. Wash your feet gently with warm (not hot) water and mild soap every day. Pat your feet and the area between your toes until completely dry. Apply moisturizing lotion to the dry skin on your feet and to dry, brittle toenails. Trim your toenails straight across. Do not dig under them or around the cuticle. Do not cut corns or calluses or try to remove them with medicine unless your doctor approves.
- If you find a minor scrape, cut, or break in the skin on your feet, keep it and the skin around it clean and dry. When you remove an adhesive bandage, be sure not to injure the skin around it. Check any wound several times a day to make sure it is healing.
- Always wear a medic-alert pendant or bracelet identifying you as a diabetic.

What Your Doctor Can Do

Although there's no cure for diabetes, your doctor can help you keep your blood sugar levels as close to normal as possible. He will recommend dietary changes and exercise and, if needed, can prescribe medication.

Prescription Drugs

If the problem stems from lack of insulin, you'll probably need to take regular insulin injections. A wide variety of slow- and faster-acting insulins are available. Among the leading brands are:

Humalog	Iletin	Velosulin
Humulin	Novolin	

For people who are still able to produce some insulin, there are a number of oral medications that either spur additional production or help the body use the available supply. They include:

Amaryl (glimepiride)	Glyset (miglitol)
DiaBeta, Glynase, or Micronase	Orinase (tolbutamide)
(glyburide)	Prandin (repaglinide)
Diabinese (chlorpropamide)	Precose (acarbose)
Dymelor (acetohexamide)	Rezulin (troglitazone)
Glucophage (metformin)	Tolinase (tolazamide)
Glucotrol (glipizide)	

Over-the-Counter Drugs

For relief of low blood sugar, glucose tablets are available over the counter.

Herbal Remedies

There are no herbs known to help diabetes.

Nutritional Support

Some people with Type 2 diabetes are able to control their condition with diet and exercise alone. A nutritionist can tailor a plan to fit your specific needs. In general, however, the following guidelines always hold true:

- Eat wholesome, balanced meals at regular, fixed times. It is best to have 3 meals a day, plus 2 or 3 snacks.
- Keep your weight normal. Lose extra pounds if you have to.
- Boost your carbohydrates to 50 percent of your calories.
- Cut fat to 30 percent of your calories.
- Make sugary foods part of a balanced meal.
- Back up your diet with regular exercise.

Alternative Treatments

Orthomolecular Medicine: Practitioners of this form of medicine use larger than usual doses of certain nutrients to prevent or cure disease. Although conclusive evidence is still lacking, some researchers have found that a daily intake of 200 micrograms of chromium picolinate can provide significant relief from diabetes, reducing the need for insulin and oral diabetes drugs.

Vegetarian Diet: Some researchers believe that vegetarians are less likely to develop diabetes than people whose diet includes meat.

Diarrhea

The Basics

Almost everyone suffers an occasional bout of diarrhea without any serious effects. The problem often results from irritation of the lining in the large intestine, which prompts food residue to rush through before excess water can be absorbed. Diarrhea can also develop when an infection or other disorder triggers an abnormal flood of fluid from the intestinal walls.

The frequent, loose, watery stools that mark diarrhea are often accompanied by cramping and gas. However, the most dangerous side effect is dehydration due to massive loss of body salts and water. If left untreated, severe dehydration can be life threatening.

Diarrhea can be caused by stress, certain foods, alcohol, and overuse of magnesium antacids and laxatives. Some drugs, particularly broad-spectrum antibiotics like ampicillin, clindamycin, and cephalosporins, can also cause diarrhea. These antibiotics can kill beneficial bacteria in the large intestine, allowing the unrestrained growth of another bacterial inhabitant called *Clostridium difficile*. This bacterium inflames the intestinal wall, making it "weep" excess water and mucus, resulting in watery stools.

Like a headache, diarrhea can be a symptom of a wide variety of underlying ailments. It's the hallmark of such chronic diseases of the large intestine as irritable bowel syndrome, inflammatory bowel disease (Crohn's disease, ulcerative colitis), and diverticulosis. Graves' disease, Addison's disease, and Legionnaire's disease can cause diarrhea. Anaphylaxis, a severe and potentially life-threatening allergic reaction, is also a cause. Diarrhea can be a sign of colon and pancreatic cancer. Severe diarrhea often accompanies the advanced stages of AIDS.

Diarrhea is also one of the chief symptoms of gastroenteritis, an intestinal disease brought on by bacteria, amoebas, parasites, toxins, certain drugs, enzymes, or allergens in food. Gastroenteritis caused by *Salmonella* is an extremely common infection—more than two million new cases are reported in the United States each year. It is usually contracted by eating contaminated or inadequately processed foods—especially eggs and poultry. Food poisoning from *Shigella* or *Staphylococcus* also causes diarrhea.

Infections by *Escherichia coli* and other bacteria living in human intestines cause a great deal of diarrheal illness in children. These infections are also prevalent among travelers to other countries, particularly those visiting Mexico, South America, and Southeast Asia. The loose, watery stools of traveler's diarrhea usually result from drinking unpurified water or eating unclean food, where bacteria, viruses, and parasites can thrive. When you swallow the infected material, the germs take up residence in the bowel, causing diarrhea.

People with mild infections recover easily. The problem generally lasts 2 to 7 days. Those with severe infections, however, require prompt replacement of lost fluid and salts in order to prevent fatal dehydration.

Call Your Doctor If . . .
■ Diarrhea lasts for more than 3 days
■ You find blood, mucus, or worms in your stool
■ You develop pain in the abdomen or rectum.
■ You have a high temperature.

Seek Care Immediately If . . .
■ You have signs of water loss, including dry mouth, extreme thirst, wrinkled skin, little or no urine, or dizziness or light-headedness.

What You Can Do
Most cases of diarrhea can be alleviated with prescription or over-the-counter anti-diarrhea medications. If you are suffering an acute attack of colitis, however, avoid these drugs; they could cause a dangerous enlargement of the bowel. If you think the problem may be due to food poisoning, see a doctor before taking a remedy. Anti-diarrhea medications are not recommended in all instances.

Most complications from diarrhea are caused by loss of water. Drink 2 to 3 quarts of fluid a day—clear liquids, such as defizzed ginger ale or cola, bottled or boiled water, hot tea, or broth during the first 24 hours or until the diarrhea stops. If you are sick to your stomach, suck on ice chips. During the next 24 hours, you may eat bland foods such as cooked cereals, rice, clear soup, bread, crackers, baked potatoes, eggs, and applesauce. Avoid alcohol and caffeine. You can return to your regular diet after 2 to 3 days.

If you have gastroenteritis, you should rest and drink plenty of fluids. You may take an anti-diarrhea medication containing bismuth, such as Pepto-Bismol.

To avoid contracting traveler's diarrhea:
■ Take 2 tablets of Pepto-Bismol 4 times a day (with each meal and at bedtime), beginning the day before you leave and continuing for 2 days after arriving home. Continue for up to 3 weeks.
■ Drink only bottled or boiled water, or canned or bottled beverages (soft drinks, beer, wine) without ice. Boil water for at least 4 minutes or use purifying tablets to treat the water.
■ Brush your teeth with mouthwash solution. Do not use tap water for this purpose or to wash off food. Always wash your hands before handling or eating food.
■ Avoid all raw fruits and vegetables except those that can be peeled. Also stay away from milk, ice cream, and other dairy products; raw meat and fish; and cold sauces, salsa, and dressings. Relatively safe foods include steaming-hot dishes, grilled foods right off the fire, and dry foods (breads, crackers).

What Your Doctor Can Do

Treatment depends on the cause. For a mild case, the doctor may prescribe an anti-diarrhea medication and suggest some dietary changes. Cases of gastroenteritis, including traveler's diarrhea, can usually be cleared up with antibiotics. If the problem is an inflammatory bowel disease such as colitis, special prescription drugs may be needed.

Whatever the cause of the diarrhea, if you have suffered excessive fluid loss you may need treatment for dehydration. For details, see the entry on this problem.

Prescription Drugs

Lomotil (diphenoxylate with atropine) and paregoric (camphorated opium tincture) are the two most common prescription medications for diarrhea. As a last resort, an antispasmodic drug such as propantheline (Pro-Banthine) can be prescribed. The doctor may also recommend small doses of a bulk-producing laxative (see "Over-the-Counter Drugs" below).

If the problem is due to infection or food poisoning, treatment with an antibiotic may be the best alternative. The drugs most commonly prescribed for this purpose are ciprofloxacin (Cipro), furazolidone (Furoxone) and sulfamethoxazole with trimethoprim (Bactrim, Septra).

For underlying inflammatory bowel disease, mesalamine or a steroid medication may be needed. See the entry on colitis for details.

Over-the-Counter Drugs

Over-the-counter medications for diarrhea include attapulgite (Donnagel, Kaopectate, Rheaban), bismuth subsalicylate (Pepto-Bismol), and loperamide hydrochloride (Diarrid, Imodium, Pepto Diarrhea Control). Do not use these medications, however, if you have a high fever.

Bulk-producing laxatives—in small amounts—can help absorb excess liquid in the bowel. Options include Citrucel, FiberCon, Konsyl, Metamucil, and Perdiem Fiber Therapy. (Avoid stimulant laxatives such as Correctol, Ex-Lax, and Senokot.)

Herbal Remedies

Herbal remedies for diarrhea include:

Agrimony	English Oak	Potentilla
Bilberry	Green Tea	Psyllium
Blackberry	Jambolan	Tormentil
Coffee Charcoal	Lady's Mantle	Uzara

Nutritional Support

Certain dietary elements tend to aggravate diarrhea in sensitive individuals. If you are lactose-intolerant, dairy products may have this effect. Copious amounts of fruit juice and fruit-flavored soft drinks can trigger the problem, as can caffeinated beverages such as coffee, tea, and cola. The magnesium in such antacids as Rolaids and Philips' Milk of Magnesia can also present difficulties.

If your diarrhea is a result of inflammatory bowel disease, you might want to try twice-daily servings of live-culture yogurt. In at least one study, it produced substantial improvement. Research also suggests that antioxidants such as beta carotene, vitamins C and E, selenium, and methionine can keep inflammatory bowel disease in remission. For details, see the entry on colitis.

To fend off dehydration, be sure to drink as much fluid as possible. While recovering, eat a bland diet, as described under "What You Can Do."

Alternative Treatments

There's nothing that alternative medicine can do for food poisoning, traveler's diarrhea, and infectious gastroenteritis. For these ailments, your best course is to see a doctor for antibiotic therapy.

However, three forms of alternative therapy have been used with some degree of success for relief of irritable bowel syndrome, one of the more common causes of diarrhea.

Biofeedback: This specialized form of training enables you to take control of otherwise involuntary bodily reactions such as spasms in the bowel.

Hypnotherapy: These treatments use the power of suggestion to modify problematic emotions, habits, and involuntary bodily responses.

Meditation: This age-old discipline promotes relaxation by emptying the mind of all outside distractions. It's a proven remedy for high blood pressure and chronic pain, and can relieve a variety of stress-related ailments.

Dislocated Joints

The Basics

Our joints are held together with extremely tough, fibrous bands of tissue called ligaments. Sometimes, however, a yank or a blow proves too much for them; they stretch or tear, and the bones they connect pop out of alignment.

You're unlikely to overlook a dislocation. The affected joint will be painful and difficult to move. It will probably look misshapen, and will quickly become swollen and red. To remedy the problem, the doctor usually must reset the bones manually (although a numbing injection will sometimes allow a dislocated jaw to pop back into place on its own).

Once the bones are back in position, you may need to wear a splint, elastic bandage, or sling to restrict movement while the ligaments heal. Pain from the injury generally begins to subside within a day or two. Healing requires 2 to 8 weeks. Dislocations tend to weaken the joint, increasing the chance of a repetition.

Call Your Doctor If . . .
■ The pain or swelling gets worse.
■ You have trouble moving the joint once the splint or sling comes off.
■ Your pain medication fails to work.
■ The joint seems to have popped out of place again.

Seek Care Immediately If . . .
■ An affected limb feels numb or cold and looks pale.
■ You have trouble breathing.

What You Can Do
■ Apply ice to the injury for 15 to 20 minutes each hour for the first 1 to 2 days. Put the ice in a plastic bag and place a towel between the bag and your skin.
■ After the first 1 to 2 days, you may put heat on the injury to help ease the pain. Use a heating pad (set on low), a whirlpool bath, or warm, moist towels for 15 to 20 minutes every hour for 48 hours.
■ To reduce the pain and swelling from a dislocated elbow, keep your arm lifted above the level of your heart whenever possible for 48 hours.
■ If you are given a splint or sling, keep wearing it until your doctor says it's okay to stop. You may need to loosen the splint if the area beyond it gets numb or tingly. Call your doctor for instructions if you don't know how.
■ If a dislocated jaw is the problem, you may need to hold it in place with a bandage for the first few days. For the first week, eat only soft foods, such as baby food, gelatin, cooked cereal, ice cream, applesauce, bananas, eggs, pasta, cottage cheese, soups, and yogurt. For about 6 weeks, do not open your mouth wide when you yawn, bite large pieces of food, shout, sing, or call out loudly. If you need to yawn, put your fist under your chin to keep your mouth from opening up too wide.
■ If the doctor prescribes pain medicine that makes you drowsy, don't drive.

What Your Doctor Can Do
Your doctor will order an x-ray of the dislocated joint. The bones will probably have to be manually popped back into place, but if you have a really bad dislocation, you may need surgery. The doctor can prescribe a strong painkiller to get you past the brief period when the pain is worst. After that, over-the-counter products are usually sufficient.

Prescription Drugs

While the pain remains severe, the doctor can prescribe a variety of pain-killing pills. Typical medications include:

DHCplus (acetaminophen with dihydrocodone)
Dilaudid (hydromorphone)
Hydrocet, Lorcet, Lortab, Vicodin, or Zydone
 (acetaminophen with hydrocodone)
Kadian, MS Contin, or MSIR (morphine)
Levo-Dromoran (levorphanol)
OxyContin, OxyIR, or Roxicodone (oxycodone)
Percocet or Tylox (acetaminophen with oxycodone)
Percodan (aspirin with oxycodone)
Talwin Nx (naloxone)
Toradol (ketorolac)
Tylenol with Codeine (acetaminophen with codeine)
Ultram (tramadol)
Vicoprofen (hydrocodone with ibuprofen)

Over-the-Counter Drugs

As the pain subsides, a nonprescription painkiller should provide satisfactory relief. Your options include:

Actron	Bufferin	Orudis KT
Advil	Excedrin	Panadol
Aleve	Excedrin, Aspirin-	St. Joseph
Alka-Seltzer	Free	Tylenol
Ascriptin	Goody's	Unisom with Pain
Bayer Aspirin	Motrin IB	Relief
BC Powder	Nuprin	Vanquish

Herbal Remedies

If you want to avoid over-the-counter drugs, there are two herbs that can help with the pain: Japanese mint and white willow.

Nutritional Support

During recovery, be sure to get an ample, balanced diet. Don't skimp on meat and dairy products, which help to supply the proteins and amino acids needed for healing.

Alternative Treatments

Magnetic Field Therapy: Advocates of this type of therapy say that it's especially good for muscle and joint pain. While the use of small magnets for this purpose is generally considered safe, its effectiveness is still under dispute.

Reconstructive Therapy: This form of treatment seeks to stimulate the growth of healthy tissue with a series of injections directly into the damaged joint. Injections usually contain the anesthetic lidocaine, an irritant such as sodium morrhuate, dextrose, phenol, minerals, amino acid supplements, and B complex vitamins. They have been found effective in several clinical trials.

Ear Infections

The Basics

Marked by nagging and often excruciating pain and pressure, these common infections stem from a variety of causes in various sections of the ear. Although they are not contagious, they are extremely common in children between the ages of 6 months and 2 years. Here's an overview of the most commonly encountered problems.

Otitis media: This is an infection of the middle ear (the area behind the eardrum). A variety of viruses and bacteria may be at fault. They gain a foothold when the tube between the ear and the back of the nasal cavity (the eustachian tube) becomes congested by a cold, a sinus or throat infection, or an allergic reaction, causing fluid to accumulate in the middle ear. In this favorable environment, the germs can quickly multiply, causing a buildup of pus and mucus behind the eardrum and inflaming the eardrum itself.

Children are especially prone to this type of infection. Most have at least one before their eighth birthday. Other frequent victims are allergy sufferers and those with broken eardrums.

Symptoms of otitis media include ear pain, a feeling of blockage or pressure, muffled hearing, ringing in the ear, headache, and fever. There may also be signs of an upper respiratory tract infection, and you may feel dizzy and have trouble walking. Some people get an upset stomach and vomit or have diarrhea. Swallowing, chewing, and nose blowing can increase the pain.

A common tip-off of otitis media in infants is tugging of the ears.

The child may cry more, seem fussier than normal, and develop a fever. In children who are just beginning to talk, speech may be unclear due to an inability to hear properly. Simply touching the ears may cause pain. Older children may say their ears feel like they are under water.

If too much pressure builds up behind the eardrum, it will break. Signs that a rupture has occurred are blood and pus draining from the ear. Although this drainage seems alarming, it does not mean that the infection has gotten worse. In fact, a small break will usually heal on its own in a few days. Do, however, have it looked at by a doctor. If it doesn't heal, surgery may be required.

If a blockage in the eustachian tube persists, a condition called serous otitis media may develop. This problem is marked by fluid oozing into the middle ear, ultimately impairing the hearing. The condition may become chronic, making the individual vulnerable to frequent infections. Chronic infection may, in turn, lead to mastoiditis, a rare complication in which the infection attacks the mastoid bone behind the inner ear. Symptoms include tenderness and a dull ache in the involved area, along with a discharge.

To prevent such complications and avert the possibility of permanent hearing loss, prompt treatment of any case of otitis media is essential.

Otitis externa: Also called swimmer's ear, this is a skin infection of the outer ear canal (the area that extends from the eardrum to the outside of the ear). The condition may be caused by either bacteria or a fungus that grows when water becomes trapped in the outer ear passageway. Swimming in dirty water or swimming frequently in chlorinated pools increases your chances of infection. You're also more likely to contract the problem if you have excess moisture in the ear, have had previous ear infections, or suffer from skin allergies. The outer ear canal also can be infected through incorrect use of cotton swabs to clean the ear. Avoid pushing swabs into the canal.

Symptoms of otitis externa include plugged ears or ear pain that becomes worse when your ear lobe is pulled. Other possible symptoms are itching, swelling, pain, a foul-smelling discharge or pus, short-term hearing loss, and fever. With treatment, the infection should be gone in 7 to 10 days.

Call Your Doctor If . . .

After treatment has begun:

- A really bad headache develops, or there's pain near the ear.
- The pain is not relieved by ear drops or heat.
- A high temperature develops.
- There is any discharge from the ear, the outer ear becomes red or swollen, or you notice swelling behind the earlobe.
- Vomiting or diarrhea sets in.
- The ear pain gets worse or the ear is still painful after 3 days of treatment.
- A rash, itching, or swelling appears.

Seek Care Immediately If . . .
- A stiff neck or dizziness sets in.
- A seizure or fainting spell occurs, or the facial muscles begin to twitch.

What You Can Do
- Do not put anything in the ear unless your doctor suggests it.
- A heating pad set on low or a warm water bottle placed on the ear may ease the pain. Alternatively, a covered ice bag over the ear may help.
- Sleeping with the head raised may help relieve pain.
- If your doctor has prescribed antibiotics, be sure to finish all the medication. If you stop treatment too soon, some bacteria may survive and cause a second infection.
- Use over-the-counter drugs to relieve pain. Your doctor may also give you eardrops to ease the discomfort.
- If the problem is swimmer's ear, keep the ear dry. Swimming is not advisable for three weeks after the infection is gone. Use ear plugs or a shower cap during showers.
- Use a cotton-tipped applicator to apply medication to the outer ear.
- A return to school or work is okay once your temperature returns to normal (98.6 degrees Fahrenheit).
- Keep the ears covered in cold weather.
- Try to stay away from people with colds, and wash your hands if you touch someone with this kind of infection.

What Your Doctor Can Do
For otitis media, the doctor will usually prescribe an oral antibiotic. Decongestant medications may also be needed to help open up the eustachian tube. In severe cases, the doctor may need to insert a pressure-equalizing tube through the eardrum in an operation called a

myringotomy. In children subject to frequent ear infections, these tubes may be left in place for several years.

Prescription Drugs

For otitis media, available oral antibiotics include:

Amoxicillin (Amoxil, Trimox, Wymox)
Amoxicillin/clavulanate potassium (Augmentin)
Ampicillin (Omnipen, Principen, Totacillin)
Azithromycin (Zithromax)
Cefaclor (Ceclor)
Cefdinir (Omnicef)
Cefixime (Suprax)
Cefpodoxime (Vantin)
Cefprozil (Cefzil)
Ceftibuten (Cedax)
Cefuroxime (Ceftin)

Cephalexin (Keflex)
Clarithromycin (Biaxin)
Erythromycin (E.E.S., E-Mycin, ERYC, Ery-Tab, Erythrocin, Ilosone, PCE)
Erythromycin/sulfisoxazole (Pediazole)
Loracarbef (Lorabid)
Penicillin V Potassium (Beepen-VK, Pen-Vee K, V-cillin K, Veetids)
Trimethoprim/sulfamethoxazole (Bactrim, Cotrim, Septra)

Your doctor also may prescribe eardrops such as Americaine, Auralgan, and Floxin.

For otitis externa, the doctor can prescribe medicated eardrops, including the following:

Acetic acid (Otic Domeboro, VoSol)
Acetic acid/hydrocortisone (VoSol HC)
Benzocaine (Americaine Otic)
Ciprofloxacin (Cipro HC)

Colistin/hydrocortisone/ neomycin (Cortisporin-TC)
Hydrocortisone/neomycin/ polymyxin B (Pediotic)
Ofloxacin (Floxin Otic Solution)

Over-the-Counter Drugs

To relieve ear pain you may take acetaminophen (Panadol, Tylenol) or ibuprofen (Advil, Motrin, Nuprin). Your doctor also may recommend decongestants such as Neo-Synephrine, Propagest, and Sudafed. Antihistamines such as Chlor-Trimeton and other hay fever remedies may also be helpful.

Herbal Remedies

There are no herbal medications for this problem.

Nutritional Support

Once an infection has set in, nutritional measures are of little assistance.

Alternative Treatments

Environmental Medicine: By fighting the allergic reactions that can contribute to congestion in the eustachian tubes, this type of therapy may help prevent repeated bouts of otitis media. Practitioners typically prescribe desensitization, diet modification, and immunotherapy. If they suggest more exotic forms of "detoxification therapy," check with a doctor before proceeding.

Eczema

The Basics

This nagging, mysterious skin disorder can come and go for years. Known medically as atopic dermatitis, it often accompanies allergic problems such as asthma or hay fever, but its specific cause is unknown.

In young children, the problem surfaces as a red, itchy, oozing, crusted rash on the face, scalp, diaper area, arms, and legs. In older children and adults the condition may take the form of dry, red, scaly patches on the eyelids, neck, and wrists. It can also appear in the folds of the elbows, knees, hands, feet, and genital area, and around the rectum. The affected area may become infected with bacteria and a course of antibiotics may be required.

The problem tends to favor people with a family history of atopic dermatitis or other allergic problems. It can be brought on by stress, food, or other irritants. Certain chemicals and fabrics may also trigger it. The disease will not spread from person to person. Doctors have no cure, but they can prescribe medications to relieve the symptoms.

Call Your Doctor If . . .

■ Itching interferes with sleep.
■ The rash gets worse or fails to improve after 7 days of treatment.
■ The rash develops pus or soft yellow scabs (signs of infection).
■ You develop a high temperature.
■ The rash flares up after contact with someone who has fever blisters (a sign of infection with herpes simplex).

Seek Care Immediately If . . .
■ The rash flares up and you begin to have difficulty breathing.

What You Can Do
■ Over-the-counter steroid creams applied 3 times daily usually provide the most relief, but they should be used very sparingly on infants. Supplement them with emollients such as white petrolatum (Vaseline). If they stop working, use emollients alone for a week or more. After this respite, the steroids may regain their effect.
■ Use warm, not hot, water when you take a bath or shower. Try to use the least amount of soap possible. Do not use any soap on the rash itself. You may add nonperfumed bath oil to the bathwater. Never use bubble bath.
■ Immediately after a bath or shower, when the skin is still damp, apply a moisturizing cream to the entire body. This will seal in moisture and help prevent dryness.
■ If you have eczema on your hands, use vinyl (not latex) gloves when doing household chores such as dishwashing.
■ Dress in clothes made of cotton or cotton blends. Avoid wool and synthetic fibers. Don't dress too warmly.
■ To relieve the problem in young children, take the following steps:
 • Keep your child's fingernails cut short. Wash the youngster's hands often. Because scratching makes the rash and itching worse, you may need to put soft gloves or mittens on the child at night.
 • If a particular food seems to cause flare-ups, remove it from the child's diet. The leading suspects are cow's milk, peanut butter, eggs, wheat, citrus fruits, and strawberries.
 • Keep the child away from anyone who has fever blisters. The herpes virus responsible for this problem can cause a serious skin infection in children with eczema.

What Your Doctor Can Do
 The doctor can prescribe creams and ointments for the rash and, if necessary, oral medications for severe itching. He can also help you identify allergic triggers that may cause flare-ups of the disease.

Prescription Drugs
 The rash and scales of eczema can be relieved with a variety of steroid creams, ointments, and lotions, including:

Aclovate (alclometasone)
Aristocort and Kenalog
  (triamcinolone)
Cordran (flurandrenolide)
Cutivate (fluticasone)
Cyclocort (amcinonide)
Decaspray (dexamethasone)
Dermatop (prednicarbate)
DesOwen or Tridesilon (desonide)
Diprolene, Diprosone, Maxivate,
  or Valisone (betamethasone)
Elocon (mometasone)
Epifoam and Pramosone
  (hydrocortisone with
  pramoxine)

Florone (diflorasone)
Halog (halcinonide)
Hytone, Locoid, Pandel, or
  Westcort (hydrocortisone)
Lidex (fluocinonide)
Maxiflor or Psorcon
  (diflorasone)
Synalar (fluocinolone)
Temovate (clobetasol)
Topicort (desoximetasone)
Ultravate (halobetasol)
Zonalon (doxepin)

For severe itching, these oral medications may help:

Atarax (hydroxyzine)
Sinequan (doxepin)

Over-the-Counter Drugs

For rash, you can choose from a number of nonprescription hydro-cortisone products, including Cortaid, Cortizone, and Nupercainal. For itching, you can try one of these oral antihistamine products:

Benadryl Allergy
Chlor-Trimeton Allergy

Dimetapp Allergy
Tavist-1

Herbal Remedies

Three natural remedies have proven especially helpful for skin problems:

Brewer's yeast
Nightshade

Red clover

Nutritional Support

Especially in children, eczema is sometimes the fault of a food allergy. Be alert for menu items that seem to be followed by an attack. If no particular food seems to be triggering the problem, you might want to ask your doctor for an allergy test.

Alternative Treatments

To the extent that an allergy is involved, you may find relief in *environmental medicine, hypnotherapy,* or a *macrobiotic diet.* There are, however, no alternative treatments specifically for eczema.

Emphysema and Chronic Bronchitis

The Basics

Known collectively as *chronic obstructive pulmonary disease (COPD),* these debilitating lung conditions plague some 16 million Americans. Their cause is well known; about 80 to 90 percent of cases are linked to smoking. Although neither disease can be cured, it *is* possible to hold back its progression. Faithful attention to medication, exercise, diet, and lifestyle can not only relieve the symptoms, but actually prolong life.

Although both disorders hinder breathing, they do it in distinctly different ways. Emphysema attacks the tiny clusters of air sacs (alveoli) that cap the end of each airway in the lungs. Blood vessels in the walls of these sacs absorb oxygen from the adjacent air. When emphysema takes hold, however, the walls begin to break down, leaving fewer, larger sacs that operate less efficiently. At the same time, the tiny airways serving the sacs start to weaken and collapse, trapping stale air inside. The end result is a declining ability to pull enough oxygen into the body and a failure to entirely rid it of waste products such as carbon dioxide.

Chronic bronchitis also produces oxygen starvation, but not by destroying the alveoli. Instead, it damages the walls of the airways, keeping them swollen, inflamed, and filled with mucus. Because the hairlike cilia that ordinarily clear the lungs also suffer damage, mucus builds up and clogs the narrowed passageways, preventing the alveoli from receiving needed air.

Both types of COPD begin with gradually increasing breathlessness during physical activity. If chronic bronchitis is the primary problem, you're also likely to be troubled by a daily cough, wheezing, and frequent lung infections. As COPD progresses through the years, breathing becomes increasingly difficult, eventually leaving victims perpetually short of breath.

Of the two diseases, chronic bronchitis is by far the more common, afflicting nearly 14 million Americans. Emphysema affects 2 million more. Both strike almost exclusively during the later years. Chronic bronchitis severe enough to cause symptoms rarely develops before age 50. Most cases of emphysema aren't discovered until the victim is over 60.

Call Your Doctor If . . .

■ Your mucus gets thicker despite your medications and ample amounts of water.

■ You cough up mucus that is bloody, yellow, or green.

■ Your nail beds turn gray or blue.

■ You develop a high temperature.

Seek Care Immediately If . . .

■ You are feeling confused, dizzy, or very drowsy; have swollen hands and feet; and find that your lips and nail beds are pale or blue.

■ You have chest pain or trouble breathing even while resting.

What You Can Do

■ Above all else, you must quit smoking. It's probably the cause of the problem, and will certainly make it worse.

■ Pace yourself. Allow for rest periods after exertion.

■ Sit down while shaving or applying makeup to conserve physical energy.

■ Avoid heavily perfumed colognes and grooming aids, as well as anything in aerosol cans. These sprays can irritate the lungs.

■ Do not wear tight clothing that constricts the chest or abdomen.

■ When cleaning house, wear a mask to reduce the amount of dust you inhale.

■ Keep your home and work space well ventilated.

■ Try eating several small meals rather than a few large ones. If there is less in your stomach, there's more room for your lungs.

■ Wear a lightweight winter coat rather than a heavy one that requires extra energy to carry around.

■ Keep a cell phone in the car in case you need help changing a tire or getting gas. Obtain a handicapped parking permit if you have trouble walking far distances.

■ Be sure to drink 8 to 10 large glasses of water each day. This helps thin the mucus, making it easier to cough up.

■ Try to avoid people who have colds or the flu. Get shots to prevent the flu and pneumonia.

■ To help keep your lungs free of infection, take 2 or 3 deep breaths and then cough. Do this often during the day.

■ A humidifier will help keep the air moist and your mucus thin. Be sure to keep the humidifier clean.

■ Stay inside during very cold or hot weather, or on days when the air pollution is high.

■ Practice deep breathing exercises for 10 or 15 minutes several times a day:

  • Relax your body, letting neck and shoulders droop.
  • Put one hand on your abdomen and the other on your chest.
  • Inhale deeply through your nose in such a way that you feel your abdomen expand.
  • Exhale slowly through pursed lips and repeat. If you feel dizzy, take a few breaths using the upper chest muscles before your next deep breath.

What Your Doctor Can Do

To pin down the diagnosis, the doctor will probably give you a pulmonary function test (spirometry), a chest x-ray and possibly a high resolution computed tomography (CAT scan) of the lungs, an electrocardiogram (EKG), and specific blood tests, including an analysis of arterial blood gases.

Depending on the type of COPD he discovers, the doctor can then prescribe drugs to expand the airways (bronchodilators) and inhaled steroids to reduce swelling and inflammation. At the first sign of infection, he'll also prescribe antibiotics. And if these medications prove insufficient, he may add oxygen therapy to assure that the body has an adequate supply.

The doctor is also likely to recommend a program of regular exercise, starting with 10 to 15 minutes of walking or biking daily or every other day, and building up to sessions that last 45 minutes to an hour. If your case is severe, enrollment in your local hospital's pulmonary rehabilitation program is another possibility.

When all else fails, you may want to consider lung-volume reduction surgery. This operation removes nonfunctioning parts of the lungs to make extra room for the portions that still work. A lung transplant is also a possibility, although there's still disagreement over how much this truly helps.

Prescription Drugs

The airway-opening drug ipratropium (Atrovent) is the first choice in most cases. Other bronchodilators used for COPD include terbutaline (Brethine, Brethaire, Bricanyl), theophylline (Respbid, Slo-bid, Theo-Dur, Uniphyl), and albuterol (Proventil, Ventolin). Steroids seem to help only about 10 percent of those with stable COPD. Inhaled preparations are preferred. The leading alternatives include beclomethasone (Beclovent, Vanceril), triamcinolone (Azmacort), and flunisolide (AeroBid).

Over-the-Counter Drugs

Nonprescription drugs, such as over-the-counter cough remedies, provide no relief from COPD.

Herbal Remedies

Herbalists may advise taking some of the herbs with expectorant, anti-inflammatory, and mucus-reducing properties that are recommended for bronchitis (see the bronchitis entry for a complete listing).

Nutritional Support

Load up on protein, vitamins, and minerals, and be sure to get plenty of liquids. Avoid milk and dairy products, which can make mucus thicker.

Alternative Treatments

Alexander Technique: This specialized form of movement training is designed to bring the muscles into natural harmony, allowing the body to revert to a healthy posture. Advocates recommend it for breathing disorders.

Hellerwork: A combination of deep tissue massage and movement reeducation, this form of therapy is also said to relieve respiratory problems.

Meditation: By relaxing the body and calming the mind—sometimes through concentrating on respiration—this discipline affords some people relief from symptoms of asthma and emphysema.

Yoga: This ancient Eastern exercise program emphasizes deep breathing. Research has documented its ability, known to improve fitness, lower blood pressure, and slow the respiratory rate.

Endometriosis

The Basics

Endometriosis—a benign but painful condition that usually strikes during the childbearing years—affects 10 to 20 percent of American women. In this disorder, clumps of the endometrial tissue that normally lines the uterus are found elsewhere in the body.

Each month these errant patches of tissue go through the same cycle as the endometrium, swelling to accept a fertilized egg, disintegrating when conception does not occur, and sloughing off during menstruation. But because this debris is not in the uterus, it can't be expelled and accumulates inside the body instead, causing pain, swelling, and irritation that can continue period after period.

Clumps of misplaced endometrial tissue are found most frequently on the ovaries, fallopian tubes, vagina, or outer uterine wall, but they can develop almost anywhere, including the abdomen, intestine, bladder, kidney, lungs, skin, surgical scars, certain nerves, the brain, and the lymphatic system. Unchecked bleeding from these clumps may create scar tissue that can spread through the pelvis, twisting and attaching organs to each other, interfering with their proper function, filling the entire cavity, and eventually producing a tumor-like mass.

While many causes have been proposed, none seem to tell the whole story. We do know, however, that the disease occurs twice as often in Japanese as in Caucasian women and is common among American blacks. Those who have a sister, aunt, or mother with endometriosis are 7 to 10 percent more likely to get it themselves.

While the condition is seldom life-threatening, it can wreak havoc on the quality of life and make conception difficult. Its foremost symptoms include painful menstrual periods with heavy irregular flow, chronic pain in the pelvis, tenderness in the abdomen, diarrhea, painful bowel movements during periods, painful intercourse, and infertility.

Call Your Doctor If . . .

■ You develop severe abdominal or back pain that refuses to go away.
■ You have heavy or unusual vaginal bleeding.
■ Your symptoms return after treatment.

Seek Care Immediately If . . .

This disorder rarely triggers an emergency.

What You Can Do

■ When you begin treatment, keep a record of your bleeding and other symptoms. This will help your doctor plan further care.

■ To relieve abdominal or back pain, use a heating pad set on "low" or a hot water bottle. Hot baths will also help relax your muscles and ease the pain.

■ If surgery has been discussed, be sure to have all of your questions answered completely before making a decision.

■ Since endometriosis can make it difficult to become pregnant, consider having children, if you want them, before the disease does too much damage.

What Your Doctor Can Do

To make a firm diagnosis, the doctor will need detailed information on the nature and location of all your symptoms. He or she will also need to do a complete pelvic examination, and may have to check certain organs with either magnetic resonance imaging (MRI), which produces three-dimensional pictures of the body's interior, or ultrasound. For a conclusive determination of the problem, you may have to undergo a laparoscopy, a technique that involves inserting a tiny lighted lens through the navel to inspect the inside of the abdomen and internal organs.

Surgery is often the best way to eliminate these abnormal growths. Surgical treatments range from burning off misplaced clumps of tissue with a laser beam to removing the affected organs themselves. For advanced endometriosis, the doctor may suggest hysterectomy and bilateral oophorectomy, in which the uterus and both ovaries are removed. This radical surgery, reserved for the most extensive and resistant cases, removes the main sources of the hormones that stimulate the errant growths.

Treatment with drugs can also shut off these hormones. Medications that suppress ovulation can create a temporary pseudomenopause (in contrast to the permanent menopause achieved surgically). Others can create a pseudopregnancy.

Prescription Drugs

Pseudopregnancy, which shuts down the menstrual cycle and inactivates the misplaced endometrial tissue, can be induced with any birth control pill. However, those with a high progesterone level are preferred. Potential side effects are the same as those that may be encountered when the pills are taken for contraception.

Progesterone-only medications also may be prescribed. Oral forms include Provera and Micronor. Quarterly injections of Depo-Provera are another alternative. These medications bring relief by shrinking endometrial tissue. Among their side effects are water retention, weight gain, and acne. As with the birth control pills, treatment usually lasts about 6 to 9 months until the problem abates.

The pseudomenopause approach relies on medications that prevent the release of two hormones that stimulate ovulation and trigger the ripening of the endometrium. Called follicle-stimulating hormone (FSH) and luteinizing hormone (LH), they originate in the pituitary gland at the base of the brain. Production of both can be shut down with drugs called gonadotropin-releasing hormone (GnRH) analogs.

Although these drugs put an end to ovulation without need for removing the ovaries, they do prompt the symptoms of estrogen deficiency, including everything from vaginal dryness to an increased risk of osteoporosis, and they are not reliable contraceptives. They come in the form of a nose spray (Synarel), as a daily or monthly injection (Lupron), or as a monthly implant beneath the skin (Zoladex). A course of treatment lasts 6 months. Similarly, a drug called Danazol will stop production of LH and FSH. Treatment with this alternative may last from 3 to 9 months.

Your doctor may also prescribe a pain reliever such as a nonsteroidal anti-inflammatory drug (Naprosyn, Feldene, Ponstel, Rufen, Clinoril, Nalfon, Dolobid, Tolectin, and Indocin) or something stronger like codeine, oxycodone, meperidine, or morphine.

Over-the-Counter Drugs

For pain, aspirin or ibuprofen (Advil, Motrin) can help.

Herbal Remedies

This condition can't be relieved with herbs.

Nutritional Support

B vitamins, especially B₆, promote the liver's ability to change estrogen to estradiol, a form of the hormone less likely to promote endometrial growths. Vitamin E is thought to counter the effects of estrogen and may break down the hormone when it is present in excessive amounts. Whole wheat, citrus fruit, and yams are reported to raise estrogen levels and perhaps should be avoided. Check with your doctor, however, before making any radical dietary changes. Remember too that diet cannot repair damaged tissues and organs and is probably useful only in early endometriosis.

One nutritional supplement to definitely keep in mind is iron. Excessive bleeding at menstruation can reduce this essential component of the blood. Exercise is also advisable, since it tends to reduce menstrual flow and, therefore, the irritations and inflammation that develop where foreign endometrial tissue is growing.

Alternative Treatments

While these treatments will not cure endometriosis, they may help relieve some of the pain:

Acupuncture: This treatment, which calls for insertion of tiny needles at specific points on the skin, is considered particularly effective for relieving pain.

Energy Medicine: This extremely controversial and unproven approach offers a variety of electrical treatments for pain relief, of which transcutaneous electrical nerve stimulation (TENS) is probably the most likely to help.

Hydrotherapy: Treatment with hot and cold compresses is often advocated for menstrual cramps and many other types of pain.

Hypnotherapy: With its ability to enhance the power of suggestion, hypnotherapy is often effective against virtually all types of pain. Like other alternative treatments, however, it won't remedy the underlying problem.

Excess Weight

The Basics

If you have trouble keeping your weight down, you're far from alone. It's estimated that about 30 percent of Americans are overweight, and that 50 million Americans go on a diet in any given year.

The reason for excess weight is obvious: too much food. But what constitutes "too much" varies from person to person, and a number of factors make weight gain more likely. The major culprits include:

■ *Dietary fat:* A high-fat diet is the single greatest source of unwanted pounds.

■ *Lack of exercise:* Our lifestyle is more sedentary than our grandparents', so we have fewer opportunities to burn excess calories.

■ *Stress:* Lack of time can lead people to grab less nutritious food, and stress often prompts us to overeat or routinely snack on junk food.

■ *Drinking:* Alcohol adds empty calories and can loosen one's self-restraint in the presence of high-fat snacks like peanuts and potato chips.

■ *Gender:* Women gain weight more easily than men. Estrogen stimulates the storage of fat in the hips, buttocks, and thighs, where it is converted to energy more slowly than fat elsewhere.

■ *Age:* For both women and men, weight tends to increase as the body's metabolism slows down with age.

■ *Genetics:* Weight problems do tend to run in families.

■ *Quitting cigarettes:* People typically gain 4 to 6 pounds when they give up smoking.

Being overweight harms more than your appearance; it can affect your health and shorten your life. Excess weight dramatically increases your chances of developing heart disease, high blood pressure, and diabetes. It has also been linked to gallstones, back pain, sleep apnea, heartburn, stroke, gout, varicose veins, osteoarthritis, carpal tunnel syndrome, and some types of cancer, including colon and prostate cancer in men and uterine, endometrial, and breast cancer in women.

Call Your Doctor If . . .

Check with your doctor before starting a diet if you have any chronic medical problems.

What You Can Do

Radical dieting is not the answer to a weight problem. Beware of claims of weight-loss miracles. If a diet claim seems too good to be true, it probably is.

Extreme dieting poses significant dangers. It can lead to nutritional deficiencies, depress the metabolism, and rob you of energy. On-again, off-again dieting, with its seesawing weight gains and losses, raises the risk of high blood pressure. Yo-yo dieting can also make your weight problem worse, leading the body to produce enzymes that increase the ability to store fat. Statistics show that almost all extreme dieters regain their weight.

To be successful, you'll need to cut back your calories moderately and burn off extra calories through exercise. Here are some tips to help you get started on your weight-loss program:

- Aim for gradual weight loss. You should not lose more than 1 to 2 pounds a week; and there may be weeks when you lose nothing at all.
- Keep a food diary. This can help you recognize an eating pattern that is sabotaging your weight-control efforts.
- Eat healthy. Increase your consumption of vegetables, fruits, and whole grains, while cutting back on empty calories and fatty foods.
- Eat slowly. Smell, taste, and savor your food. If you eat too fast, you'll overeat before you feel full.
- Burn the fat. Exercise is critical for healthy weight loss. It doesn't have to be vigorous; a brisk walk for 30 minutes every other day is enough to raise your metabolism and help burn fat.
- Be a daytime eater. While metabolism is highest during your first 12 waking hours, the typical American eats about 70 percent of the day's calorie allotment after 5:00 p.m., when the metabolism is lowest.
- Shrink and multiply your meals. Eat five or six mini-meals a day instead of three full ones.
- Look for support. Turn to friends, family, or local chapters of organizations like Weight Watchers or Overeaters Anonymous to provide the encouragement you may need when your commitment falters.
- Be flexible. Don't set rigid targets and don't let your menu dominate your life. Listen to your hunger and stop eating when it subsides.
- Drink plenty of fluids, the equivalent of 8 glasses a day. The fluids help fill you up, prevent shakiness and fatigue from dehydration, and give you something to put in your mouth.
- Don't skip meals. You'll be tempted to overeat later on.

What Your Doctor Can Do

The doctor can check for medical disorders that contribute to excess weight. Lower than normal activity of the thyroid or adrenal glands are two possibilities. However, these and other medical conditions are the culprits only 1 percent of the time.

Medical treatment ranges from dieting under a doctor's supervision to enrollment in outpatient or residential programs. To prevent you from reverting to problem eating habits, the treatment may include behavior modification counseling.

Surgery is reserved only for people who are massively obese or whose health is at risk. The two most common surgical techniques are liposuction and intestinal bypass. In liposuction, a tool is inserted under the skin to suck fat from the body. In bypass surgery, the digestive flow is routed past the intestines to reduce the amount of food absorbed. Both treatments are used only as a last resort.

Prescription Drugs

If you have a serious weight problem, your doctor may supplement your diet and exercise program with a prescription diet drug. Options include:

Adipex-P, Fastin, Ionamin, Oby-Cap (phentermine)
Bontril or Prelu-2 (phendimetrazine)
Desoxyn (methamphetamine)
Meridia (sibutramine)
Tenuate (diethylpropion)

Over-the-Counter Drugs

The nonprescription drug phenylpropanolamine is sometimes used for weight loss. Brands include Acutrim and Dexatrim. These pills can cause your weight to drop, but they won't eliminate body fat.

Herbal Remedies

There are no herbs that have been proven to reduce weight.

Nutritional Support

To lose excess weight and keep it off you'll need a well-balanced diet:

■ Eat plenty of high fiber and starchy foods such as breads, pasta, potatoes, cooked dried beans, and whole grain products. Fiber fills out the stomach and intestinal cavity, producing a feeling of fullness. If your current diet is low in fiber, increase your intake gradually to prevent bloating, cramping, and gas.
■ Eat 5 or more fruits and vegetables each day. Steam vegetables or eat them raw. Don't put sauces or a lot of margarine or butter on cooked vegetables. Snack on vegetables rather than on high-fat or high-calorie foods.
■ Switch to lower fat meats and fish, such as skinless chicken, water-packed tuna, and lean cuts of meat.
■ Bake, roast, or broil your food instead of frying. Remove all fat from meats before cooking.
■ Switch to low-fat and fat-free dairy products, salad dressings, and cheeses.
■ Stay away from candy, cookies, pastries, and other foods high in sugar.
■ Avoid high-fat snacks such as nuts, chips, and chocolate.
■ Limit alcohol. Alcoholic beverages are high in calories and low in food value.

Alternative Treatments

Fasting: Avoid total fasts, which can deplete muscle tissue as well as fat. Instead, consider a protein-sparing modified fast. Two versions are currently in use. Both are recommended only for people who are dangerously overweight. Version One calls for a daily intake of 1.5 grams of protein per 2.2 pounds of your ideal body weight, supplemented by vitamins. Version Two uses a premixed formula rich in milk or egg protein as a substitute for meat.

Hypnotherapy: This form of treatment uses the power of suggestion to alter ingrained habits—such as the tendency to overeat.

Naturopathic Medicine: A naturopathic practitioner can suggest dietary modifications and nutritional supplements to reduce weight while maintaining good health.

Vegetarianism: Meatless diets tend to be low in fat, cholesterol, and calories—and thus ideal for losing weight. Make sure, however, that the diet you adopt includes sufficient protein.

Food Allergies

The Basics

Genuine food allergies are surprisingly rare. They afflict only 1 or 2 adults in 100, and the victim is rarely allergic to more than one or two foods. Allergic reactions range from mild upsets to severe and even fatal anaphylaxis.

Immediate reactions, typical of most true food allergies, are usually dramatic, starting within seconds or up to 2 hours after eating. Delayed reactions, often the result of a milder food sensitivity, may not appear for the better part of a day. Victims may break out in a rash or hives, suffer grinding stomachaches and diarrhea, go to bed with a headache, or experience any number of other symptoms, from leg cramps to choking. While many foods can cause reactions, some of the most common offenders are nuts, shellfish, cow's milk and other dairy products, eggs, soybeans and other legumes, wheat, fruits (especially citrus fruits and tomatoes), and corn.

A true allergic reaction is a misdirected attack by the body's immune system against an ordinarily harmless substance. Other forms of food-related discomfort don't involve the immune system, but can be just as real and troubling. Some involve an intolerance or inability to digest certain foods. Others are a response to a specific chemical or additive found in the food. Whether the problem is an allergy, an intolerance, or a chemical side effect, the bottom line is the same. You need to find out what's causing the reaction and make sure it stays out of your diet.

Call Your Doctor If . . .

You think any of the following symptoms may be related to something you've eaten:

■ Your nose feels stuffed and you begin to sneeze.

■ Your skin becomes hot and itchy or breaks out in hives.

■ Your eyes tear, swell up, or itch.

■ You have an urgent need to go to the bathroom.

■ You have nausea, vomiting, diarrhea, stomach pain, or uterine cramps.

Seek Care Immediately If . . .

You develop any combination of the following warning signs. You could be in the early stages of a life-threatening anaphylactic reaction. **Call 911 or 0 (operator)** without delay.

■ You have a feeling of impending doom.

■ Your lips turn blue, starting at the edges.

■ Your tongue becomes swollen.

■ Your mouth and throat itch.

■ Your throat begins to close up.

■ You have shortness of breath or wheezing.

■ Your ears throb.

■ Your voice changes pitch or becomes hoarse.

■ Your chest feels tight and painful.

■ Your heart starts beating rapidly.

■ You feel dizzy or collapse.

What You Can Do

■ To identify an offending food, keep a diary of everything you eat and drink and note when symptoms occur.

■ If you must avoid important foods indefinitely, your nutritional status could suffer. Consult a professional for personal diet planning and advice.

■ Study the labels on every commercial food product that enters your mouth. Call the manufacturer if you are in doubt.

- Learn the many names for whatever ingredients you must avoid. For example, wheat may be listed as gluten, or egg white as albumin.
- If you are severely allergic, wear a medic-alert bracelet stating the nature of your allergy and always carry an anaphylaxis kit (Ana-Kit, EpiPen).
- If you develop itching or hives, apply cold compresses to the skin or take baths in cool water. Don't take hot baths or showers; the warmth will make the itching worse.

What Your Doctor Can Do

There's no cure for this condition, but an allergist can help you pinpoint the cause of your troubles so you can avoid it in the future. He will probably perform *skin tests* to try to determine exactly which substances you are allergic to. He can also order certain blood tests, such as the *radioallergosorbent test (RAST)*, which is done in a laboratory. He may then perform *challenge tests* with certain foods to confirm or refute skin or blood test results. He might also recommend an *elimination diet*, in which you systematically remove one food at a time to see if symptoms go away.

Prescription Drugs

To quell the symptoms of an anaphylactic reaction, the doctor may prescribe cyproheptadine (Periactin), diphenhydramine (Benadryl), or promethazine (Phenergan). Steroid medications such as cortisone (Cortone), dexamethasone (Decadron), hydrocortisone (Hydrocortone), and prednisolone (Pediapred, Prelone) are also prescribed for allergies.

For sneezing, congestion, and runny nose, antihistamines such as astemizole (Hismanal), loratadine (Claritin), and fexofenedine (Allegra) may help. Steroid nasal sprays such as beclomethasone (Beconase, Vancenase), fluticasone (Flonase), and triamcinolone (Nasacort) are another option. And if you have an asthmatic reaction, you'll probably need a bronchodilator (see the entry on asthma for details).

Over-the-Counter Drugs

To relieve the respiratory symptoms of an allergic reaction, a wide variety of antihistamines and decongestants are available over the counter; see the entry on hay fever for a complete list. Lactose intolerance, a form of food sensitivity, can be relieved with the nonprescription product Lactaid.

Herbal Remedies

A multitude of herbs are said to help symptoms such as sneezing and congestion (see the entry on colds and flu), but none seem to be able to prevent or cure an allergic attack.

Nutritional Support

Unfortunately, the only sure way to avoid an allergic reaction to a certain type of food is to avoid it. If you don't like the food, this shouldn't be too difficult, but if you do, or if it is an ingredient in a multitude of foods (such as wheat), talk to nutritional experts about finding good-tasting, nutritionally valuable alternatives.

Alternative Treatments

Sublingual Treatments: In this form of therapy, small amounts of the offending food are placed under the tongue. The idea is to inoculate the body against the food. However, this could be extremely dangerous if you have a strong allergic reaction during the treatment, and there's no proof that it works.

Provocation/Neutralization: Another type of "inoculation," this approach involves giving a person diluted doses of troublesome foods in increasing increments until a reaction is provoked and then neutralized.

Environmental Medicine: Aimed at remedying the harmful effects of pollutants and toxins in the modern environment, this style of treatment can also be applied to the harmful effects of allergenic foods.

Hypnotherapy: With its ability to enhance the power of suggestion, hypnosis has been found effective for a variety of problems that hinge on the body's involuntary responses. For some people, it appears to work against allergies.

Macrobiotic Diet: This Asian-style vegetarian diet is low in fat, emphasizes whole grains and vegetables, and restricts fluids. Because it's so limited, it may be the answer to some food allergies, but few mainstream nutritionists endorse this type of diet because it can easily cause significant nutritional deficiencies.

Food Poisoning

The Basics

Depending on the germs involved, contaminated food can trigger a reaction in as little as an hour or as long as 11 days after exposure.

Diarrhea is the most predictable symptom, and replacement fluids are the usual therapy.

(Beware, however, of botulism, the most dangerous of all food-borne illnesses. There's no diarrhea, but vomiting and weakness can quickly progress to paralysis, and without emergency hospitalization the victim may die.)

Here's a quick overview of the seven most common causes of food poisoning, along with the foods they usually infest, the symptoms they produce, and the type of treatment needed.

Campylobacter jejuni: Usually found in poultry and unpasteurized milk, this germ causes diarrhea, fever, discomfort, headache, and chills. Symptoms appear within 2 to 7 days of exposure and last 7 to 14 days. If diarrhea and fever last longer than 5 or 6 days, give replacement fluids. The doctor may prescribe antibiotics.

Clostridium botulinum: This deadly germ typically contaminates shellfish, smoked and salted fish, ham, sausage, and improperly canned foods. Symptoms range from mild discomfort to death within 24 hours. Initial warning signs are nausea, vomiting, weakness, and dizziness. Later, paralysis may set in, interfering with the ability to breathe. Hospitalization is required; mechanical breathing assistance may be needed.

Escherichia coli: Usually lurking in undercooked ground meat, unpasteurized milk, or apple cider, this germ causes watery diarrhea within 1 to 8 days of exposure. The diarrhea becomes bloody, and is accompanied by pain, nausea, occasional vomiting, and in some cases fever. In children, the disease can lead to life threatening kidney damage. Give replacement fluids; do not use antidiarrheal medications. Antibiotics usually are not needed.

Listeria: This germ can infest a wide variety of foods, including raw eggs, milk, seafood, poultry, meat, and soft ripened cheese. Especially in the very young or old, pregnant women, and people with suppressed immunity, it causes severe diarrhea, flu-like fever and headache, pneumonia, and infections of the membranes around the brain and heart. See the doctor for antibiotics.

Salmonella: Like Listeria, this bug is at home in a broad array of foods. Raw eggs, custards, unpasteurized milk, salad dressings, sandwich fillings, shellfish, poultry, fruits, vegetables, and unpasteurized cheese all can harbor this infection. Symptoms range from mild diarrhea to severe pain and diarrhea; also watery stools, nausea, vomiting, and fever. Illness develops 6 to 72 hours after eating contaminated food. Give replacement fluids. Antibiotics may be prescribed.

Shigella: Favorite hideouts include milk, uncooked tofu, and shredded lettuce and cabbage packaged for sale. The primary symptom is diarrhea, ranging from mild to life-threatening. Give replacement fluids; if the illness is severe, see the doctor for antibiotics.

Staphylococcus: This germ favors custards, sauces, cream-filled baked goods, cheeses, processed meats, and a variety of salads, including chicken, potato, ham, and egg. It causes severe cramping and abdominal pain, watery diarrhea, vomiting, perspiration, and headache. Symptoms start abruptly within 1 to 6 hours of eating the contaminated food and last 24 to 48 hours. Give replacement fluids.

Call Your Doctor If . . .
- Your symptoms last longer than a few days.
- You have a dry mouth; dry, wrinkled skin; dark urine, less urine than usual; dry eyes without tears; or unusual sleepiness. These are signs of dehydration.
- Antibiotics prescribed by the doctor cause a rash, itching, or swelling of your abdomen or legs.

Seek Care Immediately If . . .
- You can't drink fluids or keep food down.
- You have a high temperature, worsening diarrhea or vomiting, a yellow color to the skin or eyes, or a tendency to cough up blood.
- You rapidly grow weak and dizzy.

What You Can Do
If you develop food poisoning:
- Drink plenty of fluids to replace those lost through vomiting or diarrhea. A good mixture for fluid replacement is 1 teaspoon of salt and 4 heaping teaspoons of sugar in 1 quart of water.
- If you're prescribed antibiotics, continue to take them until they are all gone—even if you feel better. Stopping too soon can allow some germs to survive and cause a relapse.
- Rest in bed at least 3 days after your symptoms subside.
- Use a heating pad or hot water bottle to help relieve stomach cramps.

To prevent food poisoning:
- Clean all food—and everything it touches—scrupulously.
- Always wash your hands before preparing food.
- Keep cuts, scrapes, sores, and other hand injuries away from food.

- Keep all meat, fish, poultry, and dairy products refrigerated or frozen.
- Never thaw frozen food at room temperature. Use the refrigerator or microwave.
- Never put other food on the same surface as uncooked animal products. Wash cutting boards and knives immediately.
- Cook all meat, fish, and poultry thoroughly. Cook ground meat products until the juices run clear.
- Buy only clean, uncracked eggs. Use them within 5 weeks of purchase. Never eat raw eggs—or any batter or dressing containing raw eggs.

What Your Doctor Can Do

Your doctor can do tests to determine which organism is causing the problem, and prescribe antibiotics if necessary. If you are hospitalized, you will probably also receive an IV for administering fluids and medicine.

Prescription Drugs

The choice of antibiotics depends on the cause of the problem. Sulfamethoxazole with trimethoprim (Bactrim, Cotrim, Septra) is a typical choice for *Listeria* or *Shigella* infections. Ciprofloxacin (Cipro) or erythromycin (Eryc, PCE) are usually prescribed for *Campylobacter*.

Over-the-Counter Drugs

Check with your doctor before using a diarrhea remedy. Nonprescription choices include:

Diarrid	Imodium Advanced	Pepto-Bismol
Donnagel	Kaopectate	Rheaban
Imodium A-D	Pepto Diarrhea Control	

Herbal Remedies

There are no herbal remedies for the underlying infection, but a number of herbs have been found to help control diarrhea. They include:

Agrimony	English Oak	Potentilla
Bilberry	Green Tea	Psyllium
Blackberry	Jambolan	Tormentil
Coffee Charcoal	Lady's Mantle	Uzara

Nutritional Support

Be sure to drink plenty of liquids that have a lot of minerals and vitamins in them until the vomiting and diarrhea stop. Then eat healthy, soft, bland foods such as bananas, rice, applesauce, and toast.

Alternative Treatments

Hyperthermia: These heat treatments, usually through immersion in very hot water, are aimed at fighting infection. There are no reports, however, that they cure food poisoning.

Foot Pain

The Basics

Punished by hundreds of pounds of force with every step we take, the foot is one of nature's greatest architectural achievements. It rarely complains despite constant abuse. Yet for most of us something eventually does go wrong. Foot pain afflicts four out of five adults, even more of those in middle and older age.

Some foot problems seem to favor women. More women than men develop bunions, calluses, corns, and ingrown toenails. The primary reason is the shoes they wear: narrow, pointed, high in the heel, often flimsy, and designed for appearance rather than fit. Other ailments, such as athlete's foot and nerve pain, strike men and women equally.

The skin, bones, joints, and muscles of the foot are all prone to their own unique problems. Among the leading troublemakers are:

Pressure and friction: Constant rubbing that presses skin against bone creates calluses (large areas of thickened skin) and corns (smaller, cone-shaped versions of calluses). Another typical—and more painful—condition is an ingrown toenail. This occurs when the edge of the nail on any toe, usually the big toe, cuts through the skin sideways into the fleshy folds that cover the nail plates. Advancing age makes the foot ever more vulnerable to pressure and friction. Heel pain typically appears in middle age, as the soft pad of fat lining the bottom of the foot slowly wears down.

Fungal infections and viruses: The most common infection is athlete's foot. Presence of this fungus is often announced by a blister or rash that quickly spreads. Toenails usually become discolored, dry, and scaly, and begin to lift up from the nail bed. The infection is easily transmitted wherever people go barefoot, including pools, gyms, hot tubs, and spas. Warts also spread in public areas, but owe their existence to viruses instead of a fungus. They look like calluses but tend to be more painful and develop more rapidly. Plantar warts, which grow on the sole of the foot, hurt the most.

Skeletal problems: Most of these painful ailments are hereditary, but can be aggravated by wearing the wrong shoes. Flat feet are due to fallen arches and cause an array of problems: swollen ankles, pain on the outside of the ankles, poor shock absorption, knee and shin pain, and strained ligaments. Flat feet and other inherited deformities can lead to bunions—inflamed joints, usually at the base of the big toes, that push out to the side, away from the rest of the foot.

A joint malformation that usually can't be blamed on inherent bone structure is hammertoe—the curling of a toe into a hammer- or claw-like shape. The usual culprit is overuse of high heels or pointed shoes—which weaken the muscles and shorten the tendons that allow the toes to stretch. Other causes include diabetes, a herniated disk, sciatica, multiple sclerosis, and nerve damage.

Inflammation of the tendons and joints: The agonizing disorder known as *plantar fasciitis* results when the long tendon that connects the heel bone to the bottoms of the toes becomes inflamed. Severe pain erupts when getting out of bed in the morning or standing up after sitting for a while. A small, shelf-like growth of bone—commonly known as a heel spur—may form as the tendon continues to pull on the heel.

Excessive pressure on the joints of the metatarsals—the long bones that create the ball of the foot—can cause pain and inflammation. Anything that throws the weight of the foot forward onto the ball contributes to this condition, including high heels, hammertoes, and a tight Achilles tendon (which is anchored in the heel).

Nerve disorders: A condition called *Morton's neuroma* is the most common. This painful swelling of a nerve in the foot causes burning, numbness, and tingling. The pain usually hits in the sole of the foot under the pad of the third or fourth toe, and gets worse while walking.

Underlying disease: The most common threat is diabetes, which can lead to poor circulation and open foot sores that won't heal. Controlling this problem with proper medication and foot care is essential. For tips on what to do, turn to the entry on diabetes.

A second possible disorder is *Raynaud's disease.* This condition interrupts blood flow by causing small arteries in the foot to spasm. The skin then pales or turns a patchy red to blue. Numbness, tingling, and a burning sensation often accompany the episodes. Anything that stimulates the sympathetic nervous system—such as strong emotions or exposure to cold—can trigger these spasms.

Alleviating foot pain can be as simple as switching to flat shoes or as involved as undergoing surgery. Waiting too long to see a doctor can be a mistake. Because feet are under constant stress, even a small pain can grow larger quickly. Most people can't keep off their feet to rest them, so catching a problem early is the best solution.

Call Your Doctor If . . .
■ You develop an infection or a wart.
■ A sore or blister refuses to heal.
■ A damaged or ingrown toenail is causing pain and inflammation.
■ You have constant joint or nerve pain.

Seek Care Immediately If . . .
■ You develop numbness or weakness in your feet.

What You Can Do
To ease the pain:
■ Soak your feet in a warm solution of water and Epsom salts twice a day (refrain from this if you have diabetes).
■ Give yourself a foot massage, or get one from a professional.
■ Elevate your feet as much as possible.
■ Place a cushioned pad in your shoe to protect the offending area.

To prevent further troubles:
■ Don't wear high heels, tight shoes, or worn-out shoes with little cushioning or support.
■ Avoid going barefoot, especially in public places.
■ Use a shoe insert—preferably custom-made—or arch supports to correct structural defects.
■ Cut and file your toenails straight across.
■ Use a lotion to combat dry, cracked skin.
■ Exercise the feet to build muscle tone. Consult a doctor for the proper technique.

What Your Doctor Can Do
There are three types of doctors who frequently field foot problems: podiatrists, orthopedists, and dermatologists. The one most likely to

help is a podiatrist, a doctor who treats only problems related to the foot and ankle. Podiatrists can perform minor surgery and remove bunions, corns, and calluses. For broken bones, major foot deformities, and some bone diseases, an orthopedist might be a better choice. These doctors can treat bunions, hammertoes, and other disorders of the bones and joints. A dermatologist can help you with skin infections such as athlete's foot and warts.

Prescription Drugs

Painful joints and tendons might be injected with a steroid such as cortisone (Cortone). Athlete's foot that doesn't respond to over-the-counter products can be treated with stronger medications, including:

Exelderm (sulconazole)
Fulvicin, Grifulvin, or
  Gris-PEG (griseofulvin)
Lamisil (terbinafine)
Loprox (ciclopirox)
Lotrimin (clotrimazole)

Lotrisone (betamethasone)
Mentax (butenafine)
Naftin (naftifine)
Oxistat (oxiconazole nitrate)
Nizoral (ketoconazole)
Spectazole (econazole)

Over-the-Counter Drugs

Fungal infections can be treated with Desenex, Lamisil AT, Lotrimin AF, Micatin, or Mycelex OTC. You can try to remove warts with DuoFilm, DuoPlant, or Wart-Off.

For bunions, plantar fasciitis, and other inflammations of the joints and tendons, you can choose from a variety of nonsteroidal anti-inflammatory painkillers, including:

Actron	Bufferin	Nuprin
Advil	Ecotrin	Orudis
Aleve	Excedrin	St. Joseph
Ascriptin	Goody's	Vanquish
Bayer	Motrin	YSP
BC Powder		

Herbal Remedies

Pau d'arco is considered a remedy for fungal infections. Heartsease, mayapple, nightshade, oats, or savin tops are used for warts. There are no specific herbal remedies for foot pain, but you can check the entry on arthritis for herbs that might help relieve joint pain. As a skin rub, Japanese mint is used for muscle and nerve pain.

And white willow, an aspirin-like compound, is considered a remedy for all types of pain.

Nutritional Support
No dietary measures seem to help foot pain.

Alternative Treatments
If your problem lies in a joint, the alternative therapies listed in the arthritis entry might prove helpful. Since most foot pain is aggravated by repetitive stress to the muscles, joints, and tendons, you might also find relief from the following:

Alexander Technique: This specialized form of movement and posture training has given relief to people with a variety of musculoskeletal and repetitive stress disorders.

Aston-Patterning: This combination of physical training and massage is used to relieve muscle tension and pain, and speed recovery from injuries.

Energy Medicine: Many electrical devices promise pain relief, but few, if any, have been proven to work. Only *transcutaneous electrical nerve stimulation (TENS)* shows genuine promise for moderate, localized pain.

Massage Therapy: With systematic manual application of pressure and movement to the soft tissues in the foot, massage can relieve muscle pain and tension.

Myotherapy: This specialized form of deep-muscle massage focuses on "trigger points"—damaged, tender spots in the muscles.

Osteopathic Medicine: This branch of medicine supplements standard care with physical manipulation—ranging from light pressure on soft tissue to high-velocity thrusts on the joints. Such manipulation can be useful for joint pain, sports injuries, and repetitive stress injuries.

Gallstones

The Basics
These tiny nuggets of crystallized cholesterol can nestle in the gallbladder for years without producing any symptoms at all, then cause agonizing pain when one gets stuck in a nearby duct. It's possible to carry them through life and never experience a problem, but their presence does pose a steadily increasing risk of a painful attack. On

average, 500,000 of the 15 million Americans with gallstones require hospitalization every year.

Gallstones form when the bile stored in the gallbladder becomes so saturated with cholesterol that it begins to crystallize. Bile is produced by the liver to aid digestion—particularly digestion of fats—so if the stones begin to interfere with the normal flow of bile, digestive problems are likely to result.

People who develop symptoms typically suffer sporadic attacks of pain, usually in the stomach area. The episodes often come and go without any pattern or progression. Known medically as biliary colic, they are frequently accompanied by nausea, vomiting, fever, or jaundice (yellow skin or eyes). You also may feel bloated, find yourself unable to eat fatty food, and be troubled by constant burping.

Your chance of developing gallstones increases with age. Women are more likely to have them than men, and your odds of getting them are also greater if your parents had them. In addition, the likelihood of the problem increases if you weigh too much, have many children, take birth control pills, drink too much alcohol, and have a high-fat diet.

As long as gallstones remain symptom-free, treatment isn't necessary. Once they begin to block the ducts, surgical removal of the gallbladder is the usual remedy.

Call Your Doctor If . . .

■ You see any of the following signs that too much bile is building up in your body:
  • Yellow skin.
  • Light brown or yellow stools.
  • Dark yellow or light brown urine.
■ After surgery, you develop any of the following complications:
  • Pain from the surgery doesn't clear up or gets worse.
  • Your incision becomes swollen and red, or you see any pus. These are signs of infection.
  • Your stitches or staples come apart.
  • Your bandage becomes soaked with blood.

Seek Care Immediately If . . .

After surgery, you suffer any of the following symptoms:

■ You have a high temperature.
■ You have severe pain in the upper right side of your abdomen or between your shoulder blades.

■ You start to vomit.
■ You have shortness of breath.
■ You develop chest pain or sudden trouble breathing.

What You Can Do

For greater comfort during an attack you can take over-the-counter medications for pain, rest in bed until you are feeling better, avoid eating, and drink clear fluids. To reduce the frequency of attacks, it may prove helpful to avoid foods that give you indigestion and make sure that everything you eat is low in fat.

What Your Doctor Can Do

Gallstones that begin to cause symptoms often can be dissolved by drugs or shattered by sound waves in a procedure called lithotripsy. However, these remedies usually prove temporary; new stones are likely to develop.

The only permanent solution is surgical removal of the gallbladder (cholecystectomy). During the operation, stones in the duct that drains the gallbladder may be removed as well. There are two types of cholecystectomy:

Open cholecystectomy: This method requires a single large incision under the right rib cage. The operation takes 1 to 2 hours. Your stay in the hospital can last 2 to 5 days.

Laparoscopic cholecystectomy: This "Band-Aid surgery" technique substitutes four tiny incisions for a single large one. One is made just below the belly button. Two more are made in the abdomen above the right hip. A fourth is needed just below the ribs in the middle of the chest. A tiny, lighted scope is inserted through one incision. Miniature, remote-controlled surgical tools are inserted through the others. To give the surgeon an unobstructed view, the abdomen is inflated with carbon dioxide gas throughout the procedure. Like an open cholecystectomy, the operation takes 1 to 2 hours. However, your hospital stay may be less than a day.

Cholecystectomy is the most common abdominal surgery among American adults. The procedure is relatively safe, but like all surgery it does pose a risk of internal bleeding or infection; and blood clots could form and lodge in the lungs, making it difficult to breath.

Prescription Drugs

Ursodiol (Actigall) helps dissolve gallstones. The drug acts slowly, taking months to completely dissolve the stones. It works for between 30 and 40 percent of patients.

Over-the-Counter Drugs

For discomfort related to gallstones, you may take acetaminophen (Panadol, Tylenol), aspirin (Bayer, St. Joseph), or ibuprofen (Advil, Motrin, Nuprin).

Herbal Remedies

A huge array of herbs have been found useful for liver and gallbladder problems. They won't dissolve gallstones or effect a permanent cure, but they may offer relief from minor digestive complaints. Your options include:

Anise	Dandelion	Javanese Turmeric
Artichoke	Devil's Claw	Khella
Barberry	Dill	Milk Thistle
Belladonna	Fumitory	Peppermint
Black Root	Galangal	Rosemary
Black Walnut	Haronga	Sandalwood
Boldo	Henbane	Scopola
Caraway	Horehound	Turmeric
Cardamom	Immortelle	Wormwood
Celandine	Japanese Mint	Yarrow
Chamomile	Java Tea	Yellow Dock
Chicory		

Nutritional Support

Diets high in fat and sugar and low in fiber are most likely to promote gallbladder problems. Food sensitivities also play a role. When 69 people with gallbladder problems were placed on a diet that eliminated suspect foods, all saw their symptoms disappear. Ninety-three percent of the people experienced a return of their symptoms after they ate eggs, 64 percent after they ate pork, and 52 percent after they ate onions.

In general, if you suffer from gallstones, you should:

■ Stick to a low-fat, low-sugar, high fiber diet
■ Lose weight (if you are overweight)

■ Always eat breakfast
■ Avoid any foods that you notice cause your symptoms to flare up

If you have your gallbladder removed, you'll need to make a permanent switch to a diet high in protein and carbohydrates and low in fat. Your doctor will give you a detailed plan.

Alternative Treatments
There are no holistic or natural therapies capable of eliminating gallstones.

Genital Herpes

The Basics
Once contracted, genital herpes remains with you for life. Although the painful sores that herald its arrival usually heal within 10 days, they can reappear at any time. Later outbreaks are sparked by a variety of triggers, including surgery, illness, stress, fatigue, skin irritation such as sunburn, dietary imbalance, menstruation, hormonal imbalance, or vigorous sexual intercourse.

The disease is caused by the herpes simplex virus (HSV), a germ that's easily acquired through sexual contact with anyone who has the sores. Although genital herpes is usually the fault of the herpes simplex 2 virus (HSV-2), it can also result from infection with herpes simplex 1 (HSV-1), which usually produces cold sores in and around the mouth. Both viruses can be found in either place.

A brief period of itching and soreness precedes each attack. A reddened patch of skin then spawns a cluster of tiny blisters that erupt into a set of small circular sores. Typically quite painful, the sores are often accompanied by difficulty or pain when trying to urinate, swollen lymph glands, fever, and a generally uneasy feeling.

Although this infection has no cure, prescription drugs can speed healing of the sores and—if you suffer frequent attacks—reduce the number of outbreaks.

If you suspect that you have genital herpes, be sure to see your doctor even if the sores subside. There is a small but significant risk of complications such as inflammation of the brain, spinal cord, or bone marrow, as well as nerve pain.

Call Your Doctor If . . .
- There is any unusual bleeding from the vagina.
- You get a high temperature during treatment or you feel generally ill.
- You get a headache or start throwing up.
- Your symptoms fail to improve or become worse in the week after treatment begins.
- Your symptoms return after treatment.
- You develop any problems that may be related to your medication.

Seek Care Immediately If . . .
Herpes outbreaks do not require emergency treatment.

What You Can Do
- Tell partners with whom you had sex before you were treated that you have herpes. They also may be infected and need treatment.
- Don't have sex until all the sores clear up (about 1 month). Also avoid sex when either partner has blisters or sores. Don't have oral sex with a partner who has cold sores around the mouth.
- When it is safe to have sex, use a latex condom. In addition, the spermicide nonoxynol-9 increases protection against herpes and also helps prevent the spread of gonorrhea and other infections.
- Warm baths can help relieve pain and inflammation. Add a tablespoon of salt to the water. Applying wet tea bags or petroleum jelly to the sores may also be soothing.
- Urinating in the shower or through a tube (such as a toilet paper roll) can help women avoid pain. Pouring a cup of warm water between the legs while urinating also helps.
- Women should wear cotton panties or pantyhose with a cotton crotch. Douching is not usually recommended.
- Try to avoid stress and fatigue. They increase the chances of repeated outbreaks.
- If you're pregnant, be sure to tell the doctor that you have genital herpes. The infection increases the risk of miscarriage or early labor. Herpes also can be passed on to the baby during birth and cause serious problems, such as blindness and brain damage.

What Your Doctor Can Do
Your doctor can confirm the presence of herpes through microscopic examination of material from a sore. He can then prescribe a pill to alleviate the symptoms and speed up healing.

Prescription Drugs
There are currently three drugs available that can relieve the symptoms of genital herpes: Famvir (famciclovir), Valtrex (valacyclovir), and Zovirax (acyclovir). They can also be taken on a regular basis to reduce the number of attacks.

Over-the-Counter Drugs
Nothing available over the counter will speed healing or prevent new outbreaks. However, acetaminophen (Tylenol, Panadol) can help relieve the pain.

Herbal Remedies
No herbs have been found effective for this problem.

Nutritional Support
Maintaining a balanced, healthy diet can help to reduce the chance of repeated attacks.

Alternative Treatments
No alternative therapies have shown any promise for this ailment.

Gonorrhea

The Basics
Gonorrhea is among the most common of all sexually transmitted diseases. Some experts estimate the total number of cases at 2 million per year.

The disease is caused by bacteria that infect the sex organs (and sometimes the throat or rectum). It is spread through vaginal, oral, and anal sex, and is most common among adults between the ages of 15 and 29.

If not treated, gonorrhea can migrate to the internal sex organs, joints, skin, eyes, and heart. It can damage the uterus and the fallopian tubes, increasing the chances of a tubal pregnancy and sometimes leading to sterility. Fortunately, antibiotics provide a highly effective cure.

Typical warning signs of the infection include a discharge of thick yellow-green fluid from the penis or vagina; fever, pain or burning when urinating; the need to urinate frequently, and, in women, pain or bleeding during intercourse. The sex organs may become red, swollen, and itchy. Symptoms are much more common in men than in women. Up to 70 percent of women have no symptoms at all.

Call Your Doctor If . . .

■ You have abdominal pain, swelling of the testicles, chills, joint pain, rash, or a high temperature.

Seek Care Immediately If . . .

■ Your temperature becomes extremely high.

What You Can Do

■ Be sure to take all doses of the antibiotic the doctor prescribes. If you stop treatment too soon, some germs may survive and eventually cause a relapse.

■ Don't have sex until you have taken all the medicine. After that, use of a condom can help prevent the spread of gonorrhea and other infections.

■ Tell all partners with whom you had sex before treatment that you had gonorrhea. They may have contracted the infection, and may need treatment.

■ Wash your hands often, especially after urination or bowel movements. Do not touch your eyes with your hands.

■ If you find out you're pregnant, be sure to tell the doctor that you've had gonorrhea. The disease can be passed on to an infant during birth.

What Your Doctor Can Do

The doctor can identify the disease by taking a swab from the penis, vagina, or rectum and examining it under a microscope. He will then prescribe an antibiotic to kill the germs.

Prescription Drugs

Gonorrhea is often resistant to older antibiotics such as penicillin and tetracycline, so the doctor may chose a new drug from the cephalosporin or quinolone family. The most common treatments today include the following:

Achromycin (tetracycline)
Amoxil or Wymox (amoxicillin)
Beepen-VK, Bicillin,
  Pen-Vee K, V-Cillin K, or
  Veetids (penicillin)
Cefizox (ceftizoxime)
Ceftin, Kefurox, or Zinacef
  (cefuroxime)
Cipro (ciprofloxacin)

Claforan (cefotaxime)
Doryx, Monodox,
  or Vibramycin
  (doxycycline)
E.E.S, Eryc, Ery-Tab, or PCE
  (erythromycin)
Floxin (ofloxacin)
Minocin or Vectrin
  (minocycline)

Noroxin (norfloxacin)
Omnipen (ampicillin)
Penetrex (enoxacin)
Raxar (grepafloxacin)
Rocephin (ceftriaxone)

Spectrobid (bacampicillin)
Suprax (cefixime)
Trovan (alatrofloxacin)
Vantin (cefpodoxime)
Zithromax (azithromycin)

Over-the-Counter Drugs
A prescription is needed for all gonorrhea medications.

Herbal Remedies
Like all acute infections, gonorrhea cannot be relieved with herbs.

Nutritional Support
There are no nutritional measures that can rid you of the germs.

Alternative Treatments
Antibiotics are by far the most effective and reliable form of therapy.

Hay Fever

The Basics
Hay fever—known medically as seasonal allergic rhinitis—is a reaction to airborne irritants known as allergens. These tiny particles trigger the release of histamine in the body, causing symptoms such as itchy, watery eyes; a sore throat; and an itchy, runny, or stuffy nose. Coughing and headache may also occur. Contrary to its name, hay fever does not cause a high temperature.

Seasonal allergic rhinitis occurs only at certain times of the year (for example, the spring or fall), and is caused by pollen from weeds, grasses, and trees. Nonseasonal allergic rhinitis can affect susceptible people during any season and is caused by house dust, feathers, mold, and animals. Tobacco smoke, air pollution, and sudden changes in temperature can aggravate both kinds of allergic rhinitis.

Most people develop allergies as children or adolescents. Treatment can relieve allergy symptoms but will not cure the problem. Some people outgrow allergies as they get older.

Call Your Doctor If . . .

■ Your symptoms get worse or keep you from doing your normal activities.

■ You feel pain or pressure in your sinuses.

■ You have any problems with a medicine you are taking.

■ You develop a high temperature, headache, muscle aches, face or ear pain, severe headache, or thick, greenish-yellow drainage from your nose. These are signs of infection.

Seek Care Immediately If . . .

■ You have difficulty breathing.

What You Can Do

The best way to control allergies is to avoid or minimize exposure to the substances that cause them.

■ Keep your house as clean as possible. Get an air-cleaning filter for your heating system and have all the vents and ducts cleaned. Wear a face mask if you do the cleaning yourself. Do not touch things that are covered with dust.

■ If you find out that you are allergic to a pet, the most effective solution is to give it away. If this isn't possible, limit the animal's access to certain rooms in the house. For example, do not allow it in your bedroom.

■ If you have seasonal allergic rhinitis, stay inside with the windows and doors closed on days when the air pollution is bad or the pollen count is high; drive an air-conditioned car, and have someone else mow the lawn.

■ Don't smoke and try to avoid places that are smoky.

If your symptoms persist, you can choose from the huge variety of over-the-counter allergy medications listed below, or experiment with some of the herbal remedies that experts have judged effective. If these fail to do the job, you should see your doctor for certain other types of medication that are available only by prescription

What Your Doctor Can Do

Although most antihistamine medications are available over-the-counter, a few—such as Allegra and Claritin—require a prescription. Your doctor can also prescribe steroid pills or a steroid nasal spray to control allergy attacks.

For a really serious problem, you can get a series of skin tests to see what's causing the allergic reaction. You may need weekly or biweekly "allergy shots."

Prescription Drugs

Your doctor can prescribe the following antihistamines and steroid medications:

Allegra (fexofenadine)
Astelin (azelastine)
Atarax or Vistaril
  (hydroxyzine)
Atrohist Pediatric Suspension
  (chlorpheniramine,
  phenylephrine, pyrilamine)
Atrohist Pediatric Capsules
  (chlorpheniramine,
  pseudoephedrine)
Atrovent Nasal Spray
  (ipratropium)
Beconase or Vancenase
  (beclomethasone)
Bromfed (brompheniramine)
Codimal-L.A. or Fedahist
  (chlorpheniramine,
  pseudoephedrine)
Claritin (loratidine)
Claritin-D (loratidine,
  pseudoephedrine)
Cortone (cortisone)
D.A. II, Duravent/DA, or
  Extendryl (chlorpheniramine,
  methscopolamine,
  phenylephrine)
Decadron (dexamethasone)

Deltasone (prednisone)
Dexacort Phosphate in
  Turbinaire (dexamethasone)
Flonase (fluticasone
  propionate)
Hismanal (astemizole)
Hydrocortone (hydrocortisone)
Medrol (methylprednisolone)
Nasacort (triamcinolone)
Nasonex (mometasone)
Nasarel (flunisolide)
Nolahist (phenindamine)
Ornade (chlorpheniramine,
  phenylpropanolamine)
Pediapred (prednisolone
  sodium phosphate)
Periactin (cyproheptadine)
Phenergan (promethazine)
Prelone (prednisolone)
Rhinocort (budesonide)
Rynatan (chlorpheniramine,
  phenylephrine, pyrilamine)
Semprex-D (acrivastine,
  pseudoephedrine)
Trinalin Repetabs (azatadine,
  pseudoephedrine)
Zyrtec (cetirizine)

Over-the-Counter Drugs

Although there are dozens of allergy pills to choose from on pharmacy shelves, they all share the same few ingredients. Choose a combination that best matches your symptoms.

Antihistamines: Most allergy products include an antihistamine to relieve itchy, runny nose; sneezing; and itchy, watery eyes. Common antihistamines include brompheniramine, chlorpheniramine, clemastine, dexbrompheniramine, diphenhydramine, phenindamine, and triprolidine.

Decongestants: Many products also contain a decongestant to clear up stuffy nose and sinuses. Common decongestants include phenylephrine, phenylpropanolamine, and pseudoephedrine.

Analgesics: Most allergy products also include a painkiller such as acetaminophen, aspirin, and ibuprofen to treat the discomfort (usually a headache) associated with allergies.

Cough suppressants: Some allergy products add an ingredient to stop the cough that sometimes occurs during a bout with hay fever. Dextromethorphan is the most common cough suppressant. The antihistamine, diphenhydramine, also relieves coughs. Codeine, a very strong cough suppressant, is available in cough syrups without a prescription in some states.

Cromolyn sodium: This drug works differently from other antihistamines. Taken regularly, it can *prevent* a reaction to pollen and other allergens before the reaction starts.

Eye drops: Most over-the-counter eye drops are vasoconstrictors that shrink the size of the blood vessels in the eye. This helps to relieve the itchiness and watering that usually accompanies hay fever. If your eyes bother you, do not rub them. Rubbing will make them feel worse.

Nasal sprays: Typically, over-the-counter nasal sprays are also vasoconstrictors. They relieve congestion by shrinking the blood vessels in the nasal passages. Be sure to read the label and follow the directions carefully. If you use too much of a vasoconstricting nasal spray, your symptoms will get worse rather than better.

ALLERGY REMEDIES FOR ADULTS

Actifed Cold & Allergy
Actifed Allergy
  Daytime/Nighttime Caplets
Afrin Nasal Spray
Allerest Maximum Strength
Allerest No Drowsiness
Benadryl Allergy products
Benadryl Allergy/Cold Tablets
Benadryl Allergy Decongestant
  products

Benadryl Allergy Sinus
  Headache Caplets
Chlor-Trimeton Allergy Tablets
Chlor-Trimeton
  Allergy/Decongestant Tablets
Comtrex Allergy-Sinus
Contac
Coricidin Cold & Flu Tablets
Coricidin Cough & Cold
  Tablets

Dimetapp products
Dimetapp Allergy Dye-Free
 Elixir
Dimetapp Allergy Sinus
Dimetapp Cold & Cough
 Liqui-Gels
Dimetapp DM Elixir
Drixoral Allergy/Sinus
Drixoral Cold & Allergy
Drixoral Cold and Flu
Efidac 24 Chlorpheniramine
 Tablets
4 Way Fast-Acting Nasal Spray
Nasalcrom
Neo-Synephrine Nasal Spray
Nolahist
Novahistamine

Ryna Liquid
Ryna-C Liquid
Sinarest
Sine-Off
Singlet
Sinulin
Sinutab Sinus Allergy
Sudafed Cold & Allergy
Tavist-1
Tavist-D
Teldrin
Theraflu Flu and Cold Medicine
Tylenol Allergy Sinus
Tylenol Allergy Sinus
 Nighttime
Tylenol Severe Allergy
Vicks Sinex Nasal Spray

ALLERGY REMEDIES FOR CHILDREN

Dimetapp Cold & Allergy
Dimetapp Cold and Fever
 Suspension
PediaCare Cold-Cough
Tylenol Children's Cold

Tylenol Children's Cold Plus
 Cough
Tylenol Infants' Cold Drops
Vicks DayQuil Children's
 Allergy

Herbal Remedies

There are no herbal remedies deemed effective specifically for allergic rhinitis. However, you might want to try one of the herbs commonly used for colds, coughs, and sore throat. See the entry on colds and flu for a complete list.

Nutritional Support

Some people are allergic to certain foods or the chemicals that are added to processed foods. If you think the food you eat may be contributing to your allergy problems, you may want to consider a macrobiotic diet. This Asian-style vegetarian diet emphasizes fresh, nonprocessed whole grains and vegetables and eliminates the consumption of meats, sweets, and caffeine. Be sure to tell your doctor if you decide to try this diet, since people who follow it too strictly tend to develop nutritional deficiencies.

Alternative Treatments

Environmental Medicine: Practitioners in this field focus on pollution as the primary source of allergies and a host of other chronic conditions. Allergy relief is probably their strongest suit. They offer a wide variety of treatments, but the majority fall into four major categories:

- Nutritional therapies, such as high-dose vitamins and minerals
- Detoxification therapies to remove metals and chemicals from the body
- Immunotherapy to strengthen the immune system
- Desensitization to train the immune system not to react to allergic triggers

Hypnotherapy: With its ability to enhance the power of suggestion, hypnosis helps some people gain control over a variety of involuntary bodily responses—including allergic reactions. If you are plagued with severe, persistent allergies, it might be worth giving hypnosis a try.

Head Lice

The Basics

These tiny, gray bugs spread easily from person to person, traveling on hats, combs, or headphones. They move quickly and are hard to see, but it's easy to tell when you have them: They leave itchy red bite marks on hair-covered areas of the body.

Head lice are quick to multiply. They lay minuscule white eggs (called *nits*) in the hair near the skin, producing a new brood of bugs in about 7 days. Fortunately, the problem (known medically as *pediculosis*) is easy to treat, and should clear up in about 5 days once it has been addressed.

Call Your Doctor If . . .

- The bites become pus-filled or crusty, and the hair becomes matted and foul-smelling. These are signs of infection.
- Itching or rash returns to the scalp after treatment.
- The medication causes any kind of reaction.

Seek Care Immediately If . . .

Head lice do not constitute an emergency.

What You Can Do

- Use any lice-killing shampoo exactly as directed. Remember that although the product can kill all the lice, it may not eliminate all the nits. For this, you must use a special fine-toothed comb to physically remove them from the hair. If this kind of comb does not come with your medicine, you can find one at a drugstore.
- Removing the nits will be easier if you first soak the hair in a solution of equal parts vinegar and water. Comb the lice-infested hair thoroughly—from the skin outward—once a day until treatment is complete. You do not have to shave or cut the hair in the affected area.
- Avoid close contact with anyone until you're sure the lice are all gone.
- All clothing, bedding, and towels that have been worn or used either three days before or at any time during treatment should be machine washed in hot water and dried in a hot dryer for at least 20 minutes. Items that cannot be washed should be dry cleaned, hung outside for 2 days, or sealed in a plastic bag for 10 days.
- Soak combs, brushes, barrettes, and curlers in an antiseptic solution, rubbing alcohol, or lice-killing shampoo for 1 to 2 hours, or boil them for 5 to 10 minutes. Vacuum all rugs, mattresses, and furniture carefully.
- If a child develops the problem, be sure to tell the school or day-care center that the youngster has head lice. They will tell you when the child may return to school.

What Your Doctor Can Do

Your doctor can prescribe or recommend over-the-counter medication to get rid of the lice, and can double-check to make sure that they're gone.

Prescription Drugs

Lindane shampoo is highly effective against head lice. Be sure to use it cautiously, however. Applying it more liberally or more often than directed can result in seizures or even death, particularly in the young.

Over-the-Counter Drugs

You have a choice of several nonprescription products containing the lice-killing agents piperonyl butoxide and pyrethrine. They include:

A-200 Lice Killing Shampoo
Clear Total Lice
  Elimination System

Pronto Lice Treatment
Rid Lice Killing Shampoo

Herbal Remedies

Pyrethrum flowers (a type of chrysanthemum) are the source of the lice-killing compound pyrethrine.

Nutritional Support

There are no dietary measures that help.

Alternative Treatments

A commercial shampoo is your best bet for this problem.

Heart Attack

The Basics

Heart attack, technically known as *myocardial infarction* or *MI* for short, is the leading cause of death in America. A heart attack strikes when one of the arteries serving the heart muscle is plugged by a blood clot or closes up due to a spasm. Deprived of its supply of oxygen-rich blood, a section of the heart muscle then weakens and dies.

The most common symptom of a heart attack is chest pain. The pain may feel crushing, tight, or heavy, and may spread to the neck, jaw, shoulders, back, or left arm. It may feel like indigestion (a burning sensation under the breastbone). Other signs are trouble breathing, sweating, nausea, vomiting, pale and cool skin, and a light-headed or dizzy feeling. Some people experience no signs or symptoms at all, suffering what is called a silent MI.

Several health problems increase the chances of a heart attack, including high blood pressure and diabetes. Lifestyle factors such as cigarette smoking, excess weight, and physical inactivity also increase your risk. However, too much cholesterol in the blood presents the single greatest danger. A man with a total blood cholesterol reading of 240 is twice as likely to have a heart attack as one with a reading of 200. A level of 300 poses five times the risk.

Call Your Doctor If . . .

■ You have chest pain anytime that continues when you rest.
■ Your chest pain doesn't respond to any heart medications you've been taking.
■ You feel light-headed, dizzy, sweaty, or nauseated after taking your medicine.
■ Your blood pressure or pulse is higher or lower than usual.
■ You feel short of breath or fatigued.

Seek Care Immediately If . . .

■ You have chest pain that spreads to your arms, jaw, or back, and you feel sweaty, nauseous, and short of breath. These are signs of a heart attack. **THIS IS AN EMERGENCY.** Call **911 or 0 (operator)** to get to the nearest hospital or clinic. **Do not drive yourself.**

What You Can Do

Most experts recommend taking an aspirin tablet at the first sign of a heart attack. This drug has blood-thinning, anti-clotting properties that increase your chances of survival. It is not, however, sufficient to "cure" a heart attack. You still need to get emergency treatment as quickly as possible.

To *prevent* a heart attack, you need to adopt a long-term program of dietary and life-style measures. Key recommendations include:

■ Eat foods low in fat, salt, and cholesterol. (See the entry on clogged arteries for details.)
■ If you smoke, quit.
■ Get regular exercise.
■ Be sure to take any medications the doctor prescribes.
■ Avoid situations that cause you anxiety and learn new ways to relax, such as deep breathing, meditation, and yoga.
■ If you suffer from cardiac risk factors such as diabetes or high blood pressure, do your best to keep them under control. Follow your doctor's instructions carefully.
■ Get at least seven hours of rest each night and take a nap during the day if you feel tired.
■ Keep your weight at an age- and height-appropriate level; weighing too much makes the heart work harder.

■ If your doctor has recommended cardiac rehabilitation—a special exercise program for people who have had heart attacks—be sure to participate.

In addition, if you have just had a heart attack, ask your doctor how often you may have sex and whether you can drive. And do not lift, push, or pull anything heavy or work with your arms above shoulder level until your doctor says you may.

What Your Doctor Can Do

When you think you're having a heart attack, it's essential to get to the hospital fast. If you arrive within the first few hours after the pain begins—and you really are having a heart attack—the doctors can give clot-busting drugs to restore blood flow to the heart muscle and prevent further damage. You can also expect to be given pain medication and oxygen. Until the crisis passes, you'll be hooked up to a heart monitor (electrocardiogram), and the doctor will order a variety of tests to check your condition.

Later, if medication and lifestyle changes do not significantly improve your risk profile, your doctor may suggest *angioplasty* (insertion of a tube to clear the clogged artery) or *bypass surgery*, in which a plugged artery is literally bypassed with another vessel taken from elsewhere in your body.

Prescription Drugs

Clot Busters. These drugs can be lifesavers for many people, but can't be used if you're in danger of severe bleeding. Usually given through an intravenous injection, they include:

Abbokinase (urokinase)	Eminase (anistreplase)
Activase (alteplase)	Streptase (streptokinase)

Blood-Thinning Shots. Heparin, an intravenous drug that prevents additional clots from forming, may be given along with a clot buster when you arrive at the hospital. Aggrastat (tirofiban), a newer blood-thinner, is sometimes given after the "mini-heart attacks" labeled Acute Coronary Syndrome.

Blood-Thinning Pills. Like Heparin and Aggrastat, these drugs keep the blood from forming clots. They help provide long-term protection once the crisis is past.

Plavix (clopidogrel)	Coumadin (warfarin)

Beta-Blockers. These drugs reduce demand on the heart and can reduce the damage from a heart attack. Among them are:

Coreg (carvedilol)
Inderal (propranolol)
Lopressor (metoprolol)

Tenormin (atenolol)
Zebeta (bisoprolol)

ACE Inhibitors. These drugs lower blood pressure and spare the heart from extra work. Prime examples are:

Accupril (quinapril)
Capoten (captopril)
Prinivil (lisinopril)

Univasc (moexipril)
Vasotec (enalapril)

Nitroglycerin. This drug, often used to relieve chest pain, relaxes and expands the arteries, thus improving blood flow to the heart muscle. Leading brands of nitroglycerin include Nitro-Bid, Nitro-Dur, Nitrolingual Spray, Nitrostat Tablets, and Transderm-Nitro.

Over-the-Counter Drugs

For anyone with the clogged arteries that pose a danger of heart attack, an aspirin tablet a day can provide some degree of protection. Make sure, however, that you're using aspirin (Ascriptin Enteric, Bayer, Ecotrin, Halfprin, St. Joseph). Other over-the-counter pain-killers, such as acetaminophen and ibuprofen, do not have aspirin's blood-thinning effect.

Herbal Remedies

There are no herbal remedies that can help you *during* a heart attack. Waste no time getting to the hospital.

On the other hand, certain herbs can lower your risk of an attack in the future. For more information, see the entry on clogged arteries.

Nutritional Support

Sticking to a low-fat, high-fiber diet is one of the most important steps you can take to reduce your odds of a heart attack—or of a second attack if you've already had one. For details, see the entry on clogged arteries.

If high blood pressure is contributing to your risk of a heart attack, use salt in moderation, and make sure your diet contains plenty of potassium (found in bananas, orange juice, beans, and potatoes), calcium (found in milk, broccoli, and salmon), and magnesium (oats, bran, nuts, and legumes). Keep caffeine intake to less than 5 cups a day and keep your daily alcohol intake to less than 2 ounces of hard liquor, 4 ounces of wine, or 12 ounces of beer.

Alternative Treatments

Alternative medicine offers no help for a heart attack. A conventional emergency room should be your only destination. However, there are several alternative forms of treatment that promise to prevent attacks by keeping your arteries clear. See the entry on clogged arteries for more information

Heart Failure

The Basics

Weakening of the heart, or *congestive heart failure* (CHF), is the nation's leading cause of hospitalization for people over age 65. Hallmarks of the condition are weakness, fatigue, shortness of breath, and swelling of the ankles, feet, and fingers.

The heart is made up of four chambers: two *atria* and two *ventricles*. The atria collect incoming blood and deliver it to the ventricles. The ventricles then send it back out of the heart. Heart failure occurs when more blood goes into the ventricles than they can pump out. This usually causes fluid to back up into the lungs and veins and to leak into other tissues of the body.

There are two types of CHF: *systolic* and *diastolic*. Anything that weakens the way the heart muscle contracts is called a systolic dysfunction. When the heart's ability to expand is compromised, the situation is known as diastolic dysfunction. While both types cause similar symptoms, treatment differs for each.

CHF can result from a number of conditions, including prolonged high blood pressure, damage from a heart attack, diseases of the heart muscle, or failure of a valve. Less common causes include anemia, pregnancy, heart irregularities, thyroid disease, and toxic substances such as carbon monoxide and cocaine.

Cases of CHF range from mild (with few if any symptoms) to totally incapacitating (with symptoms present even at rest). The condition typically gets worse over time.

Call Your Doctor If . . .

■ You gain 2 or 3 pounds in a day.
■ Your blood pressure is higher or lower than usual.
■ Your pulse is faster or slower than usual.
■ You cough up yellow, green, or pink frothy sputum.
■ You find yourself wheezing.
■ You have trouble breathing, notice swelling in your feet or ankles, or feel more tired than usual.
■ You have chest pain during exercise that continues when you rest.
■ You feel light-headed, dizzy, sweaty, or nauseated after taking your medicine.

Seek Care Immediately If . . .

■ You have more trouble breathing than usual.
■ You can't sleep for lack of breath.
■ You feel weak.
■ You develop a fast or uneven heartbeat.
■ You notice increased swelling in your legs, feet, and torso, and you begin to feel dizzy.

These are signs of worsening heart failure, which constitutes an **EMERGENCY.** Call for help immediately or call **911 or 0 (operator)** to get to the nearest medical facility. **Do not drive yourself.**

What You Can Do

■ Make a point of taking all prescribed medications faithfully. Failure to take drugs for a related condition such as high blood pressure or coronary artery disease can easily trigger congestive heart failure.
■ Exercise can be a big help for people with a mild case of CHF. Try to get as much as you can handle. (Check with your doctor for the right amount.)
■ Stress puts extra demands on the heart. Try to avoid it or keep it under control.
■ Get at least 7 hours of rest each night and nap during the day if you are tired.
■ If you're a smoker, this is definitely the time to quit. A weakened heart needs every bit of help you can give it.

■ Keep your weight under control. Excess pounds put an unneeded strain on the heart.

■ Avoid really hot or cold temperatures. Dress carefully to protect yourself from extremes.

■ Do not lift, pull, or push anything heavy or work with your arms above shoulder level unless your doctor says it's okay.

What Your Doctor Can Do

To diagnose the problem, your doctor will probably request an *echocardiogram*, which uses ultrasound waves to create a video picture of the size, shape, and movement of the heart. Other tests may include a chest x-ray; blood and urine tests; an *electrocardiograph (ECG)*, which tracks the electrical currents running through the heart; and *cardiac blood pool imaging*, which gauges the contracting action of the heart.

Once CHF is confirmed, treatment typically includes a number of diet and lifestyle changes, plus medications to help relieve symptoms and slow the condition's progress. In some CHF patients, the damage is so great that a heart transplant offers the only chance for future health. A transplant is an option for someone in otherwise fairly good health, without many complications.

Prescription Drugs

ACE Inhibitors: Doctors usually prescribe a combination of drugs for CHF, but in recent years, *angiotensin converting enzyme (ACE) inhibitors* have moved to the forefront. In addition to lowering blood pressure, these drugs work at a cellular level to help prevent thickening of the ventricular wall. Common ACE inhibitors include captopril (Capoten), enalapril (Vasotec), fosinopril (Monopril), lisinopril (Zestril, Prinivil), and quinapril (Accupril).

Diuretics: These medications relieve the fluid buildup that typically accompanies CHF without reducing the output of the heart. Diuretics commonly used for CHF include furosemide (Lasix), bumetanide (Bumex), and ethacrynic acid (Edecrin).

Digitalis: If diuretics and ACE inhibitors fail to provide enough relief, digitalis may be prescribed to strengthen the heart's contractions, improve its output, and thereby ease the symptoms of CHF.

Nitroglycerin: By triggering expansion of the small blood vessels serving the heart muscle, this drug increases the heart's blood supply and improves its pumping action. Leading brands include Nitro-Bid, Nitro-Dur, Nitrolingual Spray, Nitrostat Tablets, and Transderm-Nitro.

Carvedilol (Coreg): This drug seems to improve the heart's efficiency. Combined with an ACE inhibitor, a diuretic, and digitalis, it can significantly slow the progression of the disease.

Bronchodilators: These inhaled medications open the airways and can help relieve congestive lung symptoms. But be sure to use only what your doctor prescribes. Some bronchodilators are bad for a weakened heart.

Oxygen: You may be supplied with an oxygen tank to make breathing easier.

Over-the-Counter Drugs

If clogged arteries are contributing to your CHF, your doctor may suggest you take a daily aspirin tablet to help thin the blood and prevent clots. Be sure to get aspirin. Other over-the-counter painkillers, such as acetaminophen and ibuprofen, do not have a blood-thinning effect.

Herbal Remedies

Given the vulnerability of a weakened heart, you should check with your doctor before taking *any* drugs or herbs. Among the natural remedies thought to be of some help are:

Adonis	Hawthorn Leaf	Motherwort
Belladonna	Khella	Shepherd's Purse
Camphor	Lily of the Valley	Squill
Coenzyme Q_{10}	Mate	

Nutritional Support

For people with CHF, the most important dietary guideline is always "hold the salt." By causing the body to retain fluid, excessive salt intake is often enough to trigger failure in an already struggling heart. Substitute other seasonings in cooking, watch the sodium content of all packaged foods, and ask for low-salt preparation when dining out.

You may also want to make sure your diet contains plenty of potassium, especially if you're taking a diuretic that washes potassium out of the body along with excess salt. Good sources include bananas, orange juice, beans, and potatoes.

And anyone with heart problems needs to stick with a heart-healthy, low-fat, high fiber diet that cuts down artery-clogging cholesterol levels. For details, see the entry on clogged arteries.

Alternative Treatments

Alternative medicine offers little help for people with full-blown congestive heart failure. Techniques such as yoga are said to reverse the coronary artery disease that often contributes to a CHF, but anyone with a weakened heart should approach such exercises with caution. To allay the stress, tension, and anxiety that make the heart work harder, you might also find relief in aromatherapy, biofeedback, guided imagery, hypnotherapy, and meditation.

Heartburn

The Basics

Heartburn—that burning feeling in your chest, often accompanied by a sour taste and trouble swallowing—is one of the most common of all ailments. It strikes more than 60 million adults in the U.S. at least once a month, and 25 million suffer daily. Known medically as *gastroesophageal reflux*, it's caused by stomach acids flowing back into the canal between the mouth and the stomach (the esophagus).

Acid backflow is usually the fault of a weakened lower esophageal sphincter, the muscle that ordinarily keeps the entrance to the stomach closed. We don't know why the sphincter weakens, but we do know the problem increases with age. Because heartburn also increases during pregnancy, scientists believe that fluctuating estrogen and progesterone levels may also play a role. The problem may also run in families.

Heartburn often is triggered simply by eating too much, especially if you've been indulging in fatty foods or chocolate. Alcohol, mint, and caffeinated beverages are other potential culprits, as are smoking and certain drugs such as sedatives and the blood pressure medications called calcium channel blockers. Stress, excess weight, eating on the run, and eating right before bed also can contribute to the problem.

Since part of the esophagus lies near the heart, the symptoms can be confused with angina pectoris, chest pain originating in the heart. How can you tell one from the other? It's wise to let your doctor decide. But as a general guide, it's probably heartburn when the chest discomfort is caused by eating or lying down, is accompanied by belching or regurgitating, or clears up when you take antacids. It's also probably heartburn if anti-anginal drugs don't help. But don't forget that you can have both heartburn and angina, and may need appropriate treatment for both.

Call Your Doctor If . . .

■ Your symptoms get worse or fail to improve within a few days.

■ You develop a high temperature.

■ You have extreme discomfort or pain in the digestive tract.

■ You have black stools (unless you are using a drug that contains bismuth subsalicylate).

■ You see blood in the stool.

■ You have a sudden, persistent change in bowel habits.

■ You develop abdominal swelling.

■ Your heartburn is not relieved by antacids.

■ You begin to lose weight.

Seek Care Immediately If . . .

■ You begin vomiting blood or material that looks like coffee grounds.

■ You develop severe chest pain along with nausea, sweating, or shortness of breath—you may be having a heart attack.

What You Can Do

There are a variety of very effective measures you can take to reduce the frequency of heartburn. Many are simply aimed at keeping the contents of the stomach in place and avoiding pressure on the abdomen.

■ To keep your stomach from getting too full, eat 6 small meals instead of 3 big ones. Eat slowly and chew food well, especially raw fruits and vegetables.

■ Don't eat or drink anything for 1 to 2 hours before going to bed.

■ To avoid distending the stomach, don't drink liquids just before or after a meal.

■ Avoid foods known to promote heartburn. (See "Nutritional Support" below.)

■ To help prevent heartburn at night, place 4- to 6-inch blocks under the head of your bed. This will keep your head and esophagus higher than your stomach. If you can't use blocks, sleep with several pillows under your head and shoulders.

■ Avoid bending over or lying flat after eating. Also, avoid straining during bowel movements, or when you're urinating or lifting things.

■ Don't wear clothing that constricts your chest or stomach.

■ If you're a smoker, try to quit. Smoking often causes the stomach to make more acid.

■ If you are overweight, shed the extra pounds.

What Your Doctor Can Do

Most doctors recommend treating recurrent heartburn aggressively, since stomach acid can burn the lower esophagus, causing scars that make swallowing difficult. A host of prescription and over-the-counter drugs can help. Surgery is a last resort, reserved only for people in whom nothing else works. If you're in this group, an operation to tighten the lower esophageal sphincter may relieve the problem.

Prescription Drugs

For severe heartburn, your doctor may prescribe a drug that stimulates esophageal contractions and strengthens the sphincter muscle, such as cisapride (Propulsid) and metoclopramide hydrochloride (Reglan).

To reduce the production of damaging stomach acid, several drugs called histamine H2 blockers are available, including famotidine (Pepcid), ranitidine (Zantac), and cimetidine (Tagamet). Lower-dose versions of these drugs are available over the counter.

To heal damage in the lining of the esophagus, the doctor can also prescribe lansoprazole (Prevacid) or omeprazole (Prilosec).

Over-the-Counter Drugs

An over-the-counter antacid taken 1 hour after meals can provide substantial relief. Your options include:

Aluminum hydroxide/magnesium (Maalox, Gaviscon)
Aluminum hydroxide/sodium (AlternaGEL, Amphojel)
Aluminum hydroxide/mineral oil (Nephrox)
Aluminum hydroxide/magnesium hydroxide/
  simethicone (Mylanta Liquid)
Aluminum carbonate (Basaljel)
Bismuth subsalicylate (Pepto-Bismol)
Calcium carbonate (Alka-Mints, Tums, Mylanta Lozenges, Titralac)
Calcium carbonate/magnesium hydroxide (Rolaids)
Calcium carbonate/magnesium hydroxide/simethicone
  (Di-Gel, Mylanta tablets)
Calcium carbonate/simethicone (Titralac Plus, Tums Antigas/Antacid)
Magnesium hydroxide (Phillips' Milk of Magnesia)
Sodium bicarbonate, citric acid, potassium bicarbonate
  (Alka-Seltzer Gold)
Sodium bicarbonate, citric acid, aspirin
  (Alka-Seltzer, Bromo Seltzer)

Antacids interact with a number of prescription drugs, so check with your doctor before taking them and be sure to keep doses of antacids and any other drug 2 or 3 hours apart. You also should avoid prolonged use of antacids. Depending on their ingredients, they can cause a variety of long-term side effects. Avoid sodium-based drugs if you are on a salt-restricted diet. Excessive use of calcium-based drugs can result in kidney stones. Use of aluminum-based drugs for a period of years can weaken bones. Very prolonged use of magnesium-based drugs also can cause kidney stones and heart, central nervous system, and kidney problems.

As an alternative to antacids, consider an over-the-counter histamine H2 blocker. Your options include:

Axid AR	Pepcid AC	Zantac 75
Mylanta AR	Tagamet HB	

Herbal Remedies
A wide variety of herbs soothe an upset stomach, and might help your heartburn as well. See the entry on indigestion for a complete list.

Nutritional Support
Avoiding foods that tend to relax the lower esophageal sphincter muscle can do much to solve the problem. Fatty foods and chocolate are the leading culprits. It's also wise to eliminate items that stimulate acid production, including alcohol and caffeinated beverages.

If the problem continues or gets worse, you should avoid foods and beverages that can irritate a damaged esophageal lining, such as citrus and tomato products, and pepper.

Alternative Treatments
Two alternative therapies—biofeedback and yoga—have been found especially helpful for indigestion, and could be worth trying for heartburn.

Hemorrhoids

The Basics
With symptoms that range from nonexistent to incapacitating, hemorrhoids are a universal problem in both children and adults. Also called piles, they are simply swollen veins in the rectum or anus.

You can have hemorrhoids for years without knowing it. Often they appear without warning, then vanish on their own. The typical symptoms are a swelling or soft lump at the anus accompanied by bleeding and pain. If the hemorrhoids are confined to the inside of the rectum, the only symptoms may be a mucus discharge with bowel movements and a feeling that you need to pass more stool. Itching is *not* a symptom of hemorrhoids.

Hemorrhoids are more common in people who are overweight, those who have liver problems, and older adults. Excessive straining to pass hardened stool seems to foster the problem. It also tends to develop during pregnancy, as the uterus presses on the veins of the rectum. It sometimes results merely from sitting too long on hard chairs.

Typically, hemorrhoids tend to clear up by themselves. If they persist, doctors have several simple ways of eliminating them.

Call Your Doctor If . . .

■ Your hemorrhoids cause severe pain and self-treatment fails to help.
■ Rectal bleeding is more than a trace or streak on the toilet paper or in the stool.
■ You notice a hard lump in the location of the hemorrhoid.

Seek Care Immediately If . . .

Even severe hemorrhoids do not call for emergency care.

What You Can Do

■ To reduce pain and swelling, apply an over-the-counter hemorrhoid medicine. Follow the directions on the label.
■ Clean the anal area gently with soft, moist toilet paper after each bowel movement.
■ Eat a high-fiber diet and drink plenty of liquids, at least 6 to 8 large glasses every day.
■ Sit in a tub of comfortably hot water for 20 minutes, 3 times a day.
■ If a hemorrhoid is very painful and swollen, apply an ice pack to the anal area.
■ Avoid sitting or standing for long periods of time. If the hemorrhoid is painful, lie down as much as possible.
■ You may use a stool softener to make your bowel movements easier to pass. Don't try to hurry bowel movements and don't strain.

What Your Doctor Can Do

To rule out a more serious cause of bleeding such as cancer, the doctor will examine the anal area using a short tube or a rubber-gloved finger. Bleeding can be stopped, at least temporarily, with an injection. Most large hemorrhoids can be destroyed with rubber-band ligation, which literally uses a small elastic band to cut off circulation to the offending tissue so that it dies and sloughs off. Painful and persistent hemorrhoids near the entrance to the anus may require surgical removal.

Prescription Drugs

To relieve pain and inflammation, your doctor can prescribe steroid suppositories (Anusol-HC).

Over-the-Counter Drugs

There are several nonprescription products for relief of hemorrhoidal burning, soreness, and pain:

Anusol	Nupercainal	Tucks Pads
Hemorid	Preparation H	

To prevent straining and ease bowel movements, you can choose from the following over-the-counter stool softeners, all of which contain docusate:

Colace	Dialose	Fleet Sof-Lax
Correctol Stool Softener	Ex-Lax Stool Softener Caplets	Surfak

Herbal Remedies

The following herbs have been found helpful for hemorrhoids:

Balsam of Peru	Butcher's Broom	Sweet Clover
Black Walnut	Poplar	Witch Hazel

Psyllium is an effective natural stool softener. It's available over the counter under the brand names Konsyl, Metamucil, and Perdiem Fiber Therapy.

Nutritional Support

To ease bowel movements and reduce straining, drink plenty of fluids and eat a high-fiber diet that includes fruits and vegetables, oat and bran cereal, whole-grain bread, and brown rice. Undigested fiber absorbs water, making the stool softer and easier to pass.

Alternative Treatments

There are no alternative treatments that stand out as especially helpful for hemorrhoids.

Hepatitis

The Basics

This subtle, secret illness can lie in hiding for years, causing little more than a run-down feeling while it slowly undermines the liver. Fortunately, the majority of people are able to fight it off. But for the unlucky few who develop chronic hepatitis, it can end in liver cancer or liver failure, with predictably fatal results.

Hepatitis—which literally means "inflamed liver"—is usually caused by a viral infection. There are many different types of viral hepatitis, but hepatitis A, B, and C are the most common. These infections are easily passed from person to person, and afflict hundreds of thousands of Americans each year. There is no cure for any form of viral hepatitis, but you can get protective vaccinations for hepatitis A and B.

Hepatitis A. This form of the disease, formerly known as infectious hepatitis, can be contracted from contaminated water or food. The virus appears in the stool of infected persons, and can easily be passed on by restaurant workers and food handlers who fail to wash their hands. Careless day-care workers who don't wash after changing a diaper are another source of infection. You can also catch the virus from contaminated raw shellfish.

Hepatitis A often produces no symptoms at all. When they do occur, they typically begin suddenly and last for several weeks. This period is followed by a convalescent phase of from 2 to 12 weeks. Patients usually recover completely and develop a lifelong immunity to the virus.

Symptoms usually mimic the flu, and include mild fever, fatigue, nausea, muscle and joint aches, loss of appetite, vomiting, occasional diarrhea, and vague abdominal pain. Some people also develop a yellow cast to the skin and whites of the eyes, known as jaundice, along with dark-colored urine, clay-colored stools, and itching of the skin. The liver may be enlarged and tender.

Hepatitis A is seldom severe, and does not lead to chronic hepatitis. However, in about 1 percent of cases it causes serious problems such as brain swelling and damage, long-term damage to the liver, severe liver failure, and death.

Hepatitis B. The virus responsible for this form of the disease, formerly known as serum hepatitis, infects blood and other body fluids such as urine, tears, semen, breast milk, and vaginal secretions. It is usually transmitted via blood transfusions, or through injectable-drug use. However, it is possible to catch it through a minor cut or abrasion, or during such everyday acts as brushing your teeth, kissing, or having sex.

Infants can contract the virus from the mother at birth, or from the mother's breast milk. Dental work, ear piercing, and tattooing are other ways the disease is spread. The virus is surprisingly hardy and can remain infectious for quite a while, even in dried blood, saliva, or other secretions.

Like hepatitis A, this infection frequently produces no symptoms at all. When they do occur, the flu-like first stage is followed by a second stage with jaundice. The disease pursues an unpredictable course, sometimes incapacitating a person for weeks or months and leading to complications, but usually ending in full recovery. Victims tend to be thin, weak, lethargic, and irritable, and usually have an enlarged, painful liver.

Hepatitis B is especially insidious because about 5 to 10 percent of those who catch the virus become carriers who can unknowingly spread it to others for an indefinite period. At present, there are more than a million of these silent carriers in this country.

Such individuals usually do not develop chronic hepatitis. If they do, however, they are in danger of developing cirrhosis or cancer of the liver. Cirrhosis, a progressive scarring and hardening of the liver, kills an estimated 4,000 victims of hepatitis B each year. Liver cancer is many times more likely to strike hepatitis B carriers than noncarriers.

Hepatitis C. A disease originally labeled "non-A, non-B hepatitis" is now recognized as hepatitis C. Like hepatitis B, it is contracted through contact with contaminated blood, or through household or sexual contact with an infected person. It's often picked up from a dirty needle. Sometimes the source of the infection can't be determined.

The symptoms of hepatitis C are similar to those of hepatitis B, but milder. As with other types of hepatitis, there may be no symptoms at all. Approximately 30 to 50 percent of those who contract this form of the disease end up with a chronic infection. The chronic form is usually mild, but can lead to cirrhosis in 20 percent of cases.

Call Your Doctor If . . .
- You can't drink fluids or keep food down.
- You develop a rash, itching, or swelling of your abdomen or legs.

Seek Care Immediately If . . .
- You feel confused or unusually sleepy.
- You have signs of water loss, such as dry mouth, excessive thirst, wrinkled skin, little or no urination, or dizziness or light-headedness.
- You notice that you are bruising easily.
- You have vomiting or diarrhea that lasts longer than a few days, or you develop severe abdominal pain.

What You Can Do
If you're at especially high risk of contracting this disease, see your doctor about getting shots for hepatitis A and B. If you think you've been exposed to the virus, get a shot of immune globulin to fight the disease.

There is no effective relief for the symptoms of hepatitis. Your best strategy is to keep up your strength as much as possible. You will be fatigued and tire easily for quite a while. Although you don't need to stay in bed, you should get plenty of rest. If complications set in, you may need a stay in the hospital.

You should also maintain a healthy diet, even if your appetite is poor. Eating several small meals a day may be helpful. Drink at least 8 large glasses of water each day. Don't drink any alcohol (including beer and wine) for a few weeks. Alcohol makes the liver work harder.

To avoid spreading hepatitis to others:
- Don't share dishes and eating utensils. Wash them in boiling water or an automatic dishwasher, or use disposable ones.
- Avoid close contact with other people, including kissing. Don't have any sexual contact, including oral and anal sex, until your doctor tells you it's safe.
- Wash your hands thoroughly before eating and after using the toilet. Be careful not to touch your bowel movements.
- Wash clothing and bedding at the hottest water setting.
- Clean toilets with a product that kills germs.
- If you have hepatitis A or B, warn your friends and family to get a vaccination.

■ When having sex, use a latex condom to help prevent the spread of hepatitis B and other infections.

What Your Doctor Can Do

Vaccination for hepatitis A and B can help even after you've been exposed. A shot of immune globulin (Ig) also can provide some protection after you've been exposed to hepatitis A; get it as soon as possible or within two weeks after jaundice appears. This medication is 80 to 90 percent effective in preventing the disease. Shots of hepatitis B immune globulin provide similar protection after exposure to hepatitis B. Get one shot immediately, and another a month later. This form of treatment is 70 percent effective.

Prescription Drugs

For hepatitis A, you can get a shot of a vaccine brand-named Vaqta or Havrix, or the immune globulin named Gammar P. Several vaccines are available for hepatitis B, including Comvax, Engerix-B, and Recombivax HB. Available hepatitis B immune globulins include BayHep B and HBIG.

Chronic cases of hepatitis B and C are now being treated with various types of interferon, a biotech medicine derived from the human immune system. A brand called Intron A is used for hepatitis B. Brands prescribed for chronic hepatitis C include Intron A, Infergen, Rebetron, and Roferon-A. For nausea, your doctor may prescribe a drug such as Tigan (trimethobenzamide).

Over-the-Counter Drugs

Many medications are processed through the liver. If you have hepatitis, check with your doctor before taking any over-the-counter medicines.

Herbal Remedies

A wide variety of herbs have been found helpful for liver problems, but only one—schisandra—is known to actually improve test results in cases of infectious hepatitis.

Nutritional Support

No dietary measures seem to help, but you should remember to avoid alcohol until you've recovered.

Alternative Treatments

There are no alternative therapies effective against viral hepatitis.

High Blood Pressure

The Basics

High blood pressure is often called the silent killer. You can have it for years without any symptoms while it slowly raises your odds of heart disease, stroke, kidney failure, or a heart attack. It is the most common chronic illness in America—yet less than half of its victims have it under control.

Blood pressure is simply the force your blood exerts on the walls of your veins, arteries, and heart. A blood pressure reading measures this force at two different points in time.

The first measurement is called systolic (sis-TAHL-ic). It tells the pressure as the heart contracts (during a heartbeat). A good systolic number is between 100 and 140 millimeters of mercury (mm Hg).

The second measurement is called diastolic (DI-as-tahl-ic). It gives the pressure when the heart is at rest between beats. A good diastolic number is usually lower than 90 mm Hg.

If either of these numbers is consistently elevated, you have high blood pressure (known medically as hypertension). For example, it's considered high blood pressure if your reading is 120/98, because even though the first number (systolic) is within the standard range, the second (diastolic) is above normal. Likewise, you have a problem if your reading is 180/88, because the first number is high even though the second is not.

Occasionally, high blood pressure stems from some other illness, such as kidney disease or a thyroid disorder. It can also result from pregnancy, certain medications, or excessive drinking. When the cause is known, it is called secondary hypertension.

When no specific cause can be found (which holds true in over 90 percent of all cases) the problem is labeled essential hypertension. Although there's no single cause, essential hypertension has a variety of contributing factors. It is more likely to develop if others in your family have it; if you are over 50, male, black, or overweight; and if you smoke, don't get exercise, or suffer from constant stress.

If your blood pressure is only a bit above normal, you may be able to bring it down with a few adjustments in your lifestyle. (See "What You Can Do" below.) If these changes don't work, you'll need to start taking one or more antihypertensive medications.

Call Your Doctor If . . .

■ You are dizzy and the feeling does not go away.

■ You have chest pain during exercise that doesn't go away with rest.

■ You have a fever, vomiting, or diarrhea that makes you dizzy.

Seek Care Immediately If . . .

■ Your blood pressure is higher than usual.

■ You pass out or have a seizure.

■ You have chest pain that does not go away with rest or medicine.

■ You have a headache; feel sleepy or confused; develop numbness and tingling in your hands and feet; start coughing blood; have nosebleeds; or have a lot of trouble breathing. These are signs of very high blood pressure. **Call 911 or 0 (operator)** to get to the nearest hospital or clinic. **Do not drive yourself!**

What You Can Do

There are a number of measures you can take to keep your blood pressure in check:

■ If you're a smoker, quitting is the most important step you can take. Cigarettes typically raise blood pressure sharply, as well as harming the heart and lungs. If you are having trouble stopping, ask your doctor for a medication, a nicotine patch, or a similar quit-smoking aid.

■ If you're overweight, make a concerted effort to shed some pounds. Even a small loss of weight (for instance, 10 pounds) can yield a significant drop in blood pressure—and reduce your risk of heart disease.

■ Exercise regularly. It lowers blood pressure, strengthens the heart, and keeps you healthy.

■ Avoid excessive alcohol. A couple of drinks a day don't seem to do any harm, but anything more than that is likely to raise your blood pressure.

■ Cut back on fat and cholesterol. This not only reduces your risk of clogged arteries, but lowers high blood pressure as well.

■ Try limiting the amount of salt in your diet. If you are one of the many people who prove to be salt-sensitive, this can significantly reduce your blood pressure. At the same time, make sure you're getting a sufficient amount of potassium. Ask your doctor for details.

■ Since it is hard to avoid stress, learn to control it. Try some of the stress-reduction techniques outlined in "Alternative Treatments" below. Also, don't hesitate to talk to someone about things that upset you.

If these lifestyle changes fail to do the job and your doctor put you on medication, be sure to take it faithfully. This is easier said than done, since you're unlikely to notice any difference. But unless antihypertensive medication is taken regularly, year after year, it has little chance of working. These drugs do not cure hypertension; they merely keep it under control.

What Your Doctor Can Do

If your doctor finds that you have high blood pressure, his first move will be to look for a specific cause, and remedy it if found. Otherwise, he'll begin treatment for essential hypertension. If your blood pressure is only mildly elevated, he may recommend a trial of the lifestyle changes outlined above. But if your readings are well above normal, you'll probably need a prescription antihypertensive drug from the start. Typically, the doctor will start with a single medication, then add others if necessary, adjusting the dosage of each until your readings return to normal.

Prescription Drugs

More than 100 medications are available for the treatment of high blood pressure, and they do their work in a variety of ways.

Diuretics—also called water pills—rid the body of excess water, thus reducing the amount of fluid in the bloodstream and hence the pressure on artery walls. Leading examples are:

Aldactone (spironolactone)
Diuril (chlorothiazide)

Esidrix and HydroDIURIL (hydrochlorothiazide)
Lasix (furosemide)

Beta-blockers work by throttling back the speed and force of the heart. Among them are:

Coreg (carvedilol)
Inderal (propranolol)
Lopressor (metoprolol)

Tenormin (atenolol)
Zebeta (bisoprolol)

ACE Inhibitors interfere with the production of angiotensin II, a hormone the body produces to raise blood pressure. Prime examples are:

Accupril (quinapril)
Capoten (captopril)
Prinivil (lisinopril)

Univasc (moexipril)
Vasotec (enalapril)

HIGH BLOOD PRESSURE/**189**

Angiotensin II antagonists block the action of this hormone on the circulatory system. Drugs in this category include:

Atacand (candesartan)	Diovan (valsartan)
Avapro (irbesartan)	Hyzaar (hydrochlorothiazide,
Cozaar (losartan potassium)	losartan potassium)

Calcium channel blockers work by expanding the arteries and reducing resistance to the flow of blood. They are the most widely prescribed group of drugs in the United States. Leading examples include:

Calan, Covera-HS, Isoptin,	DynaCirc (isradipine)
and Verelan (verapamil)	Procardia XL (nifedipine)
Cardizem (diltiazem)	Sular (nisoldipine)

Other drugs lower blood pressure by, in one way or another, relaxing the muscles in the walls of the arteries. Examples include:

Aldomet (methyldopa)	Loniten (minoxidil)
Apresoline (hydralazine)	Minipress (prazosin)
Cardura (doxazosin)	Tenex (guanfacine)
Catapres (clonidine)	

Over-the-Counter Drugs
None are available.

Herbal Remedies
Three herbs are thought to have a specific beneficial effect on high blood pressure. They are:

Khella
Kudzu
Onion

Nutritional Support
Cutbacks in fat, salt, and cholesterol are currently considered the most important measures. If you drink more than 5 or 6 cups of coffee a day, you might also want to try limiting your caffeine intake. And remember to avoid heavy drinking.

Alternative Treatments

Biofeedback: This technique enables patients to control otherwise involuntary reactions such as an increase in blood pressure. After applying sensors to various parts of your body and hooking them up to a computer, a biofeedback therapist will teach you mental and physical exercises that serve to bring your pressure readings down.

Hypnotherapy: With its ability to enhance the power of suggestion, hypnosis helps people gain control over a variety of involuntary bodily responses—including blood pressure. It doesn't work for everyone, but if you want to avoid taking drugs, you may want to give it a try.

Meditation is a deliberate suspension of the stream of consciousness that usually occupies the mind. Its primary goal is to induce mental tranquility and relaxation. Scientific studies have shown that it can in fact reduce high blood pressure.

Orthomolecular Medicine uses nutrients as medications. For example, recent studies have shown that increased intake of calcium, magnesium, and potassium appears to have a beneficial effect on high blood pressure.

Sound Therapy: Specially selected music can have therapeutic effects on a wide variety of ailments, reducing stress and anxiety, relieving pain—and lowering blood pressure.

Tai Chi: a fitness regimen derived from the martial arts, has been shown to reduce blood pressure and heart rate.

Yoga: This ancient discipline incorporates breathing exercises, body postures and meditation. It has been proven to lower blood pressure and may even contribute to the reversal of heart disease.

HIV

The Basics

HIV (human immunodeficiency virus) is both insidious and deadly. It can lurk in the body for years without any symptoms, then weaken the immune system to the point that it no longer can fight off disease. Stripped of its natural defenses, the body then succumbs to AIDS (acquired immunodeficiency syndrome).

The virus is spread by contact with blood or body fluids. It may infest all body fluids; but only blood, semen, discharge from the vagina, and possibly breast milk have enough of the virus to infect other people. It can be spread from male to male, male to female,

female to male, or female to female. It can be passed from a mother to her unborn child or a nursing baby.

Most people get the virus from having sex or using dirty needles to administer drugs. It doesn't matter whether you are gay or straight, and your sexual partner may not be sick or even know that he or she has the virus. You can also get HIV from an infected blood transfusion.

At first there are usually no symptoms. Typically, five or six years will pass before the immune system completely breaks down. While this period wears on, some patients begin to develop shingles, itchy skin eruptions, tuberculosis, fungal infections of the mouth, night sweats, fatigue, and swollen glands. Then, as damage to the immune system increases, severe and unusual infections set in and odd cancers begin to grow. In the end, pneumonia, brain infections, and severe diarrhea are not unusual.

Today we have a large assortment of drugs that can slow the advance of the virus and delay the arrival of AIDS. These drugs can't help, however, if you don't know they're needed. It's therefore wise to get an HIV test whenever you think you may have been exposed to the virus.

This simple blood test detects the presence of the antibodies that your system produces to (unsuccessfully) fight off the virus. A positive reading for antibodies means that the virus must be in your body. A negative reading, however, is not as conclusive. Your system can take as little as 2 weeks or as long as 6 months to produce antibodies. So a negative test now doesn't preclude the possibility of a positive test later. If you're at high risk of getting HIV or know that you were exposed, you should get another test in 6 months.

Call Your Doctor If . . .
■ You have any reason to believe you've been infected.

What You Can Do
■ Keep your risk to a minimum. Multiple sexual partners and IV drugs put you at greatest risk.
■ Don't have sex without a condom. Use one every time you have oral, vaginal, or anal sex. Always use a latex condom. Condoms made from animal skin (lambskin) will not protect you from the virus.
■ Use water-based lotions such as K-Y Jelly, Foreplay, and Wet with the condom. NEVER use oils such as Vaseline, Crisco, baby oil, or hand lotion. They could cause the condom to break.
■ Safer forms of sex include massage, hugging, masturbation, dry kissing, or oral sex with a condom.

■ If you and your partner both have HIV, you should still have safe sex. You might have slightly different strains of the virus, and you could infect each other.

■ Drug users should always use clean needles and syringes. They can be cleaned with bleach for 30 seconds and rinsed with clean water.

■ If you're getting a tattoo or having your ears pierced, make sure the operator uses a clean needle.

■ Working or living in the same house with someone who is infected with HIV is safe. Sneezing, talking, touching, handshaking, and sharing dishes or glasses, toilets, and air space does not spread the virus. You cannot get HIV from mosquito bites, from donating blood, or from touching a doorknob, table top, telephone or something else that a person with AIDS may have used.

■ Since April 1985, all donated blood has been tested for HIV. Only blood that has tested negative and has been specially treated to kill the virus is used for transfusions. There is still a small risk of HIV infection from blood, however. If you know in advance that you're going to have surgery, you may want to store a supply of your own blood. This procedure is called autotransfusion.

■ If you even suspect you've had contact with HIV, get tested. Make a special point of having the test if there's any reason to believe that a sexual partner has HIV, if you've had sex with several people, or if you've used a needle that might be infected. If you learn you have HIV, see a doctor right away. Early treatment may help.

■ If you have the virus, tell all of the people you've had sex with so they can get tested. Always tell a new partner BEFORE you have sex, then use a condom to prevent infection. Do not donate blood or organs.

What Your Doctor Can Do

Once you know you're HIV-positive, your doctor can recommend drugs and lifestyle changes to suppress the virus and delay the onset of AIDS. There are still no drugs that are certain to eliminate HIV, but researchers are making progress all the time. Be sure to discuss your medication options with your physician at every visit.

Prescription Drugs

Here are the drugs that slow the progress of HIV. Some are used alone. Others are taken as part of a "cocktail" that works better than any single part of the mix.

Agenerase	Fortovase	Sustiva (efavirenz)
(amprenavir)	(saquinavir)	Videx (didanosine)
Combivir	Hivid (zalcitabine)	Viracept (nelfinavir)
(lamivudine and	Norvir (ritonavir)	Viramune
zidovudine)	Rescriptor	(nevirapine)
Crixivan (indinavir)	(delavirdine)	Zerit (stavudine)
Epivir (lamivudine)	Retrovir (zidovudine)	Ziagen (abacavir)

Over-the-Counter Drugs
There are no nonprescription medicines that affect HIV.

Herbal Remedies
Although a number of natural medicines have been touted for HIV, few have proven effective. Laetrile, originally promoted as a cancer-fighting agent, is not only ineffective but also potentially harmful. BHT, a food preservative that advocates thought could attack HIV, also doesn't work. The soy and egg yolk product AL 721 may help maintain body weight, but won't fight the infection.

Nutritional Support
A variety of vitamins and minerals can give the immune system a boost, but it's best to avoid megadoses. Certain vitamins—especially vitamin A—can be poisonous in large amounts.

A substantial, but not overwhelming, increase in the immune-friendly vitamins is the wisest course. Here is a sample regimen prepared by the University of Miami School of Medicine. (The FDA's Recommended Daily Intake is shown for comparison.)

Vitamin A, 10,000 IU (RDI = 5,000 IU)
Vitamin B_2, (riboflavin), 9 milligrams (RDI = 1.7 milligrams)
Vitamin B_6, 20 milligrams (RDI = 2 milligrams)
Vitamin B_{12}, 50 micrograms (RDI = 6 micrograms)
Vitamin C, 360 milligrams (RDI = 60 milligrams)
Vitamin E, 60 milligrams (RDI = 30 IU)
Zinc, 75 milligrams (RDI = 15 milligrams)

Note, however, that although zinc is promising, the effect of high doses on the immune system is still under debate.

Alternative Therapies

Hyperthermia: This approach, which uses heat to treat infections, is under intensive study for HIV (which may not tolerate high temperatures as well as the body can). For example, some high-tech doctors are experimenting with extracorporeal heating, removing blood from the body, heating it, and returning it to the body at a higher temperature. To get these and other advanced forms of heat treatment, you'll probably need to check into a medical center.

Impotence

The Basics

Rarely mentioned until the advent of the drug Viagra, impotence plagues an estimated 10 million American men. Also known as erectile dysfunction, the condition is defined as the persistent inability to obtain an erection or maintain it long enough to have sex. The problem is more likely to affect older men, but is by no means an inevitable consequence of aging.

Call Your Doctor If . . .

■ You lack interest in sex or are having trouble maintaining an erection.

Seek Care Immediately If . . .

Medical assistance can safely be put off.

What You Can Do

■ Talk with your partner and take advantage of the changes in sexuality that come with age. Older men, for example, often make better lovers because of their ability to prolong the act.

■ Do an emotional housecleaning. Anger that has built up over the years is the biggest cause of diminished sexual desire.

■ Redefine "normal." Remember that no one has the physical strength, stamina, or sexual appetite at 65 that he or she did at 25.

■ Be playful and widen your sexual repertoire. Aside from ill health, sexual boredom may be the biggest threat to any long-standing relationship.

■ Poor lifestyle can affect sexual potency. Eat right and exercise. Avoid excessive alcohol, cigarette smoking, recreational drugs, and high-fat diets.

■ Be prepared; you are never too old for safe sex.

■ If necessary, seek help. In addition to your doctor, consider marriage counselors and sex therapists.

What Your Doctor Can Do

Every drug poses at least minor risks, so before prescribing Viagra (or other remedies) your doctor should rule out easily corrected causes such as medications, habits (smoking or drinking), illness, or injury. Diseases such as diabetes and multiple sclerosis, spinal cord injury, and prostate surgery can weaken the nerve impulses needed to activate the penis. Blood pressure medications, antidepressants, tranquilizers, muscle relaxants, antihistamines, and many other drugs can also have negative effects.

Most cases of impotence have a psychological as well as physical component. Anxiety, depression, or marital problems are common contributors to impotence, and about 80 percent of these cases can be overcome with the help of a professional.

If the problem persists, your doctor can recommend a number of medical treatments. If medicines don't work, two types of vascular surgery are available for impotence, although both are difficult and are offered at only a few centers. The first bypasses obstructions in the arterial blood supply to the penis, and the second reduces the amount of blood leaving the penis through the veins. If all else fails, a permanent penile implant may be the answer.

Prescription Drugs

The favorite remedy is Viagra (sildenafil), a pill that usually promotes an erection within one hour. A leading alternative is the drug alprostadil, which can be taken as an injection in the penis (brands include Caverject and Edex) or as a tiny suppository inserted in the urinary canal (brand name Muse). An older drug named Yocon (yohimbine) may also prove effective, but sometimes produces unpleasant side effects such as headache and a racing heart. Doctors have also found that a specially formulated paste of nitroglycerin, an angina drug, applied directly to the penis, produces an erection rapidly.

Over-the-Counter Drugs

There are no effective remedies available over the counter.

Herbal Remedies

Yohimbe, the original source of the active ingredient in the prescription drug Yocon, works for some men, but is not recommended due to its side effects.

Nutritional Support

Eating right and exercising are essential to a robust sex life. Smoking, excessive drinking, and an artery-clogging, high-fat diet can reduce potency.

Alternative Treatments

Aromatherapy, which uses pleasing scents to enhance relaxation and relieve anxiety, has proved for some to be an effective remedy for impotence.

Indigestion

The Basics

As often as not, indigestion is simply the stomach's way of reminding you that you've eaten too much. Symptoms range from a growling stomach, belching, bloating, and gas to a gnawing pain in or just below the chest. The problem is sometimes accompanied by loss of appetite, nausea, and a disruption in bowel habits. Antacids help diminish the symptoms. Within hours, the condition should disappear.

If you suffer from *frequent* bouts of indigestion, however, the situation may be more complex—you could be one of the six million Americans with nonulcer dyspepsia. Although half the time no underlying cause can be found for this nagging form of indigestion, it sometimes serves as a warning of gallstones, an ulcer, or even heart disease. It occasionally accompanies anxiety or depression, and is sometimes confused with lactose intolerance. Since it's not a serious condition, many of its victims don't seek medical attention. But if you have symptoms for more than 2 weeks, you should see your doctor to rule out a more serious underlying problem.

Call Your Doctor If . . .

■ Your symptoms get worse or fail to improve within a few days.
■ You have indigestion all the time.
■ Any accompanying heartburn is not relieved by antacids.

■ You have extreme discomfort or pain in the digestive tract.
■ You undergo a sudden, persistent change in bowel habits.
■ Your stool is black or streaked with blood.
■ You have abdominal swelling.

Seek Care Immediately If . . .
■ You begin to vomit blood or material that looks like coffee grounds.

What You Can Do
■ An antacid may make you more comfortable. Otherwise, wait for the problem to resolve itself.
■ To prevent indigestion:
  • Eat slowly and avoid large, heavy meals.
  • If you're a smoker, consider giving it up. Smoking increases the chances of indigestion.
  • Try to avoid stressful situations. Stress also makes the problem more likely.
  • If you're overweight, lose the extra pounds. Excess weight is associated with indigestion.

What Your Doctor Can Do
If you have persistent indigestion, the doctor will check to make sure that nothing serious is responsible for the symptoms.

Prescription Drugs
For a bad case of persistent nonulcer dyspepsia, your doctor can prescribe a digestive stimulant such as cisapride (Propulsid) or metoclopramide (Reglan).

Over-the-Counter Drugs
Antacids are the usual remedy for indigestion. You have a choice of the following varieties:

Aluminum hydroxide/magnesium (Maalox, Gaviscon)
Aluminum hydroxide/sodium (ALternaGEL, Amphojel)
Aluminum hydroxide/mineral oil (Nephrox)
Aluminum hydroxide/magnesium hydroxide/simethicone
  (Mylanta Liquid)
Aluminum carbonate (Basaljel)
Bismuth subsalicylate (Pepto-Bismol)
Calcium carbonate (Alka-Mints, Tums, Mylanta Lozenges, Titralac)

Calcium carbonate/magnesium hydroxide (Rolaids)
Calcium carbonate/magnesium hydroxide/simethicone
  (Di-Gel, Mylanta tablets)
Calcium carbonate/simethicone (Titralac Plus, Tums Antigas/Antacid)
Magnesium hydroxide (Phillips' Milk of Magnesia)
Sodium bicarbonate, citric acid, potassium bicarbonate
  (Alka-Seltzer Gold)
Sodium bicarbonate, citric acid, aspirin (Alka-Seltzer,
  Bromo Seltzer)

Antacids interact with a number of prescription drugs, so check with your doctor before taking them and be sure to keep doses of antacids and any other drug 2 or 3 hours apart.

Avoid using antacids over a prolonged period. Depending on their ingredients, they can cause a number of side effects. Avoid sodium-based drugs if you are on a salt-restricted diet. Excessive use of calcium-based drugs can result in kidney stones. Using aluminum-based drugs for a period of years can weaken bones. Very prolonged use of magnesium-based drugs can cause kidney stones and heart, central nervous system, and kidney problems.

As an alternative to antacids, you can use one of the histamine H2 blocking drugs that suppress the production of stomach acid. Over-the-counter options include:

Axid AR	Pepcid AC	Zantac 75
Mylanta AR	Tagamet HB	

Herbal Remedies

A host of herbs help soothe indigestion, including:

Angelica Root	Cinchona	Gentian Root
Barberry	Cinnamon	Green Tea
Barley	Condurango	Haronga
Bitter Orange	Coriander	Horehound
Blessed Thistle	Cumin	Iceland Moss
Bog Bean	Dandelion	Onion
Brewer's Yeast	Devil's Claw	True Unicorn
Calamus	Fenugreek	Wild Cherry
Chicory	Frostwort	Wormwood
China Orange	Galangal	Yarrow
Chinese Cinnamon	Gamboge	Zedoary

Nutritional Support

No particular *type* of food is the villain in this disorder; quantity is more the culprit than quality. However, if certain menu items usually give you trouble, it stands to reason to avoid them.

Alternative Treatments

Although many alternative therapies can calm the stress that sometimes sparks indigestion, only two are specifically recommended for the problem itself:

Biofeedback, a painless training technique that puts you in control of ordinarily involuntary physical responses, can help you relax a nervous stomach.

Yoga, an age-old set of exercises that combine prescribed postures, breathing, and meditation, is known to improve digestion.

Infertility

The Basics

If you're finding it difficult to conceive, you're far from unusual. At any given time, roughly 10 to 15 percent of American couples face problems with fertility. And about 1 in every 5 married women in the U.S. seeks medical help to conceive at some point in her childbearing years.

When should you begin to worry? It's often hard to say, since a couple with no physical problems could try to conceive for years and continually fail due to nothing more than bad timing. Nevertheless, infertility is usually defined as the inability to conceive after one year of unprotected sex.

Infertility is not necessarily an all-or-nothing proposition. For instance, *hypofertile* couples merely have trouble conceiving quickly. Their fertility may be less than ideal or they may be having problems with timing, but they can eventually conceive without special treatment. *Sterile* couples, on the other hand, are unable to conceive without medical or surgical intervention.

Infertility has many causes. A poorly functioning male reproductive system is the problem for 30 to 40 percent of infertile couples. In this group, the trouble may be a low sperm count, sperm that move too slowly through the female reproductive system, semen that is too thick, or a shortage of semen.

Another 30 to 40 percent of fertility problems are caused by a malfunction in the female reproductive system. Major culprits include the inability to release a healthy egg into the fallopian tube (the most common problem), endometriosis, infection, blocked tubes, or simply advancing age. (After about age 35 conception becomes increasingly difficult.)

In about 10 percent of cases, no cause can ever be found. Most of these couples turn out to be hypofertile and do eventually have children.

Call Your Doctor If . . .
■ You feel you need a referral to a fertility specialist.

Seek Care Immediately If . . .
No medical emergency is involved.

What You Can Do
To improve the odds of conception:
■ Remember that the best time to have sexual intercourse is the day or evening before ovulation, so that sperm will already be waiting in the fallopian tubes when the egg arrives. Ovulation occurs in mid- to late morning, usually 12 to 16 days before the next menstrual period begins.
■ Check with your doctor to find out the best position to use. For most women, the missionary position usually puts the uterus in the best position for receiving sperm, but for some women, lying on the stomach is better.
■ Lie still for about 10 minutes after intercourse to give the sperm that have entered the vagina enough time to proceed through the cervix.
■ Have intercourse at least three times during the week you expect ovulation. This raises the odds that sperm will be present in the fallopian tubes when the egg appears. Since sperm can survive in the tubes for 2 or 3 days, it's possible to have sex one day, ovulate the next day, and conceive on the third.
■ Realize that fertility may be slightly impaired for a few months after discontinuing oral contraceptives or injectable or implantable hormones. However, the effect *will* wear off.
■ Remember that alcohol, cigarettes, caffeine, and illicit drugs can decrease the number and quality of sperm.
■ Be patient. Most couples with no identifiable fertility problems do conceive unassisted within 2 years. Consider joining a support group if your patience is wearing thin.

What Your Doctor Can Do

If you consult a fertility specialist, the doctor's first goal will be to find the source of the problem. Women are usually given a complete physical exam. They are then asked to measure their *basal body temperature (BBT)* every day. The BBT is the lowest body temperature during waking hours. A measurable drop in temperature may precede ovulation by 12 to 24 hours. After ovulation, the sex hormone progesterone usually causes the body temperature to rise.

The doctor is also likely to do a semen analysis to check for the number and quality of sperm. And he'll probably order a postcoital test, performed after intercourse to assess the characteristics of the cervical mucus at the time of presumed ovulation, as well as the liveliness of the sperm that have just been deposited. Other procedures include:

Hysterosalpingography: This requires insertion of a small tube into the cervix in order to inject a dye. An x-ray of the uterus and fallopian tubes is then taken and checked for blockages or other abnormalities.

Laparoscopy: Another way of looking at the female reproductive system, this procedure calls for insertion of a tiny lens through a small incision under the navel. Looking through this scope, the doctor can examine all the abdominal organs. The operation usually requires general anesthesia and an overnight stay in the hospital.

Depending on the nature of the problem, the doctor can prescribe drug therapy to trigger ovulation or recommend surgery to correct physical problems such as adhesions (scar tissue), endometriosis, uterine fibroid tumors, or a physically abnormal uterus.

Finally, if fertility problems persist, a number of *assisted reproductive techniques* are available.

Artificial insemination: This technique calls for insertion of a syringe containing either the husband's or donated sperm into the vagina and releases the solution into the opening of the cervix.

Intrauterine insemination: Bypassing the cervix, this procedure deposits the sperm directly into the uterus.

In vitro fertilization (IVF): This technique brings sperm and an egg together outside the human body, then implants the fertilized egg into the mother's uterus.

Gamete intrafallopian transfer: This procedure is identical to IVF except that fertilization occurs in the woman's fallopian tube rather than a test tube.

Intracytoplasmic sperm injection (ICSI): This new high-tech procedure allows physicians to inject a single sperm directly into an egg.

Since a very small number of sperm are needed, ICSI offers hope for men with extremely low sperm count or sperm motility. In addition, the procedure can be used with another technique known as TESA (which draws sperm directly from the testis or the sperm duct) to restore fertility after a vasectomy or failed reversal of vasectomy.

Prescription Drugs

The number of available fertility drugs is growing steadily. Medications currently used to stimulate ovulation include clomiphene (Clomid, Serophene); bromocriptine (Parlodel); human chorionic gonadotropin (HCG) in brands such as Pregnyl and Profasi; follicle-stimulating hormone (FSH) in brands such as Follistim, Gonal-F, and Pergonal; and gonadotropin-releasing hormone (GnRH) in brands such as Supprelin and Synarel.

Over-the-Counter Drugs

There are no nonprescription medications that affect fertility.

Herbal Remedies

Researchers have yet to identify an herb that actually improves fertility.

Nutritional Support

Alcohol and caffeine have a negative effect on the quantity and quality of sperm.

Alternative Treatments

Nothing in the alternative repertoire can cure infertility.

Insect Stings

The Basics

Mosquitoes, fleas, ticks, chiggers, bedbugs, ants, bees, wasps, spiders, and other insects all can leave annoying bites or stings. Typically, you'll find a red lump (perhaps with a tiny hole at the center), often accompanied by pain, swelling, itching, or a rash. You may also develop a fever and suffer a headache, dizziness, or queasy feeling, especially if you have multiple stings.

Unless you are allergic, insect stings rarely cause a serious problem. But if you *are* allergic, the consequences can be very grave indeed. In susceptible individuals, a sting causes the body to overreact, releasing a flood of histamine and other chemicals intended to attack foreign substances. This deluge of defensive chemicals triggers severe swelling, itching, and rash, often followed by wheezing, generalized hives, angioedema (hives in the deeper levels of the skin, especially in the hands, feet, and face), and a sharp drop in blood pressure. In really severe cases, the victim may suffer chest pain, faintness, upset stomach, vomiting, cramping, or diarrhea, and may find it increasingly difficult to breathe. Without immediate treatment, such a reaction can be fatal.

Bees, wasps, hornets, yellow jackets, and fire ants inflict the most dangerous stings. Anyone with a known allergy is likely to be prescribed an emergency kit containing a shot of epinephrine, a drug that quickly reverses the worst allergic effects.

Call Your Doctor If . . .
■ The sting does not improve in a few days.
■ The area beyond the sting becomes red, warm, tender, and swollen. These are signs of infection.
■ You develop a high temperature.
■ You have symptoms of a mild allergic reaction such as swelling, itching, and a rash.
■ You've had to take epinephrine, even if symptoms fail to appear.

Seek Care Immediately If . . .
■ You have trouble breathing or develop chest pain or a tight feeling in your throat or chest. These are signs of a severe allergic reaction. You are in danger of shock and loss of consciousness. **Call 911 or 0 (operator)** to get to the nearest hospital or clinic. **Do not drive yourself!**

What You Can Do
To treat a bug bite or sting:
■ Take the stinger out by scraping it off with your fingernail, the edge of a credit card, or a knife blade. Do not use tweezers or squeeze the sting.
■ Wash the sting with soap and water, then put ice on it.
■ Raise and rest the area of the sting.
■ To help reduce swelling and itching immediately after being stung, soak a clean washcloth or towel in cold water, wring it out, and put it on the sting. Leave it in place for 10 to 20 minutes out of every hour.

- After 24 to 48 hours, a warm compress can be used to soothe the area and reduce swelling.
- To relieve pain, apply a paste made from water and either meat tenderizer or baking soda and leave it on the sting for 5 minutes.
- To further reduce the itching and swelling, use one of the over-the-counter medicines listed below.

If you are allergic to stings:
- Carry a card, or wear a medical necklace or bracelet identifying your allergy. The card or tag should list your name, your doctor's name and phone number, and the type of allergy you have.
- Be sure to carry an emergency treatment kit with you at all times and make certain that both you and your family know how to use it.
- If you're stung or bitten, give yourself the shot of epinephrine immediately. Do not wait for symptoms such as rash, itching, or swelling. Then call your doctor right away to make sure you are out of danger.
- If you're stung but don't have a self-treatment kit, get medical help immediately. **Call 0 (operator) or 911,** or go to the nearest emergency room.

Follow these suggestions to avoid getting stung:
- If you are caught in or near a swarm of bees or wasps, move away slowly. Don't swat at them. Never strike, stir up, or throw anything at a wasp nest or beehive.
- Stay away from places that may attract stinging insects. Yellow jackets nest in the ground and hornets in trees and bushes. Every type of stinging insect is attracted to flowers. Bees are more likely to sting in gloomy weather than on bright sunny days.
- Stay away from woodpiles. Be very careful when gardening or mowing the lawn. Also take precautions in picnic areas, orchards, beaches, and other places where there are exposed foods, fragrances, and bright colors.
- Use insect repellent on your skin and clothing when you go outside.
- Do not wear hair sprays, aftershave lotions, perfumes, suntan lotions, and other scented cosmetics when outdoors. Floral odors are especially attractive to bees and wasps.
- Do not wear floppy, bright-colored, or flower-print clothing outdoors.
- Protect yourself outdoors by wearing long sleeves, slacks, shoes, and socks. Wear gloves when gardening or doing other outdoor chores.

■ Check window screens for openings where insects can get in. Look around outside your home for insect nests. Keep your car windows closed when driving. Keep an insecticide spray that kills stinging insects handy at home, in your car, and whenever you are outdoors.

■ Never drink from a bottle or can that might have a hidden insect inside. Check objects for insects before touching, sitting, or brushing against them.

What Your Doctor Can Do

If necessary, the doctor can recommend medicine for minor pain, swelling, or itching. Symptoms of an allergic reaction demand emergency treatment at a hospital.

Prescription Drugs

To reduce swelling and inflammation, your doctor may prescribe an *antihistamine* like hydroxyzine (Atarax, Vistaril), loratadine (Claritin), or astemizole (Hismanal). Steroid medications also reduce inflammation. Among the options are betamethasone (Celestone), cortisone (Cortone), dexamethasone (Decadron), hydrocortisone (Hydrocortone), and prednisolone (Pediapred, Prelone).

If you have a known allergy to insect stings, your doctor will prescribe an emergency epinephrine injection device such as EpiPen or Ana-Kit.

Over-the-Counter Drugs

Itching, hives, and angioedema can be treated by taking an antihistamine such as diphenhydramine (Benadryl). Creams containing hydrocortisone or an antihistamine also can be applied to the area of the sting to relieve itching and pain. Do not use an antihistamine cream such as Benadryl at the same time that you are taking an antihistamine liquid or tablet.

Herbal Remedies

Although no herbs are recommended specifically for insect stings, a number have been found soothing for irritated skin:

Agrimony	Fenugreek	St. John's Wort
Arnica	Frostwort	Walnut
Chamomile	Heartsease	White Nettle
English Oak	Jambolan	Witch Hazel
English Plantain	Oats	Yellow Dock
Evening Primrose Oil		

Nutritional Support

There are no dietary supplements capable of providing quick relief from an insect sting.

Alternative Treatments

Apitherapy: Exposure to tiny amounts of bee venom in a desensitization program can help allergic individuals build a tolerance to the substance. But avoid all other forms of bee therapy, such as treatments with royal jelly or bee pollen, if you have even the slightest reason to suspect that you're allergic.

Insomnia

The Basics

With consequences ranging from mild frustration to outright exhaustion, sleeplessness is one of the most common disorders in the modern U.S. As many as 40 million Americans currently suffer from chronic insomnia (daily difficulty in sleeping that has lasted for a month or more), and another 25 million have endured occasional bouts of short, interrupted, or unrefreshing sleep. Women and older adults are the most likely victims.

Two types of insomnia predominate: *initial insomnia* and *early morning awakening.* Initial insomnia, or difficulty in falling asleep at bedtime, often accompanies an emotional disturbance such as anxiety or depression. Early morning awakening typically develops with advancing age, but sometimes signals depression. A third type of insomnia, *reversal of the normal sleep rhythm,* usually results from jet lag, working a night shift, sedative abuse, an injury to the brain, or sleep apnea (repeated interruptions in normal breathing while asleep).

Call Your Doctor If . . .

■ Sleepless nights are interfering with your ability to concentrate or function normally during the day.

■ The problem has gone on for several weeks or more.

■ You awake in the night gasping, or if your partner reports loud snoring or irregular breathing during the night. You could have sleep apnea.

■ You are taking a medication nightly to get to sleep.

■ You suspect an underlying medical condition is causing your insomnia.

Seek Care Immediately If . . .

Although it is an annoying problem, insomnia in itself is not life-threatening.

What You Can Do

■ Eliminate caffeine, including coffee, tea, chocolate, and caffeinated soft drinks.

■ If you smoke, try to quit. Nicotine can contribute to sleep problems.

■ Avoid alcohol; it can disrupt your sleep pattern.

■ Do not eat heavy or spicy meals right before bedtime.

■ Check the side effects of any over-the-counter cold remedies and diet pills you may be taking. Many can cause wakefulness.

■ Pursue a regular exercise routine in the morning or early evening. Exercise can improve sleep quality. (Do not, however, exercise right before bed.)

■ Limit napping during the day.

■ Set a regular sleep schedule. Go to bed and get up at the same time every day.

■ Take a warm, relaxing bath an hour or two before bedtime.

■ Experiment with relaxation techniques.

■ Try a glass of warm milk.

■ Deal with upsetting issues during the day. Keep bedtime peaceful.

■ Do not work, read, or watch TV in bed. If you have trouble falling asleep, get up and go to another room until you feel tired.

■ Try not to dwell on, or anticipate insomnia. Worrying about getting to sleep will just make it worse. Practice focusing your awareness on peaceful, pleasant thoughts.

What Your Doctor Can Do

Treatment of this condition depends on its cause. If your doctor suspects an underlying disorder such as sleep apnea, he may ask you to go to a lab for overnight sleep studies. If your insomnia stems from depression, an antidepressant drug is the most likely solution. If pain is keeping you awake, a painkiller such as aspirin, taken just before bedtime, may eliminate the problem.

Only if an emotional upset seems to be the culprit will the doctor prescribe a sleep medication. Prescription sleep aids are potentially addictive and should be used as sparingly as possible. Never take more than the prescribed dose, and don't continue taking the drug for more than 2 weeks at a time. If you do become physically dependent on one of these drugs, you'll have to work with the doctor to gradually reduce your dosage without triggering serious withdrawal symptoms.

Prescription Drugs

The most commonly prescribed sleep medications include:

Ambien (zolpidem)	Placidyl (ethchlorvynol)
Dalmane (flurazepam)	ProSom (estazolam)
Halcion (triazolam)	Restoril (temazepam)
Mebaral (mephobarbital)	Seconal (secobarbital)
Nembutal (pentobarbital)	

Over-the-Counter Drugs

Diphenhydramine is the most widely used nonprescription sleep aid. It's the active ingredient in Nytol, Sleepinal, Sominex, and Unisom Maximum Strength, and it's also found in a variety of "P.M." products such as Bayer PM, Excedrin P.M., and Tylenol PM. The drug is an antihistamine (used in a variety of allergy products, including Benadryl) that also brings on sleepiness. After 3 or 4 days, however, it may begin to lose its sedative effect.

Herbal Remedies

The herbs most commonly recommended for their sedative effects are valerian and passion flower, taken before bedtime. They may be used individually or in combination. Kava can be useful to relieve the anxiety that inhibits sleep. Studies suggest that 1 to 2 milligrams of the hormone melatonin taken shortly before bedtime also serves to promote and maintain sleep. Other natural remedies considered effective for insomnia include bugleweed, hops, lavender, lemon balm, and rauwolfia.

Nutritional Support

To foster sleepiness, eat an early dinner that is low in fat and high in complex carbohydrates. Include in your diet foods that are rich in calcium, magnesium, and the B vitamins to support healthy nerve function. Evening meals that contain foods high in the essential amino acid tryptophan (turkey, milk products, whole grains, bananas) can help make you drowsy.

Alternative Treatments

Aromatherapy: Some people find that fragrant essential oils—in a bath, applied during a massage, or sprayed in the air—provide a respite from insomnia.

Biofeedback: This specialized form of training helps people gain control over their unconscious reactions. It can relieve insomnia by enabling you to reduce involuntary muscle tension caused by stress and anxiety.

Massage Therapy: By helping to reduce anxiety and stress and relax tight muscles, massage can make it easier to sleep.

Meditation: Studies have shown that the calming mental exercises of meditation can bring an end to insomnia.

Qigong: These traditional Chinese exercises promote healthy relaxation and a sense of well-being—both of which promote normal sleep.

Sound Therapy: The soothing sound of specially selected music can reduce anxiety, relieve muscle tension, and induce sleep.

Yoga: The special breathing techniques, postures, and meditation that together form the discipline called Yoga are known to promote relaxation, reduce stress, and quiet the mind—benefits that all tend to yield a better night's sleep.

Irregular Heartbeat

The Basics

Heart rhythm disturbances are far from rare. Known medically as *arrhythmias,* they plague close to 4 million Americans. The problem grows more likely with age, and can affect any of the four chambers of the heart.

The heart's two upper chambers, called *atria*, force incoming blood to the two powerful *ventricles*, which pump it back out. The signal for the atria to contract goes out a split second before the same message reaches the ventricles. Either signal can go haywire, causing an arrhythmia in the corresponding chambers.

The heart normally operates at about 60 to 80 beats per minute. When it beats slower than that, the condition is known as *bradycardia.* If medication fails to speed it up, a temporary or permanent pacemaker may be required. When the heart beats faster than 80 beats per minute, the condition is known as *tachycardia.* Rapid beating of the ventricles, known as *ventricular tachycardia*, can quickly become dangerous, and must be corrected with drugs or a jolt of electricity.

Perhaps the most dangerous abnormal heartbeats are those that are disorganized and irregular. This can happen to either set of chambers. *Atrial fibrillation,* in which the atria twitch uselessly instead of maintaining their normal beat, can usually be stopped by drugs. *Ventricular fibrillation,* in which the ventricles quiver helplessly, can be deadly if not corrected within a few minutes, usually with the use of an electrical charge.

A variety of underlying conditions can be responsible for an irregular heartbeat:

■ Physical abnormalities of the heart itself, such as a structural defect in the valves
■ Clogged arteries (atherosclerosis)
■ Chronic high blood pressure
■ Damage resulting from rheumatic fever
■ Diseases affecting other organs
■ Mineral imbalances in the body, including high or low concentrations of potassium, magnesium, or calcium
■ The toxic effects of some drugs when levels in the bloodstream become too high

Some types of irregular heartbeat produce no symptoms and require no treatment or change in lifestyle. People with occasional *palpitations* (the feeling that your heartbeat changes in rhythm, rate, or strength), for example, usually do not have a serious condition. Palpitations can be caused by anxiety, lack of sleep, certain medicines, caffeine, or too much heavy exercise. Other arrhythmias, however, can be deadly, and may require lifelong treatment to prevent their return.

Call Your Doctor If . . .
■ You suffer repeated episodes of faintness, dizziness, or light-headedness, even if you feel fine immediately afterward.
■ You actually faint or have brief blackouts or fadeouts.
■ You have trouble breathing even at rest, have swelling in your feet or ankles, or feel more tired than usual.
■ You feel like your heart is skipping beats, fluttering in your chest, or racing.
■ You develop chest pain during exercise that continues when you rest.

Seek Care Immediately If . . .

■ You cannot move your arms or legs, feel numbness or weakness in your face or limbs, have a really bad headache, or have trouble seeing or speaking.

■ Your pulse is much higher or lower than usual after counting it for 1 minute.

■ Your heart is skipping beats or you have chest pain, especially the kind that spreads to your arms, jaw, or back and is accompanied by sweating, nausea, and difficulty breathing.

These symptoms may signal a life-threatening emergency. **Call 911 or 0 (operator)** to get to the nearest hospital or clinic. **Do not drive yourself.**

What You Can Do

■ Heart drugs must be used with extra caution. Take them exactly as directed, and never try to make up for a missed dose by doubling the next one. Check with your doctor before taking any other drugs; they could interfere with the heart medications. If your doctor prescribes digitalis or water pills for a heart problem, be sure to get your blood tested regularly.

■ Learn to count your pulse at your wrist or your neck. Teach your relatives or friends how to count your heartbeats too.

■ Make a point of exercising daily. Follow your doctor's instructions for resuming exercise after an emergency or insertion of a pacemaker.

■ Do not have sex if you are tired, have just eaten a big meal, have been drinking, or feel angry with your mate. Also avoid sex if the room temperature is too cold or hot. Stop immediately if you start to get chest pains.

■ Lifestyle issues like smoking and overeating tend to put extra demands on the heart. If you're a smoker, you should quit. If you're overweight, it's time to shed the extra pounds.

■ Seek new ways to control stress, such as biofeedback or meditation.

■ Chronic illnesses like diabetes and high blood pressure increase the risk of a heart attack. Be sure to keep them under control.

■ If you have a heart murmur, you may need to take antibiotics before dental checkups and before some types of surgery to help kill any germs that could get into your blood and cause an infection in the heart. You may also need to avoid heavy exercise or competitive sports.

■ If you have a pacemaker, be sure to inform all healthcare personnel—including dentists—and always carry an identification card.

What Your Doctor Can Do

If your heart rate is around 100 beats per minute, you may be treated in your doctor's office. But if your heart rate is faster or causing other problems, you'll need a stay in the hospital.

Your doctor will work to diagnose the cause of the problem by listening to your heart and obtaining an electrocardiogram (ECG), which monitors the heart's electrical activity. Your doctor may also ask you to wear a *Holter monitor*—a small portable device worn for 24 to 48 hours that records the heart's activity continuously. Alternatively, you may be given a *cardiac event monitor*, which you need to hold over your heart only during the occurrence of symptoms, such as palpitations.

Drug therapy is the first line of defense against arrhythmias. If the drugs prove inadequate, you'll probably be given a pacemaker to artificially stimulate the heartbeat.

Prescription Drugs

Drugs such as quinidine (Quinidex, Quinaglute, Cardioquin), procainamide (Procan SR, Pronestyl, Procanbid), and disopyramide (Norpace) work to reduce heart rate and normalize heart rhythm by slowing electrical conduction in the heart muscle.

Drugs such as lidocaine (Xylocaine), tocainide (Tonocard), and mexiletine (Mexitil) may be used for certain life-threatening ventricular rhythm problems, as may flecainide (Tambocor), propafenone (Rythmol), amiodarone (Cordarone), and sotalol (Betapace).

Digoxin (Lanoxin) and digitoxin (Crystodigin) are used to slow the heart rate and make the heart beat more forcefully.

Some drugs used to treat high blood pressure are also used to control arrhythmias, including certain beta-blockers, such as propranolol (Inderal), and calcium antagonists, including verapamil (Calan, Isoptin).

Over-the-Counter Drugs

All heart-regulating drugs require a prescription.

Herbal Remedies

Because some types of irregular heartbeat are so dangerous, you'd be wise to see a doctor for a diagnosis before attempting any form of self-treatment. Herbs that are said to help with irregular heartbeat include:

Adonis	Lily of the Valley	Shepherd's Purse
Belladonna	Mate	Squill
Camphor	Motherwort	

Nutritional Support

To prevent complications from clogged coronary arteries, you need a diet low in fat and cholesterol and high in fiber. If you are prone to palpitations, drink only decaffeinated coffee, tea, and soda; avoid chocolate, and don't smoke.

If a low potassium level is part of your problem, you may be able to clear it up by eating high-potassium foods such as potatoes with skin, bananas, and spinach. In some cases, you may have to take potassium supplements in pill or powder form.

Alternative Treatments

Biofeedback: This specialized type of training allows people to gain control over physiological reactions that are ordinarily unconscious and automatic, such as heart rate.

Hypnotherapy: With its ability to enhance the power of suggestion, hypnosis has been found effective for a variety of problems that hinge on emotions, habits, and even the body's involuntary responses.

Meditation: The calming mental exercises of meditation are a proven antidote for stress, tension, anxiety, and panic. They can slow a racing heart and relieve palpitations.

Sound Therapy: Of all the sound therapies in use today, music is the most common. It is known to reduce heart rate.

Tai Chi: More of a fitness regimen than a therapy, this slow, graceful Chinese exercise program can reduce blood pressure and heart rate. Check with your doctor, however, before undertaking this or any other exercise program.

Yoga: Practiced regularly, this age-old set of exercises can increase the efficiency of the heart, lower blood pressure, and reduce stress. But remember to check with the doctor before you begin.

Kidney Failure

The Basics

In this potentially life-threatening illness, the kidneys begin to lose their ability to filter waste products from the blood and maintain the body's balance of fluid and minerals. As the condition grows worse, poisons build up in the body, posing the danger of additional disorders including high blood pressure, seizures, and heart failure.

An astonishing variety of conditions can disrupt the kidneys. Burns, bleeding, blood infections, heat stroke, and dehydration can all bring the kidneys to a halt. So can kidney injury or disease, kidney stones, heart or liver disease, other diseases that affect the kidneys such as diabetes and lupus, infection or blockage of the urinary system, and a blockage in the arteries or veins that serve the kidneys. Long-standing high blood pressure is also a culprit, as are certain medicines.

The clearest warning of kidney failure is reduced urination. You're also likely to develop nausea, vomiting, and fatigue. Other possible symptoms include irritability, shortness of breath, a bad taste in your mouth, headache, muscle aches, numbness in the legs and feet, loss of appetite, and diarrhea. In addition, your skin may become dry, itchy and easily bruised.

Many years ago, kidney failure was inevitably fatal, but modern medicine now offers three lifesaving treatments:

Hemodialysis: In this form of treatment, an artificial kidney machine carries out the vital functions the kidneys can no longer perform. The patient is connected to the machine by plastic tubing that attaches to a specially prepared blood vessel under the skin of an arm or leg. The treatment can be done at home or at a dialysis unit.

Peritoneal Dialysis: Here, waste products from the blood are absorbed by fluid flushed through the interior of the abdomen from a tube that has been surgically placed in the abdominal wall. Once the catheter is in place, this procedure is usually done at home.

Kidney Transplantation: The major danger in a transplant is rejection of the donated organ. However, chances are good—between 80 and 90 percent—that a transplanted kidney will still be functioning one year after the operation. The exact odds depend on the quality of the match between donor and recipient.

Call Your Doctor If . . .
■ You can't eat or drink and find that you are losing weight.
■ You feel confused and irritated.
■ Your urine output for the day is considerably less than usual.
■ You are having breathing problems or muscle aches.

Seek Care Immediately If . . .

■ You have chills, nausea, or vomiting.

■ You have an extremely high temperature.

■ You are sleeping more than usual, and find it hard to wake up.

■ You notice specks of blood in your urine or stool.

■ Blood starts coming from your nose, mouth, or ears for no reason.

■ You have a seizure.

What You Can Do

■ Fluid buildup is an ever-present danger, so you may be asked to keep a record of how much liquid you drink and how much you urinate. You should also record your weight on a daily basis.

■ Be sure to take any medicines and nutritional supplements prescribed by your doctor exactly as directed. With kidney function declining, they are needed to keep your system in balance.

■ Careful attention to your diet can significantly slow the progress of this disease. Faithfully follow your doctor's advice about resting, eating, and drinking liquids.

What Your Doctor Can Do

Guided by what he finds in tests on your blood and urine, the doctor is likely to limit your fluid intake, put you on a special low-protein diet, and prescribe various medications to keep your body chemistry in balance. Depending on the severity of your condition, you may need a stay in the hospital for tests and treatment. While there, you'll probably be hooked up to a dialysis machine.

Prescription Drugs

A decline in red blood cells (anemia) is one of the most common consequences of kidney failure. To correct the problem, you'll need to take Epoetin alfa, a bioengineered form of a hormone (erythropoietin) that fosters growth of red blood cells. Anabolic steroids such as Deca-Durabolin (nandrolone) and Delatestryl (testosterone enanthate) will also help to correct anemia. If you're receiving regular dialysis, you also need to take multivitamins and iron to replace nutrients lost during the treatments.

If you receive a kidney transplant, you'll need regular doses of medications that prevent rejection. The possibilities include:

CellCept (mycophenolate)   Neoral or Sandimmune
Imuran (azathioprine)   (cyclosporine)

Orthoclone OKT3   Prograf (tacrolimus)
(muromonab-CD3)   Simulect (basiliximab)

Many transplant patients also need blood pressure medication, as well as drugs to prevent ulcers and infections.

Over-the-Counter Drugs
Nonprescription painkillers can relieve aches and pains, but there are no over-the-counter drugs that address the underlying problem.

Herbal Remedies
There are no herbal treatments for this condition.

Nutritional Support
A high-protein diet can overtax the kidneys, aggravate your symptoms, and hasten total failure. Be sure to follow your doctor's dietary instructions to the letter. Also be sure to take any vitamin/mineral supplements that he recommends. The loss of appetite that often accompanies this condition can lead to deficiencies.

The doctor may limit your water intake to an amount the failing kidneys can handle. An excessive buildup of water can lead to swelling, high blood pressure, and congestive heart failure. Because excess sodium tends to hold fluid in the body, you may need to lower your intake of salt if you're faced with water retention.

Alternative Treatments
There's nothing in the world of alternative medicine that can take the place of conventional treatment.

Kidney Stones

The Basics
Kidney stones send approximately 1 in 1,000 U.S. adults to the hospital each year. The problem strikes men more often than women. Consisting mostly of calcium, and therefore hard as a rock, the stones range is size from tiny grains to chunks large enough to fill an entire kidney.

Kidney stones travel with urine and can be found anywhere in the urinary system. They can be totally painless or thoroughly excruciating, depending on their size, their location, and whether they are blocking the passage of urine. If a stone becomes lodged in the thin, sensitive tube from the kidney to the bladder (the ureter), the pain is notoriously great.

An illness called gout can cause kidney stones, as can a blockage in normal urinary flow or the presence of a large amount of calcium in the urine. Excessive intake of calcium from food or vitamin/mineral supplements contributes to the problem.

Typical symptoms include sharp mid-back pain, blood in the urine, painful urination, nausea, and vomiting. The stones can cause long-term kidney problems that in rare cases prove fatal, but with proper treatment, they usually go away without any damage.

Call Your Doctor If . . .

■ You develop any of the symptoms summarized immediately above.

Seek Care Immediately If . . .

■ You have severe pain.
■ You are nauseous or start to vomit.
■ You have a high temperature.
■ You have stinging or burning when you pass urine, or feel a frequent urge to urinate. These are signs of infection.

What You Can Do

■ To help a stone pass and prevent others from forming, drink 3 quarts of water each day.
■ A heating pad set on low may help ease the pain.
■ Your doctor will want to analyze the stone once it passes. He may ask you to strain your urine through a special sieve or a piece of thin cloth every time you go to the bathroom. Some people find it easier to urinate into a glass jar; when the stone passes, it will be visible at the bottom of the jar.
■ Keeping active may help the stone pass. Do not stay in bed; walk as much as possible.
■ If you have a job in which sudden pain might be dangerous (such as construction), stay home from work until the stone passes.

What Your Doctor Can Do

Your doctor can diagnose the problem and locate the stone with an x-ray or ultrasound. If you are unable to pass the stone, you will probably need to be hospitalized. There, in addition to standard blood and urine tests, you may receive an *intravenous pyelogram.* This test requires injection of a dye through a vein in order to make the kidneys show up better in an x-ray.

To get rid of the stone, the doctor will probably start by trying *shock-wave lithotripsy*, a painless procedure that sends shock waves inside your body to break up the stone. If that doesn't work, you may need an operation to remove the stone.

Prescription Drugs

A number of prescription pills are available to blunt the pain, including:

DHCplus (acetaminophen with dihydrocodone)
Dilaudid (hydromorphone)
Hydrocet, Lorcet, Lortab, Vicodin, or Zydone
  (acetaminophen with hydrocodone)
Kadian, MS Contin, or MSIR (morphine)
Levo-Dromoran (levorphanol)
OxyContin, OxyIR, or Roxicodone (oxycodone)
Percocet or Tylox (acetaminophen with oxycodone)
Percodan (aspirin with oxycodone)
Talwin Nx (naloxone)
Toradol (ketorolac)
Tylenol with Codeine (acetaminophen with codeine)
Ultram (tramadol)
Vicoprofen (hydrocodone)

For repeated episodes, the drug Zyloprim (allopurinol) proves helpful in certain cases.

Over-the-Counter Drugs

Standard over-the-counter painkillers such as aspirin, acetaminophen, and ibuprofen can also ease the pain.

Herbal Remedies

A multitude of herbs have been said to help treat or prevent kidney and bladder stones, including:

Asparagus Root	Horsetail	Mate
Beans	Java Tea	Parsley
Birch	Juniper Berry	Petasite
Dandelion	Lily of the Valley	Restharrow
Goldenrod	Lovage	Stinging Nettle

Nutritional Support

You may need to change your diet depending on the chemicals in your stone. Your doctor will prescribe the right diet after tests on the stone are completed. Excess calcium often proves to be a leading culprit, for example, and you may need to limit your calcium intake. A calcium-rich diet is the preferred source of this important mineral, but if you take a calcium supplement, consider calcium citrate, which seems to make a bit more calcium available for use by the body and seems less likely to cause kidney stones than other types of calcium products.

Alternative Treatments

While none of these treatments will prevent or cure the actual stones, they may help ease the pain:

Acupuncture: This age-old Chinese treatment calls for insertion of tiny needles at specific points on the skin in order to remedy disorders elsewhere in the body. Unlikely as it seems, the technique is often quite effective at relieving pain.

Biofeedback: Through devices that measure and report certain physiological functions, biofeedback helps people control otherwise involuntary reactions. It has proven helpful for many types of pain.

Energy Medicine: Of all the electrical therapies currently available, *transcutaneous electrical nerve stimulation (TENS)* is the closest to adoption in the mainstream and can be used for any type of localized physical pain.

Hypnotherapy: With its ability to enhance the power of suggestion, hypnosis has been found effective for a variety of problems that hinge on the emotions, habits, and the body's involuntary responses. While it won't eliminate the underlying cause, it has been found effective for relieving virtually all types of pain.

Sound Therapy: While listening to music or other relaxing sounds will not cure anything, it can noticeably ease pain and anxiety.

Lupus

The Basics

This nagging, elusive, painful disease, known medically as *systemic lupus erythematosus, or SLE,* is an inflammation of the body's connective tissues. It proclaims itself through a broad range of problems. Arthritis-like symptoms are especially common, along with fever, fatigue, and rash. Mouth sores, hair loss, and chest pain are also likely, and some people develop blood abnormalities, kidney disease, headaches, seizures, and mental illness. Fatigue and pain from the disease can be overwhelming.

Severity varies: some people experience occasional mild flare-ups; others suffer frequent severe symptoms that can be life-threatening. The goals of therapy are to control symptoms and prevent progression to severe disease.

Ninety percent of patients who have lupus are women, most of childbearing age. We know that the disease develops when the immune system turns on itself, but the underlying reason for this remains unknown. Some scientists believe a genetic flaw is the culprit.

The symptoms of lupus come and go, often disappearing for years at a time. The disease *can* eventually prove fatal, but early diagnosis has increased the 10-year survival rate to better than 95 percent in most developed countries.

Call Your Doctor If . . .
■ You experience chest pain.
■ You develop a fever and sore throat.
■ You experience swelling in your legs.

Seek Care Immediately If . . .
Fortunately, even a major flare-up rarely requires emergency attention.

What You Can Do
■ Be sure to tell your doctor about every drug you are taking, since some drugs can cause a reversible lupus-like reaction.
■ Some of the medications used to treat lupus have potentially serious side effects that you must be monitored for. Be sure to have blood tests and eye exams done whenever they are recommended.
■ Limit your exposure to direct sunlight and wear a sunscreen when you go outside.

What Your Doctor Can Do
Your doctor can prescribe medications to ease your symptoms and slow the progression of the disease. The choice of drugs depends on the severity of your condition.

Prescription Drugs

For a mild case of lupus, the usual prescription is nothing more than a nonsteroidal anti-inflammatory drug to relieve joint pain. The leading options include:

Actron, Orudis, or Oruvail (ketoprofen)
Anaprox, Naprelan or Naprosyn (naproxen)
Cataflam or Voltaren (diclofenac)
Motrin (ibuprofen)
Ponstel (mefenamic acid)

Drugs originally used to fight malaria have also proven very helpful. Leading choices include:

Aralen (chloroquine)
Plaquenil (hydroxychloroquine)

Severe flare-ups are usually treated with steroid medications to fight inflammation. Since long-term use of these drugs can cause serious side effects, the doctor will probably use the lowest effective dose and periodically discontinue the drug. Dosage must be slowly tapered off, so don't attempt to quit taking the drug on your own. Typical choices include:

Cortone (cortisone)
Decadron (dexamethasone)
Deltasone or Orasone (prednisone)
Hydrocortone (hydrocortisone)
Pediapred or Prelone (prednisolone)

Drugs that suppress the immune system are often added to steroid therapy. The two you are most likely to encounter are:

Cytoxan or Neosar (cyclophosphamide)
Imuran (azathioprine)

Over-the-Counter Drugs

For mild cases of lupus, nonprescription anti-inflammatory drugs are often all that's needed. Your options include aspirin, ibuprofen, ketoprofen, and naproxen—but not acetaminophen. Leading brands include:

Actron	Backache Caplets	Goody's
Advil	Bayer	Motrin IB
Aleve	BC Powder	Nuprin
Alka-Seltzer	Bufferin	Orudis KT
Ascriptin	Excedrin	St. Joseph

Herbal Remedies

There are no herbs specifically recommended for lupus. However, you might want to experiment with some of the remedies for joint pain listed in the entry on arthritis.

Nutritional Support

Although concrete scientific evidence is lacking, some medical experts believe that inflammatory reactions such as lupus are sometimes caused by food allergies. Grains, dairy products, and red meat are leading suspects.

If you think that a certain food is aggravating your symptoms, try eliminating it from your diet for 6 weeks at a time. If this seems to make a difference, discuss the situation with your doctor. A radical change in your diet could lead to deficiencies, particularly when you are dealing with a chronic disease.

Alternative Treatments

Alexander Technique: This movement-training program is designed to bring the body's muscles into natural harmony. People with lupus use it for pain management.

Lyme Disease

The Basics

Named for the town in Connecticut where it first surfaced, Lyme disease is a vague, elusive ailment that's sometimes confused with flu or arthritis. A recently discovered germ named *Borrelia burgdorferi* is the cause. It is spread only by tick bites, and cannot be passed from one person to another. A vaccine to prevent the infection is now available.

The ticks that carry this bug usually live on deer, rabbits, and mice, but also can be found on dogs. Infections are most frequent in the late spring and summer. You can get sick anywhere from 3 days to a month after being bitten. Some people never realize they've been exposed.

Soon after an infected bite, a small red bump may appear and then grow bigger, usually with a clear area in the middle that looks like a bull's-eye. The bump may (or may not) turn into a rash after a few days or weeks. The rash is typically accompanied by flu-like symptoms, including muscle pain, headache, stiff neck, fever, chills, and tiredness. If not treated early, the infection may spread to other parts of the body. Weeks, months, or even years later, roughly half of those who fail to get treatment develop repeated bouts of joint pain. A smaller number of victims suffer neurological problems within a few weeks or months after the bite. A few even develop heart problems.

Call Your Doctor If . . .

■ You get any new symptoms.

■ You develop a rash, itching, or swelling after taking prescribed antibiotics.

Seek Care Immediately If . . .

■ You get a stiff neck, a really bad headache, shortness of breath, or a fast heartbeat.

What You Can Do

■ Take antibiotics exactly as directed until they are all gone. Don't stop taking them as soon as you begin to feel better. Some of the germs may survive and cause a relapse.

■ To avoid infection:

• During tick season, stay out of woods and fields likely to have ticks, if possible. If you know you'll be exposed to ticks, see your doctor for immunization with the Lyme disease vaccine.

• In the woods, wear long pants, socks pulled up over the bottom of your pants legs, and shirts with long sleeves. Keep your shirt tucked in. Use a lotion or spray to keep bugs and ticks away.

• Check for ticks every 2 to 3 hours while you are out and again after you go inside. Be sure to check your head, neck, armpits, and crotch. Also check your pets for ticks and have them wear tick collars.

• If you find a tick, take it off with a pair of tweezers. Don't use your fingers. Hold the tick behind the head and slowly pull it out. Ticks that are taken off within 18 hours are not likely to cause Lyme disease.

What Your Doctor Can Do

Lyme disease is a difficult illness to diagnose, since not all infected patients notice a tick bite or develop the telltale bull's-eye rash. Blood tests can aid in the diagnosis, but are not exact and cannot confirm or rule out Lyme disease. Doctors are often forced to make a judgment call, deciding on the basis of clues from your symptoms whether they are caused by Lyme disease or some other ailment.

If the verdict is Lyme disease, you'll need to take antibiotics for up to 3 weeks to stamp out the infections. The medicine is usually taken by mouth, but in severe cases may need to be taken intravenously. Any complications, such as arthritis, will be treated separately.

Prescription Drugs

Amoxicillin, doxycycline, and tetracycline are the antibiotics most frequently prescribed for this ailment. Specific options include:

Achromycin V (tetracycline)
Amoxil (amoxicillin)
Ceftin (cefuroxime)
Declomycin
 (demeclocycline)
Doryx, Monodox, or
 Vibramcyin (doxycycline)
Dynacin, Minocin, or Vectrin
 (minocycline)
Terramycin (oxytetracycline)

Over-the-Counter Drugs

For the aches and joint pains that often accompany Lyme disease, aspirin and other nonprescription anti-inflammatory drugs are the usual recommendation. Your options include:

Actron
Advil
Aleve
Alka-Seltzer
Ascriptin
Backache Caplets
Bayer
BC Powder
Bufferin
Excedrin
Goody's
Motrin IB
Nuprin
Orudis KT
St. Joseph
Vanquish

Nutritional Support

No nutritional measures are known to relieve this disease.

Herbal Remedies

The following remedies are used for pain:

Japanese Mint
White Willow

Alternative Treatments

Alexander Technique: This form of movement training brings the body's muscles into natural harmony. People with Lyme disease use it for pain management.

Manic Depression

The Basics

Manic depression is typified by moods that seesaw between mania (overexcitement, overactivity, and unreasonably good feelings) and depression (extreme sadness). These repeated swings between two emotional poles have earned the illness the name bipolar disorder.

Believed to result from chemical changes in the body and brain, bipolar disorder is sometimes triggered by a stressful event. It currently affects 3 million people in the United States. Your odds of developing the problem are higher if:

■ Someone else in your family has had a mood disorder, especially a bipolar disorder.
■ You are in your late teens or early twenties.
■ You are under a lot of stress.

Symptoms usually begin suddenly, but occasionally develop gradually. The mood swings may be obvious to other people before you become aware of them. During both the manic and depressive phases, there may be changes in your:

■ Eating or sleeping habits
■ Weight
■ Energy level
■ Feelings about sex
■ Desire to be with other people
■ Feelings about the future

Some people with this disorder develop impulses to hurt themselves or others.

During periods of mania, you may find yourself:

- Abusing drugs or alcohol
- Becoming preoccupied with sex
- Having hallucinations
- Saying things that don't make sense
- Showing bad temper
- Spending too much money
- Talking too fast
- Thinking very highly of yourself

During periods of depression, you may:

- Cry a lot
- Eat too much or too little
- Have difficulty making decisions
- Have thoughts of suicide
- Have trouble concentrating
- Prefer solitude
- Sleep a lot or not at all
- Suffer low self-esteem

The standard treatment for this disorder is the drug lithium, with an antidepressant sometimes added during low periods. A potent tranquilizer may be necessary to control manic episodes. In severe cases, hospitalization may be necessary.

Call Your Doctor If . . .
- You feel an intense mood swing coming on.
- You're unable to sleep well or find that you are sleeping more than usual.
- You undergo a change in appetite.
- Your medicine makes you drowsy, dizzy, or sick to your stomach.

Seek Care Immediately If . . .
- You begin to have thoughts of suicide or homicide.
- Your medicine causes an allergic reaction (swelling or trouble breathing).

What You Can Do
- Be sure to take the prescribed medication regularly, even if it seems to have no effect at the start. Take no more lithium than prescribed;

extra doses can cause lithium poisoning. Since lithium can affect judgment and coordination and some antidepressants can make you drowsy, be cautious when using machinery or driving until you know how the drugs affect you. Check with your doctor before taking any other drugs, either prescription or over-the-counter.

■ Avoid alcohol and recreational drugs while taking antidepressants. They may interact badly.

■ Since it's hard to avoid stress, learn to control it with such techniques as deep breathing, muscle relaxation, meditation, or biofeedback. (See "Alternative Treatments" below.) Try not to bottle up your feelings; talk to your doctors, family, or friends and let them help you. You may also want to join a support group.

■ Encourage those close to you to talk to your doctor. He can give them tips on how to deal with your illness.

What Your Doctor Can Do

Before treatment begins, the doctor may order blood tests, an x-ray, EKG, or a CT scan to rule out other illnesses.

At first, you will probably need to visit a clinic or doctor's office 1 to 4 times a month. If you suffer from extreme mood swings, you may require hospitalization, so it's important to seek drug therapy—and stick with it. Patients who present a danger outside the hospital can be involuntarily hospitalized for up to 3 days by the police or a doctor.

If medication doesn't work for you—or isn't fast enough—the doctor may recommend electroconvulsive therapy. This form of treatment can be very helpful. Also known as ECT or shock therapy, it applies a mild electric current to the brain. Although the treatment temporarily disrupts the memory, full recall typically returns within two weeks.

Prescription Drugs

The drugs typically prescribed for bipolar disorder include the following:

Depakote (valproic acid)
Eskalith, Lithobid, and
  Lithonate (lithium)

Sinequan (doxepin)
Thorazine (chlorpromazine)

To relieve severe depression, the doctor may also prescribe a standard antidepressant. See the entry on depression for details.

Over-the-Counter Drugs

Nothing available without a prescription is effective for this problem.

Herbal Remedies

No herbs are known to remedy bipolar disorder.

Nutritional Support

There are no nutritional strategies known to help.

Alternative Treatments

None of the many alternative treatments currently available will cure bipolar disorder. However, to the extent that stress aggravates the problem, stress-reducing therapies may prove helpful. Consider the following:

Alexander Technique: A system of movement and posture training
Aromatherapy: Treatments with concentrated herbal oils
Aston-Patterning: A specialized form of physical training and massage
Guided Imagery: A mind/body therapy involving focused visualization
Hellerwork: A combination of deep massage and movement training
Massage Therapy: Relaxing bodywork to relieve tension
Qigong: Chinese exercises that improve fitness and reduce tension
Reflexology: A specialized foot massage said to relieve stress
Rolfing: A forceful deep-massage technique
Sound Therapy: Use of specially selected music to relieve stress
Yoga: A program of breathing exercises, body postures, and meditation with a proven calming effect

Measles

The Basics

Highly contagious, measles can take hold in anyone who hasn't already had the disease or has failed to get a shot. Although it favors preschool children, it can also attack teenagers and young adults.

Measles is caused by the rubeola virus. It infects the throat, airways, and lungs, as well as the skin. It takes 1 to 2 weeks for the illness to develop once you've been exposed.

The first symptoms are a high fever (up to 105 degrees), a loud cough, a runny nose, and red eyes. These are followed in 2 to 4 days by the appearance of tiny, white spots in the mouth and throat. A day or two after that, a rash breaks out on the forehead, then spreads around the ears and down onto the body. The rash lasts 4 to 7 days. Complications include ear infections, croup, bronchitis, and pneumonia.

By the time symptoms appear, nothing can be done to cure the disease. Antibiotics have no effect. However, if you know you've been exposed, a shot within the next two days can prevent the illness. (If you can't take the vaccine due to pregnancy or a weak immune system, a dose of gamma globulin may help.)

Call Your Doctor If . . .

■ Your child's temperature goes up after a day or two in the normal range.

■ The child coughs up thick, brown, green, or gray sputum, or the cough lasts for more than 4 or 5 days.

■ The child has a really bad headache.

■ An earache develops.

Seek Care Immediately If . . .

■ The child has trouble breathing or starts breathing very fast.

■ The child develops a headache, drowsiness, stiff neck, and vomiting all at once.

■ The child has a seizure.

■ The child develops a very high temperature.

What You Can Do

■ Keep a sick child away from people who have never had measles or the measles vaccine. Notify your child's school or day-care facility so that other children can be monitored for the development of the disease. The child should stay out of school or daycare until the fever and rash are gone. This usually takes about 7 days.

■ You may give acetaminophen for fever. Do NOT give aspirin to a child with measles. This could lead to an illness (Reye's syndrome) that causes brain and liver damage. Be sure to check for aspirin on the label of any over-the-counter medicines you buy.

■ To relieve coughing, use a cool-mist humidifier to increase air moisture. Do not use hot steam. You also may give your child honey, corn syrup, cough drops, or a cough medicine.

■ Make sure the child gets as much rest as possible and has plenty of sleep.

■ The child's eyes may be sensitive to light for a few days. Wipe them often with a clean, wet cotton ball. It will also help for the child to wear sunglasses or stay in a darkened room.

What Your Doctor Can Do

The doctor can vaccinate your children against measles with an MMR shot. (MMR stands for measles-mumps-rubella.) Children usually receive their first shot at about 15 months of age and a booster shot either before entering kindergarten or at age 11 or 12.

Once the disease takes hold, there's little the doctor can do other than watch for complications such as bronchitis or pneumonia. The illness usually runs its course in 7 to 10 days.

Prescription Drugs

None available.

Over-the-Counter Drugs

For fever, use only NON-ASPIRIN products such as Advil, Motrin IB, Panadol, and Tylenol. For cough, consider one of the following children's cough products:

Benylin Pediatric Cough
  Suppressant
Halls Juniors
Pertussin CS

Robitussin Pediatric Cough
  Suppressant
Vicks 44 E, Pediatric

Herbal Remedies

No herbal medications are known to speed recovery from measles. However, there's a wide variety of natural remedies that can ease some of the symptoms:

COUGH

Anise	Dill	Hemp Nettle
Balsam	Echinacea	Horehound
Balsam of Peru	Elder	Horseradish
Blue Mallow	English Ivy	Iceland Moss
Brewer's Yeast	English Oak	Japanese Mint
Camphor	English Plantain	Khella
Caraway	Ephedra	Knotweed
Cardamom	(Ma Huang)	Larch
Chamomile	Eucalyptus	Licorice
Chinese Cinnamon	Fennel	Linden
Cinnamon	Galangal	Lungwort
Cloves	Garlic	Marshmallow
Couch Grass	Gumweed	Meadowsweet

Mullein	Primrose	Star Anise
Mustard	Radish	Sundew
Nasturtium	Red Clover	Thyme
Niauli	Sandalwood	Watercress
Onion	Sanicle	White Nettle
Peppermint	Seneca Snakeroot	Wild Cherry
Pimpinella	Soapwort	Wild Thyme
Pine Oil		

FEVER

Anise	Cloves	Japanese Mint
Ash	Couch Grass	Larch
Balsam	Dill	Mustard
Balsam of Peru	Echinacea	Onion
Caraway	English Oak	Peppermint
Cardamom	English Plantain	Pine Oil
Chamomile	Galangal	Radish
Chinese Cinnamon	Garlic	Sandalwood
Cinnamon	Iceland Moss	

Nutritional Support

Give your child plenty of fluids, including water, juice, and clear soups.

Alternative Therapies

There are no alternative therapies that have any significant effect on this—or any other—viral infection.

Menopause

The Basics

Menopause—the time in a woman's life when menstrual periods stop—is typically accompanied by a variety of troublesome symptoms. Often called the "change of life" or the "change," it typically begins around age 50, but can happen from age 35 to 59. It usually lasts 1 to 2 years.

During menopause your ovaries slowly stop making the hormones that trigger ovulation, in particular estrogen and progesterone. Declining levels of these hormones are responsible for many of the symptoms that arise in the course of the change. Once menopause is over, lack of the hormones increases your risk of heart disease and fosters development of the brittle-bone disease, osteoporosis.

As menopause begins, your periods will become irregular, then eventually stop completely. You're likely to suffer hot flashes, night sweats, and vaginal dryness. Your skin will tend to become drier, your hair may become thinner, your breasts may lose some of their fullness, and you'll begin to lose muscle tone. Many women develop a mildly overactive bladder.

Other symptoms reported around this time include anxiety, cold hands and feet, constipation, depression, diarrhea, dizziness, fast heartbeat, fatigue, headaches, inability to concentrate, insomnia, irritability, memory loss, muscle and joint aches, nausea, nervousness, palpitations, and weight gain. These problems are thought to stem largely from emotional reactions to the change, rather than the actual loss of hormones.

Call Your Doctor If . . .

- You have heavy vaginal bleeding.
- Your period lasts longer than usual.
- You notice spotting (blood) between periods.
- You have a period after 6 months or more without one.
- You feel a burning sensation when urinating.
- You have trouble urinating.

Seek Care Immediately If . . .

- You have severe abdominal pain.

What You Can Do

The changes of menopause can be substantial and disconcerting, but they need not disrupt your life. Unpleasant symptoms can usually be controlled with medications, and your emotional response depends on your outlook. Try to view menopause as the beginning of a new and promising period of your life, free from former obligations, instead of regarding it as an ending. To minimize your problems, keep the following points in mind.

- If you are having hot flashes and sweating, wear your clothing in layers. Choose cotton if sweating at night is a problem.
- Vaginal dryness may make sex uncomfortable. Your doctor can prescribe an estrogen cream to use in and around the vagina. You can also use a water-based lubricating jelly.

- You CAN get pregnant while going through menopause. You are not free from the possibility of pregnancy until you have gone a year without a menstrual period. To avoid pregnancy, keep using birth control during this time.
- Exercise regularly. This will slow down bone loss due to lack of estrogen, strengthen your heart, and keep your weight and appetite under control. It will also make you feel better.
- You may go through menopause with no mood changes. But if you're one of the many women who become nervous, irritable, tired, or mildly depressed, let your doctor know about it. Talking to your partner or a close friend can also help.
- The danger of heart disease rises after menopause. Get a head start against it by adopting a low-fat, high-fiber diet, exercising regularly, and watching your weight. If you're a smoker, menopause makes quitting more important than ever.
- Be sure to visit your doctor each year for a routine checkup. If you are taking estrogen, you should have a Pap smear every 12 months.

What Your Doctor Can Do

During and after menopause, estrogen replacement therapy is often prescribed to prevent heart disease and osteoporosis and to relieve symptoms such as hot flashes and vaginal dryness. The estrogen is usually supplied in a pill or a patch. To reduce the risk of uterine cancer, the doctor can prescribe combined therapy with estrogen and progestin.

If you have a family history of cancer and can't take hormones at all, you can still fend off osteoporosis with other types of medication. See the entry on osteoporosis for more information.

Prescription Drugs

Products used in estrogen replacement therapy include the following:

Alora, Climara, Estrace, Estraderm, Estring, FemPatch, and Vivelle (estradiol)
Cycrin and Provera (medroxyprogesterone)
Estratab and Menest (esterified estrogens)

Ogen and Ortho-Est (estropipate)
Premarin (conjugated estrogens)
Premphase and Prempro (conjugated estrogens and progesterone)

Some doctors prescribe the osteoporosis drug Evista (raloxifene) as an alternative to estrogen replacement therapy. Evista is said to offer the benefits of estrogen on bones and the heart without the slightly increased risk of cancer that long-term use of estrogen may pose.

Nonhormonal medications that can help reduce hot flashes include Catapres-TTS (clonidine) and Narcan or Talwin Nx (naloxone).

Over-the-Counter Drugs

There are no nonprescription remedies for hot flashes. However, for vaginal dryness you have a choice of KY Lubricating Jelly or Replens.

Herbal Remedies

There are two herbs that experts have judged helpful to relieve hot flashes: black cohosh and greater burnet.

Nutritional Support

Modern nutritional science offers a variety of strategies for easing the symptoms of menopause and preventing its long-term effects.

- Incorporating foods abundant in plant estrogens may help moderate your body's hormonal fluctuations during menopause. These foods include: alfalfa, apples, barley, carrots, cherries, chickpeas, garlic, green beans, oats, peas, sweet potatoes, rye, tofu (soybean curd), and yams.
- To stem the loss of calcium that inevitably results from lower estrogen levels, doctors now recommend a calcium intake of between 1,000 and 1,500 milligrams per day for women over 50. Calcium is found in milk and dairy foods, nuts, seafood, and green leafy vegetables. Your doctor may also recommend calcium pills.
- Caffeine-containing beverages such as coffee, tea, and cola can increase the number and intensity of hot flashes. Simply omitting these items from your diet can be a remedy in itself.
- Alcohol is suspected of aggravating hot flashes, and excessive alcohol intake definitely increases the risk of osteoporosis. Your best course is to use alcohol only in moderation.
- Vitamin D enhances calcium absorption. To be sure you're getting enough vitamin D, get regular exposure to the sun or take a vitamin D supplement.
- Vitamin E may help hot flashes and vaginal dryness. Take a supplement or boost your intake of whole grains, green vegetables, beans, and nuts.
- Weight gain is common during menopause, and excess weight increases your risk of heart disease, high blood pressure, and diabetes. To

maintain your former body weight, you may need to cut your calorie intake by 10 to 15 percent, while increasing your activity level.

■ Because menopause prompts an increase in your risk of heart disease, it's the ideal moment to adopt a heart-healthy diet. That means cutting back on artery-clogging cholesterol and fat, and increasing your intake of cholesterol-fighting fiber. Cutting down on salt is also warranted. Excessive sodium encourages high blood pressure in some women, and can increase your calcium loss as well.

Alternative Treatments

The world of alternative medicine offers no relief for symptoms such as hot flashes and vaginal dryness. However, you may find comfort in one of the many treatments that relieve tension and stress. They include various forms of bodywork and massage, aromatherapy, guided imagery, qigong exercises, sound therapy, and yoga.

Menstrual Cramps

The Basics

Known medically as *dysmenorrhea* (dis-men-oh-REE-uh), this problem plagues as many as half of all menstruating women. During the shedding of the lining that builds up in the uterus each month, its muscular walls contract to expel tissue and blood. This action can be accompanied by sharp cramps in the lower abdomen right before the menstrual period or when bleeding begins. Pain may be accompanied by nausea, vomiting, diarrhea, dizziness, headache, tension, and occasionally, faintness. Fatigue and irritability can also be a problem. The pain may spread to the upper legs and lower back. The cramps usually subside after 1 or 2 days.

Not to be confused with dysmenorrhea is the dull, aching pain in the lower abdomen that some women experience about 2 weeks before they menstruate. This problem is less severe than the pain that occurs with bleeding and is caused by the release of an egg from the ovary.

Menstrual cramps range from mildly annoying to severely incapacitating. Doctors classify them as primary or secondary. The term "primary dysmenorrhea" means there is no underlying physical abnormality causing the pain. "Secondary dysmenorrhea" means that an infection or growth is the cause.

Call Your Doctor If . . .

■ Your pain is not controlled by medication or lasts more than 3 days.
■ You have pain with urination or bowel movements, or pain that is located on only one side.
■ There is any chance you could be pregnant.

Seek Care Immediately If . . .

■ You have a high temperature, vomiting, diarrhea, rash, dizziness, or muscle aches during your menstrual period.
■ The pain is very severe. (For example, if you have trouble walking.)

What You Can Do

Applying heat to your abdomen or back helps ease the pain. Do this for about 20 minutes once or twice a day. Use a heating pad set on low or a warm water bottle, or take a warm bath for 10 to 15 minutes.

Stay as active as possible. Exercise often helps relieve pain. You don't need to stay in bed.

What Your Doctor Can Do

Your doctor will look for an underlying cause, such as an infection or growth. If he finds one, you'll receive treatment accordingly. Otherwise, a pain medication is the most likely answer.

Menstrual cramps are associated with high levels of prostaglandins, substances your body makes which can cause both painful cramps and contractions of the uterus. A variety of medications inhibit prostaglandins, thereby relieving menstrual discomfort. They are called nonsteroidal anti-inflammatory drugs. Some are available over-the-counter, others only by prescription.

If these drugs fail to provide relief, the doctor may try prescribing oral contraceptives (birth control pills), which are sometimes used to treat painful periods and PMS.

Prescription Drugs

Anaprox (naproxen)	Naprelan	Ponstel
Cataflam	(naproxen sodium)	(mefenamic acid)
(diclofenac)	Oral contraceptives	Voltaren
Motrin or	Orudis or Oruvail	(diclofenac)
Rufen (ibuprofen)	(ketoprofen)	

Over-the-Counter Drugs

Actron
Advil
Aleve
Ascriptin
Bayer Aspirin
BC Powder
Bufferin
Excedrin
Excedrin, Aspirin-
  Free

Goody's
Midol Menstrual
  Formula
Midol PMS
  Formula
Midol Teen
  Menstrual Formula
Motrin IB
Nuprin
Orudis KT

Pamprin Maximum
  Pain Relief
Pamprin
  Multi-Symptom
Panadol
St. Joseph
Tylenol
Unisom with Pain
  Relief
Vanquish

Herbal Remedies

There are no herbal remedies specifically for menstrual cramps. However, you can try such general pain relievers as Japanese mint and white willow (which contains a natural form of aspirin).

Because the hormonal changes that occur during a woman's monthly cycle can cause other symptoms known collectively as premenstrual syndrome, you might also want to try one of the herbs recommended for that problem. For details, turn to the entry on PMS.

Nutritional Support

Magnesium may reduce prostaglandin-induced menstrual pain. You should also try limiting your intake of caffeine-containing beverages, such as cola, coffee, and tea.

Alternative Treatments

Acupuncture: This form of therapy is based on the belief that specific points on the exterior of the body are associated with a corresponding internal organ, and that stimulation of these external sites with tiny needles can relieve internal symptoms. Although acupuncture won't cure an underlying ailment, it seems effective for many types of pain—including menstrual cramps.

Energy Medicine: Transcutaneous electrical nerve stimulation (TENS) attempts to interrupt the travel of pain signals from their point of origin to the brain. During the treatments, electrodes are stuck on the skin and a small electronic unit delivers pulsed currents through the electrodes to the nerves. TENS may also stimulate the production of endorphins, the body's natural painkiller, and may reduce prostaglandin-induced menstrual pain.

Hydrotherapy: The application of hot and cold compresses to the body, with or without electrical stimulation, is sometimes used to treat menstrual cramps.

Hypnotherapy: Through enhanced power of suggestion, a hypnotist can help you change the way you perceive problems such as pain and help you discover new ways to respond to them.

Migraine

The Basics

Migraine headaches are common: 17.6 percent of women and 5.7 percent of men suffer at least one migraine a year. The problem tends to run in families. Most victims have a close relative with migraines.

Migraine headaches typically affect one side of the head. They can last anywhere from a few hours to a few days. Some people have them weekly, others have less than one a year. The problem usually surfaces sometime between the teen years and the age of 40.

At the onset of a migraine, the blood vessels in your head first shrink, then swell, causing pain that can last for days. Scientists have identified a brain chemical called serotonin that plays a major role in the development of migraine headache. Bright lights, emotional upset, fatigue, loud noises, missed meals, strong smells, tension, and weather changes all can trigger a migraine. The headaches can also be brought on by certain foods and beverages. (See "Nutritional Support.") Many women get migraine headaches before or during their monthly period.

Migraine can be classified as either classic or common.

■ *Classic migraines* begin with warning signs such as a sensation of flashing lights or colors, nausea, vomiting, and sensitivity to noise, light, or smells. You may feel as though you are looking through a tunnel. One side of your body may feel prickly, hot, or weak. These warning signs, called an aura, last about 15 to 30 minutes. They are followed by pain.

■ *Common migraines* do not have the same warning signs. However, you may feel tired, depressed, restless, or talkative for 2 or 3 days before the headache starts.

There are a number of over-the-counter and prescription medications for the treatment of headache and migraine. Some prescription medications need to be taken every day to prevent migraine. Others should be taken as soon as the aura or headache starts. You should discuss your medication options with your physician.

Call Your Doctor If . . .

■ Your medication causes any side effects.

Seek Care Immediately If . . .

■ You have a headache that gets worse or lasts more than 24 hours despite treatment.
■ You develop a high temperature.
■ You faint or develop weakness, numbness, double vision, difficulty with speech, or neck pain or stiffness.

What You Can Do

■ Overuse of pain medication can cause rebound headaches, so be sure to tell your doctor the name of every medication that you take and how often you use it.
■ At the first sign of a headache:
  • Apply cold compresses or ice packs to your head, or splash cold water on your face.
  • Lie down in a quiet, dark room for several hours. You may sleep, meditate, or listen to music. Do not read. Rest during the attack.
■ To help prevent migraines:
  • Keep a headache diary to help you identify foods and situations that trigger your attacks. Write down the names of medications you took during the attack and document whether or not they helped.
  • Try to learn how to deal with stress. Yoga, biofeedback, or relaxation therapy may be helpful.
  • If the headaches first appeared after you began taking birth control pills, you may want to talk to your doctor about changing to a different method.

What Your Doctor Can Do

Before prescribing a migraine medication, your doctor will examine you to make sure your headaches aren't caused by some other underlying problem.

If you suffer from frequent migraines, the doctor may prescribe a daily medication to prevent them from occurring. You must remember to take this medication faithfully, even when you are feeling well. It may take several weeks before you notice an improvement.

The doctor will probably give you a prescription for medication to relieve a headache once it occurs. You may have to try several different medications before you find the one that works for you. Migraines are often accompanied by nausea and vomiting. If this is a problem, you may have to use an injectable medication, a nasal spray, or a rectal suppository instead of a pill.

Many of the drugs used to treat migraine interact with each other. Check with your doctor before combining any migraine medications, including those available over-the-counter.

Prescription Drugs

Drugs prescribed to prevent frequent migraines include:

Blocadren (timolol)   Inderal (propranolol)
Depakote (divalproex)

Drugs prescribed for relief of the headache itself include:

Amerge (naratriptan)   Maxalt (rizatriptan)
Cafergot or Wigraine (caffeine,   Midrin (acetaminophen,
 ergotamine)   dichloralphenazone,
DHE 45 and Migranal   isometheptene mucate)
 (dihydroergotamine)   Zomig (zolmitriptan)
Imitrex (sumatriptan)

Over-the-Counter Drugs

Standard nonprescription headache medications may also provide relief. Only one of these products—Excedrin Migraine—has been approved specifically for migraines. However, standard Excedrin Extra Strength contains exactly the same ingredients.

Actron   Excedrin   Nuprin
Advil   Excedrin, Aspirin   Orudis KT
Aleve   Free   Panadol
Alka-Seltzer   Excedrin Migraine   St. Joseph
Ascriptin   Goody's   Tylenol
Bayer Aspirin   Motrin IB   Vanquish
Bufferin

Herbal Remedies

Feverfew

Nutritional Support

Certain foods can trigger a migraine attack. Common offenders include alcohol, artificial sweeteners, beans, canned soup, cheese, chocolate, coffee or tea, hot dogs, lunch meat, nuts, pickles, raisins and red wine. Keep a record of the times when you eat these foods and the onsets of your migraine attacks. Give up any item that turns out to be a trigger.

Remember that hunger may also be a trigger. Try not to skip or delay meals.

Alternative Treatments

Acupuncture: The use of acupuncture to treat painful conditions such as headache dates back thousands of years. The treatment is based on the belief that specific points on the exterior of the body are associated with a corresponding internal organ, and that stimulation of these external sites with tiny needles can relieve internal symptoms. Today scientists suspect that acupuncture may alter the body's production of certain chemicals, including serotonin, a neural messenger associated with migraine.

Alexander Technique: This system of muscle relaxation and movement training is considered especially helpful for arthritis and muscle strains, but it can also provide relief from a variety of other ailments, including migraine.

Biofeedback: A technique that enables patients to control otherwise involuntary reactions, biofeedback may help you fight off the blood-vessel spasms that trigger a migraine. After applying sensors to various parts of your body and hooking them up to a computer, a biofeedback therapist will teach you mental and physical exercises that can short-circuit an attack.

Energy Medicine: Transcutaneous electrical nerve stimulation (TENS) attempts to disrupt pain signals in the nerves. During the treatments, electrodes are stuck on the skin and a small electronic unit delivers pulsed currents through the electrodes to the nerves. TENS may also stimulate the production of endorphins, the body's natural painkiller.

Hydrotherapy: Two types of hydrotherapy are used to treat migraine headaches. In constitutional hydrotherapy, hot and cold compresses are applied to the body and mild electrical stimulation is delivered to various muscle groups. Hot fomentation is like constitutional hydrotherapy, but does not use an electrical current.

Hypnotherapy: Through enhanced power of suggestion, hypnotherapists have proven surprisingly successful at relieving all kinds of pain. This approach doesn't work for everyone, but is certainly worth a try.

Mononucleosis

The Basics

Famed for the run-down feeling it fosters, mononucleosis is a viral infection that attacks the lungs, liver, and lymph system (a key part of the immune system). The virus, known as *Epstein-Barr*, favors people between the ages of 12 and 40 years. A mild case of infectious mononucleosis may clear up in as little as a week, while more severe cases can drag on for months.

Often called the "kissing disease," mononucleosis is spread mainly through saliva. Infected droplets sprayed into the air by sneezes and coughs can also transmit the disease. The virus is more likely to take hold if you are tired, under stress, or have another illness. Symptoms include fever, sore throat, swollen glands, headaches, body aches, fatigue, loss of appetite, swollen liver, swollen spleen, and occasionally yellow skin and eyes.

There is no remedy for this illness. About half its victims recover on their own within 2 weeks, although feelings of fatigue can linger for 3 to 6 weeks after the other symptoms are gone. In rare cases, the throat may become so swollen that breathing is difficult. Liver damage, nervous system infections, lung complications, and blood abnormalities are also rare possibilities.

Although some experts have speculated about a connection between mononucleosis and chronic fatigue syndrome, doctors have failed to find any proof of a link.

Call Your Doctor If . . .

■ Your fever lasts more than a few days or surpasses 105 degrees Fahrenheit.
■ You still have symptoms after several weeks.
■ You have yellowing of the skin (a sign of liver problems).

Seek Care Immediately If . . .

■ You develop severe pain in your abdomen or shoulder.
■ You have trouble swallowing or breathing.
■ You feel dizzy or confused.

What You Can Do

■ Anyone under 18 should NOT take aspirin during this illness. Aspirin increases the risk of a serious complication called Reye's syndrome, which can damage the brain and liver. Be sure to check the label of any over-the-counter medicines you use. Acetaminophen is a safe alternative to relieve fever and pain.

■ Gargling may help relieve sore throat. Use warm salt water (1 teaspoon of salt in 1 cup of water) or double-strength tea. Sucking on hard candy also helps.

■ Rest until your temperature returns to normal (98.6 degrees Fahrenheit). Get plenty of sleep and don't try to push yourself too hard. You may gradually resume your regular activity after your fever is gone, but be sure to rest when you are tired.

■ For 4 to 5 weeks, it's best to avoid physical activity such as heavy lifting, strenuous exercise, or sports. These activities could injure your spleen.

■ While you have symptoms, remember to avoid close contact with those who are most likely to catch it from you: infants and people who are already ill.

What Your Doctor Can Do

Although there is no specific treatment for mononucleosis, you should see your doctor throughout the illness so you can be watched for the rare occurrence of spleen, liver, or nervous system damage.

Prescription Drugs

Nothing will cure the disease. For severe complications, such as difficulty breathing, the doctor can prescribe steroid medications such as prednisone.

Over-the-Counter Drugs

For relief of symptoms such as fever and pain, use acetaminophen (Panadol, Tylenol). To ease the sore throat that usually accompanies mononucleosis, try one of the following nonprescription lozenges and sprays:

Cepacol Sore Throat Lozenges	Sucrets
Cepacol Sore Throat Spray	Vicks Chloraseptic Cough &
Cepastat Sore Throat Lozenges	Throat Drops and Lozenges
Halls Cough Drops	Vicks Chloraseptic Sore Throat
N'Ice Sore Throat and Cough	Spray
Lozenges	Vicks Cough Drops

Herbal Remedies

Although herbs, like all other medicines, are ineffective against the underlying illness, a large number have been found helpful for relieving a sore throat. Usually, they are taken as a soothing tea. Possibilities include:

Agrimony	Couch Grass	Onion
Anise	Dill	Peppermint
Balsam	Echinacea	Pine Oil
Balsam of Peru	English Oak	Potentilla
Bilberry	English Plantain	Radish
Blackberry	Galangal	Rhatany
Blackthorn	Garlic	Rose Flower
Brewer's Yeast	Iceland Moss	Sage
Caraway	Jambolan	Sandalwood
Cardamom	Japanese Mint	Slippery Elm
Chamomile	Knotweed	Tormentil
Chinese Cinnamon	Larch	Usnea
Cinnamon	Marigold	White Nettle
Cloves	Mustard	Witch Hazel
Coffee Charcoal	Myrrh	

Nutritional Support

Although you may not feel like eating while you are ill, try to maintain a balanced diet. Drink at least 8 glasses of fluids each day, especially while you have a fever.

Alternative Therapies

Nothing in the realm of alternative medicine can rid you of this disease.

Obsessive-Compulsive Disorder

The Basics

Unrelenting, unwelcome thoughts, plus an urge to repeat senseless rituals, define the strange illness known as obsessive-compulsive disorder (OCD). By some estimates, this problem afflicts as many as one person in 50 at some point in life.

Obsessions are unwanted—even abhorrent—ideas, words, or images that repeatedly invade a person's consciousness. They may be fleeting and focus on one subject or persistent and broad-ranging. Among the more common obsessions are fear that harm may come to oneself or to a loved one, an unreasonable belief that one has a terrible illness, and persistent thoughts of repugnant sexual acts.

Compulsions are repeated acts performed to quell obsessions. Most seem absurd and are usually performed against one's will. Common compulsive rituals include counting, repeated hand washing, hoarding, and endlessly rearranging objects to keep them in precise alignment with each other.

While the disorder can surface at any age, it usually begins during adolescence and early adulthood. Recent research indicates that one-third of cases actually originate during childhood. The disorder tends to last for years, even decades, but its course varies from person to person.

While OCD was once thought to be a purely psychological illness, there is now growing evidence of a neurologic basis. OCD patients respond well to medications affecting the neurotransmitter serotonin, suggesting that an imbalance in brain chemistry is responsible. In addition, research employing *positron emission tomography (PET)* demonstrates that brain activity in people with OCD is distinctly different from other people's, again pointing to a true physiologic basis for the disorder.

Call Your Doctor If . . .
■ You find that obsessive thoughts are taking up a notable amount of your time, are hard to control, interfere with your life, and cause you significant distress.

Seek Care Immediately If . . .
■ You feel an urge to hurt yourself or someone else.

What You Can Do
The first and most important thing you can do is to get help. Many people with OCD do not seek care because of embarrassment or shame. But remember: With so many people suffering at least some form of OCD, your own symptoms are unlikely to be surprising.

Start with your family physician. He or she can help you determine whether your symptoms are caused by an anxiety disorder, another medical or psychological condition, or both, and can refer you to a mental health professional, if necessary.

When choosing a therapist, make sure you feel comfortable with the proposed treatment strategy and feel a sense of confidence in the therapist. You may also want to explore the options of group therapy and self-help groups to complement treatment. Other things you can do include:

■ Stay fit: Exercise at least three times a week, get plenty of rest, and eat a balanced diet.
■ Talk things over with your family and friends. Don't waste energy trying to hide your worries.
■ Try to deal with your problems one at a time instead of lumping them into one huge dilemma. Smaller problems cause less anxiety.
■ Take a short time-out period during the day when you feel stressed. Close your eyes and take deep breaths.
■ Try using muscle relaxation. Start with the muscles in your face: Tense them, hold them this way for a few seconds, and then relax. Repeat this with the muscles in your neck, shoulders, hands, belly, back, and legs.
■ Make time for fun and remember to take time to relax.
■ Be sure to provide your doctor with a complete rundown of any medications—over-the-counter and prescription—that you are taking, as well as your eating and drinking habits. All have a bearing on your treatment.
■ Give any medication you've been prescribed an ample chance to work. Drugs for this disorder usually take at least a month to make a difference.

What Your Doctor Can Do

If your doctor suspects OCD, he or she may recommend that you see a psychotherapist or psychiatrist because a combination of behavioral therapy and medication is often the best course of treatment; neither treatment is 100 percent effective on its own.

In the behavioral therapy called exposure and response prevention, the patient is first exposed to the feared object or idea, either directly or through the imagination, then discouraged or prevented from carrying out the usual compulsive response. For example, a compulsive handwasher will be asked to touch something dirty, then not wash his hands. This treatment works best when the therapist is specifically trained in this technique, the patient is motivated to succeed, and the patient's family is cooperative. After repeatedly confronting a feared object without a compulsive response, the patient becomes less anxious and can begin to resist the compulsion. This therapy alone often solves most of the problem.

Prescription Drugs

Though OCD is considered an anxiety disorder, tranquilizers don't relieve it. Instead, it responds best to drugs that raise the level of serotonin in the brain. The serotonin boosters Anafranil (clomipramine) and Luvox (fluvoxamine) are marketed specifically for OCD. In addition, several antidepressants that lift serotonin levels are helpful for this disorder as well. The options include Prozac (fluoxetine), Paxil (paroxetine), and Zoloft (sertraline).

Over-the-Counter Drugs

There's nothing for this problem available over the counter.

Herbal Remedies

The antidepressant herb St. John's wort appears to work in part by boosting the amount of serotonin available to the brain. It has not, however, been tested for OCD.

Nutritional Support

The essential amino acid tryptophan is the raw material for serotonin. It's especially plentiful in bananas, dried dates, milk, meat, fish, turkey, and peanuts; and supplements are available by prescription. There's no research, however, on this nutrient's effectiveness against OCD; and a proven serotonin booster probably has a much better chance of success.

Alternative Treatments

Hypnotherapy, with its ability to enhance the power of suggestion, has been found effective for a variety of problems that hinge on emotions and habits, including phobias and compulsions.

Osteoporosis

The Basics

Osteoporosis—the dreaded brittle-bone disease that strikes some 25 million Americans in their later years—gets its start during middle age. Throughout life, our bones are continuously rebuilding themselves, shedding old calcium deposits and replacing them with new. But from about age 35 onward, the balance gradually begins to tip, with calcium leaching out of the bones faster than it can be replaced.

The problem is especially serious for postmenopausal women. Estrogen produced during the childbearing years promotes dense, healthy bones, and when it declines after the change of life, bone loss can speed up dramatically. Caucasian, Hispanic, and Asian women are more likely to develop the problem. Smokers and childless women are also at greater risk, as are those with a delicate frame and a history of osteoporosis in the family.

Medical conditions such as diabetes, kidney or liver disease, chronic diarrhea, lactose intolerance, and celiac disease tend to promote osteoporosis. Certain medications, including steroids, thyroid hormone, and the seizure drug Dilantin, also weaken the bones. Insufficient calcium in your diet will make the problem worse, as will a deficiency of vitamin D. Because weight-bearing exercise strengthens the bones, lack of exercise is an important contributing factor.

Too often, the first sign of osteoporosis is a broken bone. However, there are often earlier warnings. Tooth loss during midlife is one signal. Backache (due to gradual collapse of the spinal bones) is another. A loss of height is further evidence of crumbling in the spine, eventually followed by a dowager's hump, a protrusion of the upper back and a shortening of the chest area.

Although osteoporosis was once considered unstoppable, we now have medications that can slow its progress and even reverse its effects. We also know how exercise and diet alone can delay its onset and minimize its severity.

Call Your Doctor If . . .
■ You develop new, unexplained symptoms. They may be related to a medicine you are taking.

Seek Care Immediately If . . .
■ You develop sudden, severe pain in your back.
■ You have pain after an injury or fall.

What You Can Do
■ If your back is affected, a firm mattress may help you sleep.
■ To pick up objects, bend at the knees rather than from the waist.
■ Eat a balanced diet, high in calcium and vitamin D, with lots of green vegetables and milk.

■ Ask your doctor to suggest a good weight-bearing exercise program. Exercise will not cure osteoporosis, but it can help you preserve the bone mass you have, strengthen your back and hips, maintain flexibility, and steady your gait. Within only 6 months, a regular exercise program can reduce your risk of bone fractures.

■ To relieve pain, you may use over-the-counter painkillers such as aspirin, acetaminophen, and ibuprofen.

■ Falls are especially dangerous if you have osteoporosis. To avoid them:
  • If you are unsteady on your feet, use a cane or have someone help you walk.
  • Remove loose rugs and long electrical cords from your home.
  • Keep your home well lighted at night.
  • Avoid icy streets and wet or waxed floors. Hold the railing when using stairs.

What Your Doctor Can Do

Your doctor will probably do a test to check the level of your bone density. The most popular and accurate test is dual-photon absorptiometry (DPA), which takes about 20 to 40 minutes. A faster, less expensive test, the p-DEXA, takes only 10 minutes, but doesn't measure density in the spine and hip, the most serious fracture sites. If the test reveals osteoporosis, your doctor can prescribe a variety of medications to halt and reverse deterioration.

Prescription Drugs

Fosamax (alendronate) can prevent and even reverse the bone loss associated with osteoporosis. This once-a-day pill must be taken with a full glass of water first thing in the morning, at least 30 minutes before your first food, beverage, or other medication. To avoid digestive problems, be sure not to lie down for at least 30 minutes after taking Fosamax.

Evista (raloxifene) is a relatively new drug that offers estrogen-like effects on bone and cholesterol levels without the risk of uterine cancer (and the possible risk of breast cancer) posed by estrogen therapy. It does not, however, relieve menopausal symptoms.

Calcitonin is a natural hormone that can prevent loss of bone mass in women with osteoporosis. Synthetic forms of the hormone can be taken as an injection (Calcimar or Miacalcin) or as a nasal spray (Miacalcin). If you take the injection, your doctor will teach you how to inject the medicine yourself. If you use the nasal spray, you should alternate nostrils each day.

Estrogen replacement therapy, which relieves menopausal symptoms and helps prevent heart disease, can also stop or even reverse the bone loss of osteoporosis. Estrogen increases the risk of uterine cancer, so it's prescribed along with protective doses of progesterone for those who have not had a hysterectomy. Medicines available for replacement therapy include the following:

Alora Patch (estradiol)
Climara Patch (estradiol)
Cycrin (medroxyprogesterone)
Estrace (estradiol)
Estraderm Patch (estradiol)
Estratab (esterified estrogens)
Estring (estradiol)
FemPatch (estradiol)
Menest (esterified estrogens)

Ogen (estropipate)
Ortho-Est (estropipate)
Premarin (conjugated
  estrogens)
Premphase, Prempro
  (conjugated estrogens and
  progesterone)
Provera (medroxyprogesterone)
Vivelle Patch (estradiol)

Over-the-Counter Drugs

You'll probably need a calcium supplement if you're unable to include large amounts in your diet. Calcium citrate is often the preferred formulation because it's easily absorbed. A less expensive alternative is a calcium-based antacid such as Tums or Titralac.

Herbal Remedies

No herbs are known to relieve this problem.

Nutritional Support

Whether or not you take prescription medications for this condition, you need to optimize your intake of several important bone-building nutrients:

Calcium: Women over the age of 50 should increase their calcium intake to between 1,000 and 1,500 milligrams of calcium per day. Calcium is found in milk and dairy foods, nuts, seafood, and green leafy vegetables.

Vitamin D: This vitamin helps your body absorb calcium and promotes its uptake into the bones. The recommended dose is 400 international units (IU) per day. Vitamin D is present in such foods as egg yolk, certain fish, fish liver, and butter. It is also added to bread, milk, cereal and other foods. An 8-ounce glass of milk contains 100 IU. Exposure to 15 minutes of sunshine per day can also trigger the body's formation of vitamin D.

Magnesium: This important mineral helps your body utilize calcium and vitamin D. Your daily magnesium dose should be at least half the amount of calcium you consume on a daily basis. For example, if you take 1,200 milligrams of calcium, you need 600 milligrams of magnesium.

Phosphorous: For maximum benefit from calcium, you need an amount of phosphorus equal to your calcium intake. Too much phosphorous, however, speeds up bone loss and increases urinary calcium levels. Most Americans get too much phosphorous by eating excessive quantities of red meat, white bread, processed cheese, and soft drinks. To keep your phosphorous intake in line, avoid consuming large quantities of food labeled as containing sodium phosphate, potassium phosphate, phosphoric acid, pyrophosphate, or polyphosphate.

Excess consumption of protein, sodium, sugar, alcohol, and caffeine has also been shown to decrease absorption of calcium from your diet.

Alternative Treatments

Tai Chi: The slow, graceful Chinese exercise program known as Tai Chi increases strength and muscle tone, improves range of motion and flexibility, and enhances balance and coordination. Since it is a weight-bearing exercise, it is helpful for preventing osteoporosis.

Parkinson's Disease

The Basics

There are few people who don't know at least one individual afflicted with Parkinson's disease. An estimated 500,000 to 600,000 Americans suffer the tremors, slowness, and stiffness of this progressive nervous disorder.

The odds of getting Parkinson's rise with age. The first symptoms typically appear between the ages of 50 and 70 years, although a quarter of those with Parkinson's first notice a problem between the ages of 30 and 50. The hallmarks of the disease are tremors (in 70 percent of cases) and a slowdown in movement. After many years, mental ability may also begin a slow decline.

Doctors do not know what triggers this disease. It's not hereditary and not contagious. What they do know is that, as Parkinson's sets in, cells in the region of the brain that governs movement and balance begin to slowly deteriorate, producing less and less of a chemical messenger called dopamine. The shortage of dopamine results in diminished control of the muscles.

The first symptoms of Parkinson's are subtle and come on very gradually. Typical early warning signs include fatigue, weakness, a stiff neck or back, tight muscles, and quivering hands. These symptoms may mean Parkinson's—or may mean nothing at all.

Tremors are the most distinctive symptom of Parkinson's. Typically, they start in an arm or leg on one side of the body. In time, they spread to the other side of the body, and may eventually affect the jaw, neck, and tongue. Tremors alone do not mean you have Parkinson's. Certain medications and other health conditions also cause the problem. Nor does an absence of tremors mean you don't have Parkinson's disease. About 30 percent of the people afflicted with other symptoms never develop the well-known tremors in the hands.

As the disease progresses, movement becomes slower. People find that motions are hard to start, difficult to control, and a challenge to complete. Muscles become stiffer than usual. Tightness in the back and neck may force the victim to stoop. Rigid facial muscles produce a blank, staring appearance. Gestures get jerky. Walking turns into a shuffle. Falls become likely.

In most people, the muscles in the mouth and throat eventually become involved. Speech becomes soft, indistinct, and monotonous. Victims may stammer, run words together, or repeat the same thing over and over. They may develop a tendency to drool. Swallowing may be impaired, and there's a danger of losing the cough reflex that normally protects people when food goes down the windpipe.

In the more advanced stages of the disease, memory loss and confusion may set in. A decline in mental ability, however, may be caused by a medication or depression, so if this problem surfaces ask your doctor whether changing medication or starting an antidepressant might be advisable.

Although there is no cure for Parkinson's disease, a variety of medications can dramatically slow its advance. Different drugs work better at different stages of the disease, and many therapies eventually produce side effects that partly offset their benefits. Treating Parkinson's is therefore a constant balancing act—a trial-and-error effort to identify which drug or drugs best control the most symptoms with the fewest side effects at any given moment.

Call Your Doctor If . . .

■ You get nauseous. This is a common side effect when you begin taking Parkinson's medications.

■ You develop hallucinations—hearing, feeling, or seeing things that aren't there. This is another potential side effect.

■ You feel dizzy. This too may be caused by your medication.

■ You begin to feel you cannot cope with the illness.

Seek Care Immediately If . . .

■ You find yourself contemplating suicide.

■ You undergo a big change in behavior (for example, becoming very confused or excited).

■ You become frightened or find you can't stay calm.

What You Can Do

■ Maintain a healthy diet. You may find it easier to eat frequent small meals. To avoid swallowing problems, cut your food into small pieces. Drink liquids with every meal; use a straw, if necessary. Tie a bib or napkin around your neck to keep food off your clothes. Eat slowly.

■ Do not carry hot foods if your hands shake badly. The food could spill and cause a burn. To keep your food warm, you may want to use a warming tray. Put a Lazy Susan on the table or counter to hold frequently used items so you won't need to collect them before every meal. Use a cart with wheels to move items from room to room.

■ If you begin to have difficulty speaking, ask your doctor about seeing a speech therapist. Faithfully practicing speech exercises can help remedy the problem. Muscle exercises can also help relieve swallowing problems.

■ Be sure to follow a regular exercise program. Exercise can relieve pain caused by rigid muscles, cramps, and a stooped posture. It can also prevent deterioration due to contractures (muscles and joints that become frozen in certain positions). Try massage to relax stiff muscles.

■ When Parkinson's disease begins to interfere with balance and movement, your chances of falling increase. A stooped posture contributes to the problem, as does the tendency to "freeze" when you try to start walking. At home, you can reduce freezing problems by putting tape strips along routes you use often. The tapes make it easier to move.

■ To keep from falling, make wide turns when you walk. You may feel safer with a 4-prong cane or a walker. Remove loose carpeting from the floor. If you have trouble getting up from a sitting position, use chairs with side arms and hard cushions.

■ Using a raised toilet seat will make it easier to get up. Grab-bars on the walls beside toilets and inside showers and bathtubs will also make getting up easier and prevent falls. A special chair inside the shower is another option. Use a wash mitt instead of a washcloth.

■ Allow extra time or get help for bathing, dressing, eating, or other personal needs. Use an electric razor to avoid shaving cuts. Choose clothes or shoes with Velcro closures.

■ You may find it difficult to turn in bed or find a comfortable sleeping position. A firm mattress may help. Bed rails or wearing silk or satin pajamas will facilitate movement in bed.

■ Stop drinking liquids 3 to 4 hours before going to bed. Urinate just before lying down so you won't have to get up during the night. Keep a night light on in the bathroom.

■ If your eyes become dry from lack of blinking, try using artificial tears, available at pharmacies and supermarkets.

■ If you feel depressed, check with your doctor. He can prescribe medications that help.

What Your Doctor Can Do

Medications are the first line of defense, but for advanced cases there are a few surgical alternatives. Such treatments tend to be exotic, controversial, and very much on the cutting edge of science. Among the techniques being tried are fetal tissue transplantation, transplantation of genetically engineered cells, and operations such as *pallidotomy* (risky surgery on the *globus pallidus* region of the brain), and *thalamic stimulation or reduction* (surgery on the *thalamus* portion of the brain).

Prescription Drugs

For the mild symptoms of early Parkinson's, your doctor may prescribe the following:

■ *Spasm-controlling drugs* such as Akineton (biperiden), Artane (trihexyphenidyl), Cogentin (benztropine), Kemadrin (procyclidine), and Levsin (hyoscyamine)

■ *Drugs that mimic the effects of dopamine,* including Mirapex (pramipexole) and Requip (ropinirole)

■ *Symmetrel* (amantadine), which relieves tremors, rigidity, and slowness of movement

■ *Benadryl* (diphenhydramine), an antihistamine that often controls tremors
■ *Norflex* (orphenadrine) to control tremors

By far the most effective drug for treating Parkinson's is *levodopa*, also called L-dopa. It is usually prescribed in combination with carbidopa, in brands such as Sinemet and Atamet. It corrects the shortage of dopamine in the brain. Doctors tend to hold back from using it immediately because it has a limited lifespan—working well for several years and then losing its effectiveness.

Selegiline, in brands such as Eldepryl or Carbex, may be given to boost the effectiveness of levodopa. *Parlodel* (bromocriptine), *Permax* (pergolide), and *Tasmar* (tolcapone) may be combined with levodopa therapy to reduce the amount of levodopa that is needed and smooth out fluctuations in levodopa's effectiveness.

Over-the-Counter Drugs
Nothing available over the counter is effective for Parkinson's disease.

Herbal Remedies
No herbs are known to be effective for this disorder.

Nutritional Support
Hopes that vitamin E might combat Parkinson's have not panned out. No nutritional measures are known to make a difference.

Alternative Treatments
The world of alternative medicine has nothing to offer in this area.

Phlebitis

The Basics
In a typical case of phlebitis, a vein near the surface of a limb (almost always the leg) becomes painfully inflamed. The affected vein generally feels like a cord that is warm and tender to the touch. It can become troublesome in a matter of hours or gradually worsen over a period of 1 to 2 days. It usually clears up in 1 to 2 weeks.

Although phlebitis is uncomfortable, it usually isn't harmful—

unless blood clots start to form. If this happens, and the clotting moves into deeper veins (a condition known as *deep venous thrombosis* or *deep vein thrombophlebitis*), the situation can become dangerous.

Clots in the deeper veins can block part or all of a limb's circulation. Worse yet, unlike clots near the surface, they can break away from the vein wall and lodge in a lung, causing the potentially fatal condition known as a pulmonary embolism. Prompt treatment of deep vein thrombophlebitis is therefore extremely important.

The danger of clotting increases when blood is allowed to sit undisturbed in a vein for an extended period. Prolonged bed rest, or even a protracted trip in an airplane or car, can allow the blood in the lower legs to settle and start to clot. Tip-offs of a deep-vein clot include swelling, pain, and redness in the area of the clot (usually in the ankle, calf, or thigh). Walking may be painful.

Call Your Doctor If . . .

■ You are being treated with blood thinners and find that you are bruising easily and often.

■ You begin bleeding from your gums or nose, or have blood in your urine or stools.

■ You notice increased swelling or pain in the calf of your leg. This often signals a serious clot.

Seek Care Immediately If . . .

■ You suffer sudden chest pain, have trouble breathing, or begin coughing up blood. These are signs of a pulmonary embolism. **Call 911 or 0 (operator)** to get to the nearest hospital or clinic. **Do not drive yourself.**

What You Can Do

■ Apply warm compresses over the inflamed vein to ease the discomfort.

■ To keep from getting blood clots:

- Move your legs as soon as possible after surgery or during long periods of bed rest.
- Exercise your legs every 1 or 2 hours while on long car or airplane trips.
- Do not smoke if you are taking birth control pills. This combination increases the chance of clots.
- Avoid crossing your legs at the knee or ankle.
- If you are told to wear tight, elastic stockings on your legs, do so.

Constricting the veins helps to keep blood flowing and clots from forming.
• Do not wear tight garters, girdles, or knee-high hose.
■ If you are taking a blood thinner:
  • Wear a medic-alert bracelet that says you are taking a blood thinner. Ask your doctor how to get one.
  • Tell your dentist that you are taking this type of medication.
  • Watch for bleeding from your gums or nose, and for blood in your urine or stools.
  • Since you will bruise more easily, avoid contact sports that can cause injury.

What Your Doctor Can Do

For simple phlebitis, a prescription for a nonsteroidal anti-inflammatory drug is probably all you'll need. But if a clot is involved, you may have to go to the hospital. There you'll be given tests to identify the exact location and size of the clot. One of these tests is essentially an x-ray of the veins taken after injecting a dye. Another uses ultrasound (inaudible sound waves) to build a picture of the affected vein on a television-type screen. Depending on the severity of the condition, the doctor may give you a clot-busting drug or a less potent blood-thinning medication. If drugs fail to dissolve the clot, you may need to have it removed surgically. The earlier you are treated, the less likely you are to end up with a clot in your lung.

Prescription Drugs

For phlebitis, the best remedy is a nonsteroidal anti-inflammatory drug. The leading choices include:

Anaprox and Naprosyn
  (naproxen)
Cataflam and Voltaren
  (diclofenac)
Clinoril (sulindac)
Daypro (oxaprozin)
Dolobid (diflunisal)
Ecotrin (aspirin)
Feldene (piroxicam)

Indocin (indomethacin)
Lodine (etodolac)
Motrin (ibuprofen)
Nalfon (fenoprofen)
Naprelan (naproxen sodium)
Orudis and Oruvail
  (ketoprofen)
Relafen (nabumetone)
Tolectin (tolmetin)

In the hospital for deep vein thrombophlebitis, you may be given the clot-busting drug Streptase (streptokinase) through an IV (a tube placed in your vein for giving medicine or liquids). You may also receive IV doses of the blood-thinning drug heparin. Later you may be prescribed blood-thinning pills such Coumadin (warfarin).

Over-the-Counter Drugs

To prevent further clotting, the doctor may recommend one of the most effective and popular blood-thinning medications of all: simple aspirin. Be sure to take only aspirin, not other over-the-counter pain-killers such as acetaminophen or ibuprofen, which do not have a blood-thinning effect. If aspirin upsets your stomach, check with your doctor before using it on a regular basis.

Herbal Remedies

Taken orally, an extract of butcher's broom can relieve inflamed veins and help treat the lower-leg discomfort caused by throm-bophlebitis. Applied externally, witch hazel also soothes inflamed veins. Squill is also considered useful for vein problems, and horse chestnut and sweet clover are said to improve poor circulation in the veins. Do not rely solely on any of these herbs, however, if you have signs of a severe clot, such as swelling and pain in the calf. This dan-gerous situation demands evaluation by a doctor.

Nutritional Support

Omega-3 fatty acids—which are abundant in fish oils and fatty fish—may have important blood-thinning properties, although ex-perts are not entirely sure how they work. Check with your doctor before taking fish oil capsules, however. Combined with other blood-thinners, they could cause excessive bleeding.

Alternative Treatments

Hydrotherapy, in the form of warm water-soaked compresses, will ease the discomfort of phlebitis. Indeed, use of warm and cold com-presses to manage the pain and swelling of soft tissue injuries and burns is standard medical practice, and has been proven effective in a variety of well-controlled clinical trials.

Pneumonia

The Basics

Despite major medical advances, pneumonia is still a major killer, particularly among people over age 65. Technically an inflammation of the lungs, pneumonia is dangerous because it is typically accompanied by a buildup of fluid that plugs the tiny sacs (alveoli) where oxygen is pulled from the air and transferred to the bloodstream. Without oxygen, the body dies.

There are many types of pneumonia. The most common culprits are bacteria such as *Streptococcus pneumoniae, Staphylococcus aureus, Haemophilus influenzae*, and the mycoplasma group. The disease is also classified by its effects. "Atypical" pneumonia, for example, is often milder than other forms and is commonly referred to as "walking pneumonia." "Nosocomial" or "hospital-acquired" pneumonia is a major problem; nearly 18 percent of all infections caught in the hospital are pneumonia, and this type is usually more severe than other forms and more resistant to treatment.

A number of factors increase your risk of getting pneumonia. If your immune system has been weakened by another disease (such as a heart condition, diabetes, AIDS, cancer, and other lung conditions), poor diet, or lack of exercise, pneumonia can more easily take hold. Cigarette smoking and high alcohol intake definitely increase your risk. And prolonged use of certain drugs can make it easier for the infection to develop. Leading offenders include some anticancer drugs, methotrexate, minocycline (Minocin), nitrofurantoin (Macrodantin, Macrobid), and amiodarone (Cordarone).

Many of the signs of pneumonia are similar to that of a cold or flu, including fever, coughing, shortness of breath, or rapid breathing. The key factors to keep in mind are the severity and length of the illness. Other less specific symptoms may include weakness, fatigue, weight loss, and a generally ill feeling.

Call Your Doctor If . . .

■ You have a high temperature.

■ Your medicine does not relieve your chest pain in a few days.

■ You get nauseated or have vomiting or diarrhea.

■ You are coughing up pink, frothy, or bloody sputum.

■ You have problems such as a rash, itching, swelling, or stomach pain that may be caused by your medicine.

■ Another family member shows signs of pneumonia.

Seek Care Immediately If . . .

■ You have a lot of trouble breathing, or have blue or pale skin, lips, or nail beds.

■ You have a severe headache, neck stiffness, or feel confused.

■ You continue to have fever and chills and feel worse even when taking your medicine.

What You Can Do

■ If you are diagnosed with pneumonia and your doctor prescribes antibiotics, be sure to take all of them. Stopping once symptoms subside is a good way to invite a relapse.

■ Get plenty of bedrest and drink plenty of fluids.

■ If you are coughing up sputum and milk seems to make it thicker, avoid milk products temporarily.

■ Often during the day, take 2 or 3 deep breaths and then cough. If it hurts when you cough, hold a pillow against your chest or try lying on your side.

■ Use a humidifier to keep air moist and sputum thin.

■ Stay inside during very cold or hot weather and when air pollution is high. This will aid your breathing and help control your cough.

■ Rest at home until you feel better. You may return to work or school when your temperature is normal, but expect to feel tired for up to 6 weeks after your illness.

■ If you have chest pain, apply a heating pad or warm cloths to your chest for 10 to 20 minutes, 2 to 3 times per day.

■ Pneumonia can make you prone to other lung infections. Avoid people who have colds or the flu, and get shots against flu and pneumonia.

■ If you smoke, this is an ideal time to quit.

What Your Doctor Can Do

Your doctor will begin by performing a thorough physical exam and listening very carefully for specific chest sounds to determine whether you do, in fact, have pneumonia. If it seems likely, your doctor will want you to get a *chest x-ray*, a picture of your lungs, which may reveal the fluid build-up in the lungs. He may also order lab tests to identify the germ causing the infection; and perhaps a *bronchoscopy*, a procedure in which a tube is inserted through the windpipe into the bronchial tubes, allowing the doctor to collect a tissue sample for diagnostic purposes.

Prescription Drugs

Today, pneumonia can almost always be cured. If it's the result of a bacterial infection, the doctor will prescribe a broad-spectrum antibiotic such as one of the penicillins, cephalosporins, erythromycins, or quinolone antibiotics. Tetracycline or sulfa drugs may also be used.

If the problem is due to a viral infection, antibiotics won't help. However, there are a couple of antiviral medications that can provide some relief: Symmetrel (amantadine) and Flumadine (rimantadine). To make breathing easier, you may also be given oxygen and medications to open the bronchial passages.

Over-the-Counter Drugs

Painkillers, such as ibuprofen (Advil, Motrin), acetaminophen (Tylenol), and aspirin, can be useful for relieving body aches and pain and bringing down a high fever. Expectorants, such as guaifenesin, found in many over-the-counter cough remedies, can make it easier to bring up sputum.

Herbal Remedies

Countless herbs are said to help coughs and fever; see the entry on colds and flu for a complete list. A variety of herbs are also helpful for inflamed bronchial passages, and you can find this group listed in the entry on bronchitis. However, even a mild case of pneumonia can occasionally progress to a severe disease, so don't put off seeing the doctor. Herbs will have little effect on the underlying infection, while prescription medications from the doctor will usually bring it to a quick end.

Nutritional Support

As with any infection, a well-balanced diet will improve your resistance and help fight off the germs. Also be sure to keep yourself well hydrated with plenty of fluids.

Alternative Treatments

The best—and certainly the safest—bet for this type of infection is a course of conventional prescription drugs. However, a form of treatment called *hyperthermia* is advocated for respiratory infections by many natural practitioners. The most common approach is immersion for about 20 minutes in water heated to as high as 108 degrees Fahrenheit. The temporary fever that this procedure induces is thought to help kill the invading germs.

Premenstrual Syndrome

The Basics

This distressing group of symptoms plagues many women for a week or two before the start of their period. Officially dubbed premenstrual syndrome, it is better known as PMS. Medical science has yet to find a cure, but we do have ways of reducing some of the symptoms.

The exact cause of PMS is unknown, although the symptoms are thought to be related to the wave of hormones that washes through the body prior to menstruation. PMS becomes more common with age. About half of all women can expect to have it at some point in their lives. We do not know why some cases are more severe than others, but stress seems to encourage the problem.

PMS produces a wide range of symptoms. Fortunately, most women have only a few. Potential problems are both emotional and physical:

■ *Changes in how you act or feel:* Feelings of anger, tension, anxiety, loss of control, or depression; hunger; mood swings; crying spells; cravings for foods like chocolate, sugar, or salt. Some women simply want to be left alone. Others have trouble thinking or concentrating. Some feel very tired. Others can't sleep.

■ *Changes in your body:* The most common physical symptoms are weight gain and swollen breasts, belly, ankles, hands, and face. Acne and headaches can also occur. Some women feel dizzy, and can actually faint. Constipation or diarrhea may develop. Some women find that they are not urinating as often as usual.

Call Your Doctor If . . .

■ You have difficulty coping with your symptoms.

Seek Care Immediately If . . .

Emergency care is rarely needed.

What You Can Do

■ Write down when your periods start and end and what your symptoms are each day. Do this for at least two or three menstrual periods. Knowing exactly when you are likely to have PMS symptoms will help you plan your activities to keep the time as free from stress as possible.

■ Try exercising daily. Many women find that regular exercise relieves their symptoms. Try some stress-reduction programs as well. A variety are listed under "Alternative Treatments" below. If you feel totally overwhelmed, a counselor may be able to help you learn to lessen stress and handle possible conflicts in your life. Ask your doctor for sources of help or look in the telephone book under Mental Health Services.

■ Pay careful attention to your nutrition (see below). It has a major impact on this condition.

■ Learn as much as you can about PMS. Books on the subject can be found in bookstores and libraries. Look for PMS support groups in your community or on the Internet.

What Your Doctor Can Do

At the outset, your doctor can make sure that the symptoms aren't caused by some other problem. Fibrocystic breast disease, endometriosis, a pelvic infection, diabetes, thyroid disease, allergies, and certain emotional disorders are all possibilities. If PMS is the only culprit, diet and exercise may be the best remedies, but the doctor can prescribe certain medications to relieve severe symptoms.

Prescription Drugs

Medicines that help the body get rid of water (diuretics) can reduce the swelling that often marks PMS. Hormones (birth control pills) and related medicines work for some women. Specific possibilities include:

Diuretics such as Aldactone (spironolactone) and HydroDIURIL (hydrochlorothiazide)	Parlodel (bromocriptine) Ponstel (mefenamic acid) Progesterone injections

Over-the-Counter Drugs

Several nonprescription products can help relieve cramps, aches, and bloating. They include:

Lurline PMS Tablets Midol PMS Formula	Pamprin Multi-Symptom

Herbal Remedies

Bugleweed Evening Primrose Oil Potentilla	Shepherd's Purse Vitex

Nutritional Support

■ Avoid foods that have a lot of salt. Excessive salt contributes to water retention and bloating. Check the sodium listing on the Nutrition Facts label. Keep your intake below 3,000 milligrams a day.

■ Try to avoid foods and beverages that have caffeine in them, including coffee, colas, tea, and chocolate. Too much caffeine can make you feel nervous and moody, and are known to make PMS symptoms more intense.

■ Eating a low-fat diet based on grains and vegetables while reducing your intake of red meat—especially during the 2 weeks prior to the beginning of your period—may help to control your PMS symptoms.

■ Increasing your calcium intake to 1,300 mg per day may reduce irritability and physical symptoms such as backache.

■ Nicotine and alcohol can also intensify PMS symptoms. Don't drink alcohol or smoke for 1 week before your period.

Alternative Treatments

Two types of alternative therapy have been found especially helpful for PMS:

Hydrotherapy: Advocates of these treatments believe that it helps bring the body back into balance. In constitutional hydrotherapy, hot and cold compresses are applied to the body and mild electrical stimulation is delivered to various muscle groups. Hot fomentation is like constitutional hydrotherapy, but does not use an electrical current.

Meditation: The goal of meditation is to induce mental tranquility and physical relaxation by deliberately suspending the stream of consciousness that usually occupies the mind. Meditation seeks to alleviate the harmful effects of tension and stress—factors that are known to aggravate a number of medical conditions, including PMS.

There are a number of other stress-reduction treatments that may also be helpful. They include:

Alexander Technique: A system of movement and posture training
Aromatherapy: Treatments with concentrated herbal oils
Aston-Patterning: A specialized form of physical training and massage
Guided Imagery: A mind/body therapy involving focused visualization
Hellerwork: A combination of deep massage and movement training
Massage Therapy: Relaxing bodywork to relieve tension

Qigong: Chinese exercises that improve fitness and reduce tension
Reflexology: A specialized foot massage said to relieve stress
Rolfing: A forceful deep-massage technique
Sound Therapy: Use of specially selected music to relieve stress
Yoga: A program of breathing exercises, body postures, and
  meditation with a proven calming effect

Prostate Problems

The Basics

For men, a prostate problem is one of the most common of all the ailments that plague the later years. The prostate, a walnut-sized gland that surrounds the exit from the bladder, produces the fluid in semen. From the age of 40 onward, this gland displays a tendency to grow larger. After age 60, this problem is joined by an increased risk of prostate cancer.

Because of the prostate's location, most symptoms of an enlarged prostate involve the body's ability to rid itself of urine. Typical difficulties include:

- A need to urinate frequently, especially at night
- A weak or interrupted stream when urinating
- A feeling that you cannot empty your bladder completely
- A feeling that you must urinate right away
- Urinary dribbling
- Trouble starting the flow of urine or holding it back
- Painful urination

These troublesome symptoms can be warning signs of cancer, or merely the result of prostate enlargement. Here's a quick overview of these problems:

Benign Prostatic Hyperplasia: More often than not, prostate symptoms are the result of the noncancerous prostate growth known as benign prostatic hyperplasia (BPH). As the new tissue swells the prostate, the enlarged gland begins to obstruct the flow of urine, increasing the frequency and difficulty of urination. BPH is very common in men over age 40, and affects all races equally. Left untreated, urinary retention caused by BPH can lead to urinary tract infections and serious kidney problems.

Prostate Cancer: Men in their 60s and 70s face a one-in-eight chance of developing this disease. The problem is usually discovered during a routine rectal exam, or through a PSA (prostate-specific antigen) screening test. Any enlargement or significant tumor (lump) can be detected during the rectal exam. If the cancer has not yet produced a lump, a high level of PSA may still give it away. Transrectal ultrasound can also detect cancers too small to show up on physical examination. Sometimes early cancer is detected when men undergo surgery to correct BPH.

Scientists haven't discovered what triggers prostate cancer. However, they do know that it tends to run in families, and that it's more common among African American men. Other factors associated with the disease include smoking and a high-fat diet.

Prostate cancer is the next-to-most common form of cancer in men (after skin cancer), with well over 100,000 new cases reported each year. Fortunately it tends to grow very slowly, and is therefore one of the most curable forms of the disease. When the cancer is discovered and removed while still confined to the prostate, the chance of a five-year cure is 94 percent.

Call Your Doctor If . . .

■ You find blood in your urine.
■ You have difficulty urinating.
■ Your urine becomes cloudy and foul smelling, or you experience pain or burning when you pass urine. These are signs of infection.

Seek Care Immediately If . . .

■ You cannot urinate at all and your bladder is painfully full. If this happens, the bladder must be emptied by inserting a small tube (a catheter) into the urinary canal (urethra).

What You Can Do

Regular physical exams and prostate cancer screening can help ensure that any prostate problems are detected early enough to be eradicated with the least extensive surgery and the fewest complications. The American Cancer Society now recommends screening for all men aged 40 and older.

To cope with an enlarged prostate:
■ Don't let your bladder get too full. Urinate as much as you can whenever you feel the urge.

■ Whenever possible, sit on hard chairs instead of soft ones.

■ Avoid exposure to cold temperatures or dampness.

■ Do not eat spicy foods; they often irritate the urinary tract.

■ Frequent sex reduces the risk of a urinary blockage. However, you should avoid becoming sexually aroused without ejaculating.

If you have had a prostate operation:

■ Apply ice for pain or swelling for the first 24 to 48 hours after surgery; then apply heat.

■ While confined to bed, exercise your legs frequently to keep blood clots from forming.

■ If bowel movements are difficult, don't strain. Walk to help stimulate the bowels. Eat foods rich in fiber to help restore regularity. Drink plenty of liquids.

■ Eat healthy foods to encourage healing and boost energy.

■ Don't sit for a long time in a car—or anywhere else. Sitting like this promotes bleeding.

■ Do not lift anything heavy until your doctor says it's okay.

What Your Doctor Can Do

If the problem is prostate cancer:

The choice of treatment is based on age, general health, size of the tumor and how quickly it is growing, and whether the cancer is confined to the prostate or has spread to adjacent tissue or other parts of the body. You may need surgery, hormone treatment, radiation, or a combination of these treatments.

Surgery: For men under age 70, if the tumor has not spread outside the prostate, a *prostatectomy* (surgical removal of the prostate) is typically recommended. Radical prostatectomy—removal of the entire prostate, adjacent lymph nodes, seminal vesicles, and a portion of the bladder neck—offers excellent results.

Studies have reported 15-year survival rates in up to 93 percent of men with localized disease who were treated with radical prostatectomy. However, this procedure is likely to cause impotence and, to some extent, urinary incontinence, either temporary or permanent. To improve the chances of avoiding these side effects, a nerve-sparing prostatectomy technique is now available in certain hospitals. It's not, however, suitable for every patient.

Hormone therapy: If the cancer has spread beyond the prostate, its growth can be at least temporarily controlled by eliminating the male hormone testosterone, which promotes the growth of prostate cancer cells. There are several medicines that can block production of testosterone. For advanced cancer, another option is surgical removal of the testicles (the source of 95 percent of the body's testosterone). Both approaches—surgery and medications—are sometimes combined in an all-out effort to rid the body of all testosterone.

In 85 percent of men receiving hormonal therapy, tumor size, urinary obstruction, and symptoms such as bone pain are reduced. However, potential side effects include weight gain, blood clot formation, cardiac failure, painful breast growth, hot flashes, impotence, and loss of sex drive. And within about 3 years, most men become resistant to any given hormonal therapy.

Radiation: This form of therapy can be administered through an external beam directed at diseased tissue, or as small radioactive pellets implanted in the gland and left there for life. Radiation may be used instead of surgery if the tumor is small. It is also used after surgery to kill any cancer cells that may have been missed.

The treatments are not without side effects, often including inflamed bladder, diarrhea, increased frequency of urination, skin rashes, and urinary tract and rectal symptoms such as pain, inflammation, and bleeding. Your doctor can prescribe medication to treat these side effects.

Watchful waiting: Because prostate cancer is slow to develop and spread, doctors sometimes recommend no treatment at all. This "watchful waiting" approach is most often adopted when a man is already in his 70s or beyond, has no symptoms, and suffers from a localized, relatively nonaggressive form of the cancer.

If the problem is benign prostatic hyperplasia:
Working with tiny surgical devices advanced up the urethra, a surgeon can relieve pressure from an enlarged prostate by either cutting away a section of the constricting prostate tissue (transurethral resection of the prostate or TURP) or making slits in the tissue (transurethral incisions) that allow the urethra to spring open. Recently, a procedure has been introduced that obliterates excess prostate tissue with microwaves. Laser prostatectomy is also being explored. And for men who cannot tolerate surgery, doctors have been experimenting with permanent insertion of a tube (stent) to brace open the walls of the urethra. Finally, since there's a 10 percent chance that the condition will improve on its own, watchful waiting is often recommended for mild cases.

Prescription Drugs

For benign prostatic hyperplasia, your doctor can prescribe Proscar (finasteride), a drug that shrinks the prostate, or a drug that relaxes muscles in the bladder and prostate, allowing urine to pass. Choices in this category include Cardura (doxazosin), Flomax (tamsulosin), and Hytrin (terazosin).

To eliminate testosterone in cases of advanced prostate cancer, the doctor can select among drugs such as Nilandron (nilutamide), Eulexin (flutamide), Megace (estrogen and megestrol), Lupron Depot (leupro-lide), and Zoladex (goserelin).

Over-the-Counter Drugs

There are no nonprescription drugs for prostate conditions.

Herbal Remedies

Researchers have found that urinary difficulties caused by prostate enlargement can be relieved by four herbal products: pumpkin seed, pygeum, saw palmetto, and stinging nettle. Remember, however, that if the underlying cause is cancer, none of these remedies will provide a cure.

Nutritional Support

Some studies suggest that the odds of prostate cancer can be reduced by following a diet low in fat and high in vitamin D and antioxidants (especially vitamin A, selenium, and possibly fish oils). Although fat doesn't seem to trigger prostate cancer, it does promote the growth of tumors once cancer gets started. If you're in a group at high risk of prostate cancer, it's therefore wise to keep fats—especially saturated fats—to a minimum.

Alternative Treatments

There are no holistic or natural therapies deemed capable of curing this problem.

Psoriasis

The Basics

The thick, scaling, silvery plaques that mark psoriasis tend to cluster on the scalp, elbows, knees, buttocks, and back. The plaques result from overproduction of skin cells—with the cells typically maturing in three to four days instead of the usual 28 to 30—but we still don't know what triggers this rampant growth. Psoriasis can also appear in the eyebrows, armpits, and groin, and sometimes affects the nails, causing thickening and crumbling of the nail plate and separation of the nail from the nail bed. A form of the disease called *pustular psoriasis* causes blisters instead of plaques, either on the palms and soles or all over the body.

The problem usually surfaces gradually, typically between ages 10 and 40. The plaques come and go, but the underlying condition is likely to hang on permanently. A typical mild case of psoriasis poses no danger to your health. However, a severe complication called *psoriatic arthritis* can be painful and crippling, and another serious form known as *exfoliative psoriatic dermatitis* can cover the entire body, leading to general disability.

Call Your Doctor If . . .

■ Your symptoms make it difficult to sleep.
■ You experience a worsening of symptoms.

Seek Care Immediately If . . .

Psoriasis, even at its worst, is rarely an emergency.

What You Can Do

■ Your treatment regimen for psoriasis may be very complicated and messy. To get the best results, you need to set aside time each day to apply the recommended lotions and creams. Some products are best applied after bathing, when the skin is still damp. Others should be applied a short time before bathing, then washed off. It is also important to know which medications should be covered with a dressing and which should be left exposed to the air.
■ Exposure to sunlight can help get rid of the plaques, but be careful not to get sunburn.
■ If your doctor prescribes the potent drug methotrexate, be sure to have the recommended blood tests to monitor the function of your blood cells, kidney, and liver.
■ Because some psoriasis medications are very dangerous during pregnancy, be sure to discuss your reproductive plans with your physician before starting any new treatment.

What Your Doctor Can Do

There is no cure for psoriasis, but treatment can reduce the frequency and severity of flare-ups. You may have to experiment with a variety of treatment plans to find out what works best for you.

A typical, mild case of psoriasis can usually be handled with creams and ointments. More extensive cases are often helped by *psoralen ultraviolet light A* (PUVA) therapy. Patients undergoing these treatments take a drug called methoxsalen and, after a waiting period, are exposed to long-wave ultraviolet light. This procedure can prolong the time between flare-ups, but increases the risk of skin cancer.

For severe, disabling cases, the doctor can prescribe more potent (and toxic) drugs to be taken by mouth.

Prescription Drugs

The usual treatment calls for application of lubricating creams, coal tar products, and preparations of anthralin or vitamin D. Leading options include Anthra-Derm, Drithocreme, and Micanol (anthralin); Dovonex (calcipotriene); and DHS (coal tar). Steroid creams and ointments can be used along with or in place of these products. Aristocort and Kenalog (triamcinolone) are often recommended.

Medications for more severe cases include the powerful cancer and arthritis drug methotrexate, a potent analog of vitamin A called Accutane (isotretinoin), and the immune-system suppressant Neoral (cyclosporine).

Over-the-Counter Drugs

A variety of lubricants, steroid creams, and coal tar preparations are available without a prescription. Leading examples include:

Aqua Tar	Fototar	Packer's Pine Tar
Balnetar	Hydrogenated	Petroleum Jelly
Cortaid	Vegetable Oil	Polytar
Cortizone	Medotar	Polytar Bath
Cutar Bath Oil	MG217 Medicated	PsoriGel
Emulsion	Neutrogena T/Derm	Taraphilic
Doak Tar	Oxipor VHC	Tegrin for Psoriasis
Estar	P&S Plus	Zetar Emulsion

Herbal Remedies

Although a number of herbs have been found helpful for simple skin inflammation, none of them seem to relieve psoriasis.

Nutritional Support
No special dietary measures are known to help.

Alternative Treatments
Light therapy, considered experimental and alternative for many ailments, is an accepted remedy for psoriasis.

Rash

The Basics
Sometimes serious—but often trivial—the red, itchy skin eruptions that we label a rash can be the tip-off of a major infection, or evidence of nothing more than a minor irritation.

Allergies are often the cause: Poison ivy, oak, and sumac are frequent culprits; medications are sometimes to blame; and many common foods and household products can also provoke an allergic response. Persistent dampness and rubbing—the problems underlying diaper rash—are other potential causes.

Occasionally, however, the source is more sinister. A seemingly innocuous rash can proclaim the arrival of infections ranging from chickenpox to typhoid fever. Among the many serious disorders marked by a rash are Lyme disease, measles, rheumatic fever, ringworm, Rocky Mountain spotted fever, scarlet fever, shingles, strep infections, syphilis, other sexually transmitted diseases, and toxic shock syndrome.

If there's any reason—such as accompanying symptoms—to suspect that a broader problem underlies a rash, your wisest course is to see the doctor. Even if the rash is due to an allergy, it may signal the need for medical attention. A severe allergy to a food, insect venom, or substance such as latex can close up your throat and put your life in danger.

Call Your Doctor If . . .
■ You develop a fever, headache, coughing, muscle aches, sore throat, chills, or fast heartbeat.
■ You develop a rash after starting a new prescription or over-the-counter medication.
■ The rash seems to spread.
■ The rash makes you very uncomfortable.

■ A diaper rash develops crusting, pus, large blisters, or additional redness, or fails to disappear within 7 days.
■ A baby with diaper rash develops white spots in the mouth. This could signal an infection called thrush. Your doctor can give you medicine to treat the problem.

Seek Care Immediately If . . .
■ You have difficulty breathing.

What You Can Do
■ Minor skin rashes can usually be treated with over-the-counter medications.
  • Agents such as calamine lotion help dry up the rash.
  • Antihistamines can help relieve the itching. An antihistamine cream, such as diphenhydramine, may work on its own. If it doesn't, you can take the antihistamine in a pill form. Be careful when driving, however; antihistamine pills can make you drowsy.
  • Hydrocortisone cream also helps stop itching and makes the rash go away.
  • Oatmeal baths (such as Aveeno) are helpful for relieving the itch caused by a rash, especially in children.
■ If you have poison ivy, oak, or sumac, be sure to wash your bed linens every day and your bath towels after each use. To keep from spreading the rash, do not share your bath towels with anyone else.
■ If you develop a rash, be sure to note the date, what it looked like and how long it took to go away. If you get sick a few weeks after having the rash, this information may give your doctor important clues about your illness.

To remedy diaper rash:
■ Most rashes improve in 3 days with proper care. Keep the diaper area clean and dry to help the rash clear up.
  • Check the child's diaper about once an hour. Wake the youngster up one time during the night to change the diaper until the rash improves. Change the diaper right away if it is wet or soiled from a bowel movement.
  • If the child has a bowel movement, use a mild soap with warm water to clean the diaper area. Gently rinse the area to remove any soap. Plain warm water and cotton balls or baby wipes also can be used.
  • Before closing the diaper, be sure the area is completely dry.

- Leave the child's bottom open to air as much as possible during naps or after bowel movements. To protect the bed, put a towel or diaper under the child.
- Diaper creams and ointments usually are not needed. However, an ointment such as zinc oxide can be helpful if the diaper area is dry and cracked, or the child has diarrhea. Make sure the area is clean and dry before applying any ointment.
- Do not use plastic pants until the rash improves.
- Punch small holes in disposable diapers to let air in. This will help the rash heal faster.
- After washing cloth diapers, rinse them twice to get rid of extra soap. Don't use fabric softeners if they make your baby's skin red or rashy.
- If the youngster's bottom stays bright red and raw-looking, or has small red dots, check with your doctor. There may be an infection.

What Your Doctor Can Do

Your doctor will determine if your rash is a minor skin irritation or the sign of a more serious illness. Treatment of the underlying cause may be necessary. To relieve itching and irritation, the doctor can prescribe a steroid ointment, cream, or lotion, or recommend an over-the-counter remedy.

If the rash is severe, your doctor may prescribe a steroid medication that you need to take by mouth for a few days. The dosing schedule is sometimes complex, requiring a different number of pills each day. Be sure to follow the treatment plan carefully, and do NOT stop taking the medication if the rash goes away.

Prescription Drugs

For severe rash and skin inflammation, the following prescription products are available:

Aquanil HC and Hydrocortone
  (hydrocortisone)
Celestone and Diprolene
  (betamethasone)
Chloresium (chlorophyllin
  copper complex)
Cortone (cortisone)

Cutivate (fluticasone)
Decadron (dexamethasone)
Dermatop (prednicarbate)
Pediapred (prednisolone)
Solu-Medrol
  (methylprednisolone)
Vistaril (hydroxyzine)

Over-the-Counter Drugs
For relief of minor rash, you can use the following nonprescription products:

Aveeno	Caladryl	Cortizone
Benadryl	Cortaid	

Remedies for diaper rash include:

A + D Original Ointment	Desitin Creamy
A + D Ointment with Zinc	Desitin Ointment
Balmex Ointment	Moisturel Cream
Desitin Cornstarch Baby Powder	

Herbal Remedies
The following herbs have been found helpful for symptomatic relief of skin inflammation. (They do not address any underlying problems.)

Agrimony	Fenugreek	St. John's Wort
Arnica	Frostwort	Walnut
Chamomile	Heartsease	White Nettle
English Oak	Jambolan	Witch Hazel
English Plantain	Oats	Yellow Dock
Evening Primrose Oil		

Nutritional Support
Remember that the sudden eruption of a rash may be the first sign of an allergic reaction to food. A severe food allergy can trigger a life-threatening anaphylactic reaction. Without fast treatment, the throat swells, closing off the airway and leading to suffocation. Meanwhile, blood pressure falls until the victim goes into shock.

The foods most likely to cause an anaphylactic reaction are peanuts and peanut products such as peanut butter; tree nuts; shellfish, especially shrimp and crab; and other fish. Other reported incidents have involved milk, soybeans, wheat, barley, rice, corn, potatoes, spinach, bananas, melons, tomatoes, citrus fruits, and chocolate.

Alternative Treatments
There are no alternative treatments specifically aimed at rash.

Seizures

The Basics

Few medical problems are as dramatic as a seizure, yet the majority of these attacks are relatively harmless. The result of a sudden excessive discharge of nerve cells in the brain, seizures rarely last more than a few minutes, and are often over in seconds.

If seizures occur regularly, the condition is called epilepsy. An astonishing array of minor neurological problems qualify as forms of this disorder, but the convulsive attacks that usually bring the word to mind are a type of generalized seizure that results from nerve cells misfiring across the entire brain.

Generalized seizures come in two varieties. In *petit mal* attacks, the victim loses consciousness and stops moving for 10 to 30 seconds, but doesn't suffer uncontrolled twitching or jerking. In *grand mal* attacks, the victim loses consciousness and falls to the floor with muscles jerking purposelessly. Control of the bladder and bowels may be lost during the attack, which typically lasts 2 to 5 minutes. Victims generally have no symptoms between episodes, but may feel a sudden change in mood just before an attack and suffer a headache, muscle soreness, and sleepiness immediately after.

About 1 person in 50 will have a seizure at some point in life, but only 1 in 200 has epilepsy. In the majority of cases, for which no underlying cause can be found, the attacks begin between ages 2 and 14. Seizures before age 2 are generally related to developmental defects, birth injuries, or metabolic diseases affecting the brain. Seizures that begin after age 25 are usually related to brain injury, tumors, or brain disease. Petit mal seizures are typically limited to children, and never begin after age 20. Grand mal seizures can strike at any age.

Seizures tend to run in families. They are more likely in mentally retarded children and individuals with cerebral palsy. They can also be triggered by head injury, withdrawal from alcohol or other drugs, a high fever (febrile convulsion), tetanus, a brain tumor, an overdose of insulin, or an infection.

Call Your Doctor If . . .

- A seizure victim does not wake up shortly after the attack.
- The victim develops new problems (such as difficulty seeing, speaking, or moving).

Seek Care Immediately If . . .

■ An injury occurs during a seizure.

■ The victim develops a high temperature.

■ The victim throws up and inhales the vomit.

What You Can Do

If you are a seizure patient:

■ Take your prescribed medication exactly as directed. Do not stop taking the medicine without talking to your doctor first.

■ Avoid activities in which a seizure would cause danger to yourself or to others. Do not operate dangerous machinery, swim alone, use ladders, or climb in high or dangerous places such as roofs or girders. Do not drive until your doctor says it's okay.

■ Wear an emergency medical identification bracelet with information about your condition. If you have a seizure, people around you will be able to tell what's wrong and get appropriate help.

■ If you have any warning of the onset of a seizure, lie down in a safe place where you can't hurt yourself.

■ Teach your family and close friends what to do if you have a seizure.

If you are with someone who is having a seizure:

■ Stay calm. To keep the person from falling onto hard or sharp objects, move these potential hazards out of the way.

■ DO NOT force anything into the person's mouth or try to open clenched jaws. Turn the victim on his or her side when the violent movement stops or vomiting begins.

■ When the seizure is over, the victim may be confused or drowsy and may need reassurance that everything is all right. Help him or her to rest and relax.

What Your Doctor Can Do

Your doctor will try to determine the underlying cause of the seizure, using tools such as blood tests, electroencephalograms to measure brain activity, and diagnostic imaging with CT scans or an MRI. If necessary, he will prescribe medication to prevent a recurrence.

Prescription Drugs

Drugs prescribed for seizures include the following. The doctor will select according to the type of seizures involved.

Atretol, Carbatrol, Epitol, or
    Tegretol (carbamazepine)
Celontin (methsuximide)
Depaken (valproic acid)
Depakote (divalproex)
Diamox (acetazolamide)
Dilantin (phenytoin)
Felbatol (felbamate)

Klonopin (clonazepam)
Lamictal (lamotrigine)
Meberal (mephobarbital)
Mysoline (primidone)
Neurontin (gabapentin)
Phenobarbital
Valium (diazepam)
Zarontin (ethosuximide)

Over-the-Counter Drugs
There are no nonprescription drugs for seizures.

Herbal Remedies
There are no herbs known to be effective for this problem.

Nutritional Support
Seizure disorders have never been linked to nutrition, and no special dietary measures are recommended.

Alternative Treatments
Biofeedback: This form of therapy appears to reduce the severity and frequency of seizures in some people with epilepsy. It provides you with training in the control of normally involuntary ("automatic") physical reactions, employing sensors that give you feedback on the functions you are trying to control.

Sepsis

The Basics
Sepsis—and its deadly offspring, septic shock—develop when bacteria from a small, localized infection enter the bloodstream and spread throughout the body, causing a widespread infection. The infection can begin anywhere, including the teeth, urinary tract, or even a cut. Signs that it has spread include fever, chills, and digestive problems (nausea, vomiting, or diarrhea). Tests may reveal bacteria in the blood.

In healthy people with good resistance, the infection usually clears up on its own without the need for treatment. However, in the chronically ill and those with weak immune systems, it can blossom into septic shock. This life-threatening condition develops when an especially virulent strain of bacteria such as staph begins to overwhelm the body with harmful toxins.

As the toxins take effect, they prompt fluid to leak from blood vessels out into the tissues. They may also weaken the heartbeat. Together, these reactions lower blood pressure. As blood pressure declines, less blood reaches the tissues. The body and its organs become deprived of oxygen, while waste products accumulate. Eventually organs such as the lungs, heart, or kidneys may come to a halt.

Fortunately, septic shock usually occurs only in hospitals, where invasive medical procedures provide powerful germs with easy access to the bloodstream. Patients with underlying medical conditions such as diabetes, cirrhosis, leukemia, lymphoma, and cancer are especially at risk, as are those undergoing surgery or delivery. The problem is more likely in the elderly and newborns.

If septic shock does strike outside the hospital, it's a signal to get to the emergency room fast. Without immediate treatment, it's usually a killer.

Call Your Doctor If . . .
■ You have a high temperature.
■ You have fever, swelling, pain, or redness while you are being treated. These are signs of continuing infection.
■ You plan to have surgery or work on your teeth after you have had sepsis. You may need to start taking antibiotics first.
■ You have a rash, swelling, hives, or trouble breathing. These could be a reaction to the antibiotics taken to fight the infection.

Seek Care Immediately If . . .
■ You or a family member develops these symptoms of septic shock: fever, chills, fast breathing, fast heart rate, dizziness, confusion, and low urinary output.

What You Can Do
It is important to take proper care of small infections so they won't have a chance to spread. Symptoms of a small infection in one part of the body are redness, swelling, and tenderness.

If you develop sepsis, your doctor will aggressively treat the infection with antibiotics. In addition, you should:

■ Get lots of rest. Slowly restart your usual activities as you feel better.
■ Finish taking all the antibiotics you've been prescribed even if you

begin to feel better. If you stop taking the drug too soon, some bacteria may survive and cause a relapse.

■ To keep from getting sick again, stay away from people who have illnesses that can spread. Also, get shots against pneumonia and the flu.

■ Eat healthy foods to help keep up your resistance to infection.

■ Wash your hands after going to the bathroom and before eating. This will keep you from spreading the infection or becoming infected by germs that live in body wastes.

What Your Doctor Can Do

If you develop septic shock, you'll need to be treated in the hospital with antibiotics, IV (intravenous) fluids, oxygen, and drugs to bring your blood pressure up to normal. Surgery may be necessary to drain fluid from infected areas of the body.

Prescription Drugs

For septic shock, you'll need specialized antibiotics given intravenously. A pressure-raising drug such as dopamine may also be given by IV. Once the infection is under control and the body can take care of itself, this medicine can be stopped.

Over-the-Counter Drugs

To reduce infection-induced fever, your doctor may recommend medications such as acetaminophen (Tylenol) or ibuprofen (Advil, Motrin, Nuprin).

Herbal Remedies

There are no herbs capable of dealing with this type of emergency.

Nutritional Support

Good nutrition can boost your resistance and protect against infection, but it won't overcome septic shock.

Alternative Treatments

Hyperbaric Oxygen Therapy is a generally accepted supplementary treatment for destructive soft tissue infections. During hyperbaric oxygen therapy, patients inhale 100 percent oxygen under pressure. The oxygen has an antibacterial effect. By itself, however, it can't halt the ravages of septic shock.

Sickle Cell Anemia

The Basics

Painful, debilitating—and presently incurable—sickle cell anemia is limited almost exclusively to people of African descent. It's estimated that from 1 to 3 African-Americans in every 1,000 has this congenital disease. To be afflicted, you must inherit the sickle cell gene from both parents.

The disease works its mischief by deforming some of the red blood cells, turning them sickle-shaped instead of round. This makes them more likely to jam together and block small blood vessels; and it reduces the blood's ability to carry needed oxygen to the body's tissues. The disease usually surfaces at about the age of 6 months. Although there is no cure, your doctor can relieve some of the symptoms.

Pain in the bones is common among sickle cell victims, and children typically suffer from pain in the hands and feet. Attacks called sickle cell crisis are marked by joint and back pain, often accompanied by severe abdominal pain and vomiting. Blood clots may develop in the lungs, kidneys, brain, and other organs. Stubborn sores may develop on the legs.

Other possible symptoms include shortness of breath, paleness, fatigue, weakness, difficulty walking, and liver problems (jaundice). Victims may also suffer from abnormal bone growth, and are liable to severe infections that further deplete the supply of red blood cells. Urinary tract infections are twice as common in women with the sickle cell gene and those infections must receive prompt treatment.

Because of the blood's limited ability to store oxygen, you may need to take special precautions when traveling to higher elevations or taking an airplane flight.

Call Your Doctor If . . .

■ You develop the painful symptoms of a sickle cell crisis.
■ You have a sore that won't get better.

Seek Care Immediately If . . .

■ You have severe chest pain, with or without a cough.
■ You have severe stomach pain, abdominal pain, or constant vomiting.
■ You have severe pain in a bone or joint.
■ You have blood in your urine or urine that appears cloudy.
■ You have fainting spells.

What You Can Do

- Always wear a medic-alert bracelet or necklace stating you have sickle cell anemia.
- Drink at least 8 glasses of water a day—more if you have a fever. This helps keep the cells from blocking blood vessels.
- During a pain crisis:
  - Stay warm.
  - Apply warm compresses to painful parts of your body.
  - Rest in bed.
- To prevent a crisis:
  - Avoid high altitudes. Don't drive in the mountains or use air travel. If you have to fly, take oxygen while you are in the air.
  - Avoid activities that may cause injury.
  - See your doctor immediately if injury or infection occurs.
  - If you become pregnant, see your doctor regularly.
  - Avoid difficult exercise.
  - Avoid cold temperatures.
  - Make sure you and your child have had all the necessary shots, especially the shot protecting you against pneumonia.

What Your Doctor Can Do

To treat sickle cell crisis, the doctor will probably prescribe painkillers, give you oxygen, and have you drink a lot of liquids. Blood transfusions are necessary only when you've suffered a severe loss of red blood cells (often as a result of a severe infection). Pregnant women, however, may need transfusions every 1 to 3 weeks, starting in the first trimester; and a transfusion may help cure the leg sores that sickle cell disease sometimes provokes.

Prescription Drugs

While the pain remains severe, the doctor can prescribe a variety of pain-killing pills. Typical medications include:

DHCplus (acetaminophen with dihydrocodone)
Dilaudid (hydromorphone)
Hydrocet, Lorcet, Lortab, Vicodin, or Zydone (acetaminophen with hydrocodone)
Kadian, MS Contin, or MSIR (morphine)
Levo-Dromoran (levorphanol)
OxyContin, OxyIR, or Roxicodone (oxycodone)
Percocet or Tylox (acetaminophen with oxycodone)

Percodan (aspirin with oxycodone)
Talwin Nx (naloxone)
Toradol (ketorolac)
Tylenol with Codeine (acetaminophen with codeine)
Ultram (tramadol)
Vicoprofen (hydrocodone with ibuprofen)

Over-the-Counter Drugs

Minor aches and pains can be controlled with standard nonprescription painkillers such as aspirin, acetaminophen, or ibuprofen.

Herbal Remedies

There are no herbs known to be helpful for this disease.

Nutritional Support

Supplements such as iron, cobalt, and vitamin B_{12} relieve some forms of anemia, but can't fight sickle cell disease.

Alternative Treatments

A number of alternative therapies have been used effectively to treat chronic pain. They might offer you some relief from the painful symptoms of sickle cell anemia, though they won't remedy the underlying cause.

- *Acupuncture* is often effective for short-term pain relief. It requires the insertion of tiny needles at specific acupoints on the skin. Scientists suspect that the needles trigger the release of natural painkillers within the body. The ancient Chinese believed that they enhanced the flow of vital energy.
- *Biofeedback* captures information about your body's involuntary response to pain, then relays it back to you so you can learn to modify counterproductive reactions.
- *Energy Medicine* preys on desperate patients with a variety of unproven devices. However, there is one technique—transcutaneous electrical nerve stimulation (TENS)—that has been found effective in at least a few trials. It is thought to work by "drowning out" pain signals. It seems most effective against moderate, localized pain.
- *Hypnotherapy* uses the power of suggestion to blunt all forms of chronic pain. Although it doesn't work for everyone, it has proven highly effective for some.
- *Massage Therapy* uses pressure on the body's soft tissue to promote

the flow of blood, relieve pain-induced tension, stimulate the nerves, and loosen muscles and connective tissue.

■ *Meditation,* with its calming mental exercises, is a proven antidote for stress, tension, anxiety—and chronic pain.

■ *Sound Therapy,* in the form of soothing music, can boost the effectiveness of pain medications and further relieve your discomfort.

■ *Therapeutic Touch* is a controversial "laying on of hands" that is sometimes administered by nurses to provide temporary pain relief for hospitalized patients.

Sinusitis

The Basics

The painful symptoms of sinusitis are caused by swelling and irritation in the sinuses (the air spaces behind and above the nose), especially the sinuses located behind the forehead and cheekbones. Typically, you'll have pain, pressure, or swelling around the forehead, cheeks, or eyes that sometimes gets worse when you bend over. You may have a headache, sore throat, fever, chills, a dry cough, or tooth pain. The discharge from your nose may be thick and yellow or green in color.

Sinusitis usually starts when a common cold leads to swelling of the mucous membranes and increased production of mucus. As the sinus passages become swollen and blocked, trapped mucus tends to build up, offering bacteria an inviting breeding ground. Without treatment, the resulting infection will continue and could cause long-term problems.

Sinusitis is not always the fault of a cold. It can also be caused by smoking, hay fever, swimming in dirty water, tooth infection, staying outside in cold, damp weather, or spending a lot of time in dry, indoor heat.

Call Your Doctor If . . .

■ You develop a high temperature.

■ You get nosebleeds.

■ You have a really bad headache that is not eased by over-the-counter medication.

■ You notice swelling over the forehead, eyes, side of the nose, or cheek.

■ Your vision becomes blurred.

Seek Care Immediately If . . .

■ You have trouble breathing and develop a rash, itching, or swelling after taking your medicine. These are warnings of an allergic reaction that can become quite severe.

What You Can Do

■ Use a cool-mist vaporizer or humidifier to add moisture to the air. This will help thin the nasal discharge, allowing it to drain more easily. Steam inhalation also will promote drainage of the sinuses.

■ Be sure to drink 8 to 10 large glasses of water each day. This too keeps the nasal discharge thin.

■ To help ease the pain, put heat on your face and nose with a warm washcloth or an electric heating pad (set on low).

■ Blow your nose gently. In very young children, use a bulb syringe to empty the nose. First, place your thumb on top of the bulb and squeeze it down. Then, still holding the bulb down with your thumb, insert the tip of the syringe into the child's nose. Slowly release your pressure on the bulb. Repeat this 2 or 3 times in each nostril. Do not hold the child's nose closed over the syringe.

■ To help prevent future attacks, wash your hands after touching a person who has a cold and avoid swimming in dirty water.

What Your Doctor Can Do

Your doctor will probably prescribe an antibiotic to kill the bacteria causing the infection. The doctor may also recommend decongestants to help the sinuses drain normally and painkillers to ease your symptoms.

If you have sinusitis frequently, it should prompt your doctor to search for an underlying cause, such as structural abnormalities, allergic rhinitis, or immune deficiency.

Prescription Drugs

Doctors use a variety of antibiotics to eliminate sinus infections. You must finish all the medication prescribed, even if the infection starts to clear up. If you stop treatment too soon, some bacteria may survive and cause a second infection. The most common choices for sinusitis are:

Achromycin V or Sumycin (tetracycline)
Augmentin (amoxicillin)
Biaxin (clarithromycin)
Ceftin (cefuroxime)
Cefzil (cefprozil)

Cipro (ciprofloxacin)
E.E.S., E-Mycin, Eryc, Ery-Tab, Erythrocin, Ilosone,
  or PCE (erythromycin)
Levaquin (levofloxacin)
Lorabid (loracarbef)
Omnipen, Principen, or Totacillin (ampicillin)
Pen-Vee K (penicillin V)

To help drain the sinuses, the doctor may also prescribe one of the following:

Congess or Syn-Rx (guaifenesin, pseudoephedrine)
D.A. II, Duravent/DA, or Extendryl (chlorpheniramine,
  methscopolamine, phenylephrine)
Duravent, Entex LA, or Exgest LA (guaifenesin, phenylpropanolamine)
Fedahist or Kronofed-A (chlorpheniramine, pseudoephedrine)
Nolamine (chlorpheniramine, phenindamine, phenylpropanolamine)
Rynatan (chlorpheniramine, phenylephrine, pyrilamine)

Over-the-Counter Drugs

A number of nonprescription drugs will help drain the sinuses and relieve painful pressure, although they cannot cure the underlying infection. They include:

Afrin	Otrivin	Sinutab
Benzedrex	Privine	Sudafed
Drixoral Nasal	Propagest	Vicks Sinex
Decongestant	Triaminic AM	
Neo-Synephrine	Decongestant	

Some over-the-counter drugs treat both sinus pressure and the pain of sinusitis. These combination medicines include:

Actifed Sinus	Dimetapp Allergy	Sudafed Sinus
Advil Cold and	Sinus	Theraflu Sinus
Sinus	Drixoral	Triaminicin
Benadryl Allergy	Allergy/Sinus	Tylenol Allergy
Sinus Headache	Sinarest	Sinus
Comtrex Allergy-	Sine-Aid	Vicks DayQuil
Sinus	Sine-Off	Sinus Pressure &
Coricidin 'D'	Sinutab Sinus Allergy	Pain Relief

Check with your doctor before taking any sinus medicines if you have heart disease, high blood pressure, thyroid disease, diabetes, glaucoma, enlarged prostate, or breathing problems.

Herbal Remedies

There are no herbs capable of curing a sinus infection, and none that are specifically recommended for sinus inflammation.

Nutritional Support

There are no nutritional strategies specifically recommended for sinusitis.

Alternative Treatments

Environmental medicine sometimes helps nasal congestion and sinus headaches. This medical approach aims to relieve disorders that its practitioners blame on pollutants and toxins in the modern environment. The majority of environmental medicine treatments fall into four categories:

- Nutritional therapies, which use oral and intravenous vitamins, minerals, and other important nutrients.
- Detoxification, which calls for the removal of metals and chemicals from the body.
- Immunotherapy, which involves treatments to strengthen the immune system.
- Desensitization, which is the process of retraining the immune system to eliminate allergies.

Sore Throat

The Basics

Sore throat is one of the most common of all medical complaints. The condition is sometimes a disease in its own right. More often, however, it is just one of a number of problems accompanying an illness such as influenza or a cold.

Typical symptoms include pain, swelling, redness, and a tickle or lump in the throat, a cough, and swollen glands in the neck. You also may have a fever, headache, muscle and joint pain, or ear pain. People with a really bad sore throat may drool, have a constant urge to swallow, or have trouble swallowing and talking. The problem usually clears up in a few days unless there is a more serious underlying disorder.

Ninety percent of the time, sore throat stems from infection with a virus. Allergies or irritation from smoking, alcohol use, or chemical fumes also can cause sore throat. Various bacteria and fungi are other possible culprits.

The streptococcus bacterium, responsible for strep throat, is a common *nonviral* cause of sore throat. Children between the ages of 5 and 10 years get strep throat most frequently—mainly from October through April. Typical symptoms of strep throat include a fever, severe pain and difficulty swallowing, inflamed tonsils, a sore and red throat, a strawberry appearance of the tongue, enlarged lymph nodes, loss of appetite, weakness, malaise, and abdominal discomfort. Left untreated, a strep infection can lead to rheumatic fever.

Call Your Doctor If . . .

■ Your throat pain gets worse or fails to get better in a few days.

■ You develop a high fever.

■ You get a rash anywhere on your skin or the inside of your mouth.

■ You have swollen, tender lumps in your neck.

■ You have a thick discharge from your nose.

■ You have a really bad headache.

■ You cough up green, yellow, brown, or bloody sputum.

Seek Care Immediately If . . .

■ You have trouble breathing or swallowing.

■ You have really bad throat pain or start to drool.

What You Can Do

■ Rest and drink plenty of fluids.

■ Gargle with mouthwash or warm salt water (1 teaspoon salt in 1 cup of water) several times a day. DO NOT SWALLOW the mouthwash or salt water.

■ Sucking on throat lozenges or hard candy may ease the pain. You also can take over-the-counter pain medications, such as acetaminophen and ibuprofen, and use a nonprescription antiseptic throat spray.

■ You can use a cool-mist humidifier (vaporizer) to increase air moisture and help relieve the tight, dry feeling in your throat. Do not use hot steam.

■ Do not smoke or drink alcoholic beverages until the condition clears up.

■ You may be more comfortable if you limit your diet to soft foods or liquids.

■ Do not share food, drinks, or eating utensils while your throat is sore.

What Your Doctor Can Do

Your doctor may have tests done for the presence of bacteria. If a bacterial infection is the cause, the condition can be cured with an antibiotic. However, in the more likely event that a virus is the cause, an antibiotic would be useless and is rarely prescribed.

Prescription Drugs

For strep throat and other bacterial infections, the doctor can choose from a variety of antibiotics. The selection depends on which bacteria are causing your infection, your medical history, and the severity of the infection. Whatever the prescription, be sure to finish it completely. If you don't, a few bacteria may survive and you may suffer a relapse.

Biaxin (clarithromycin)
Ceclor (cefaclor)
Cedax (ceftibuten)
Ceftin (cefuroxime)
Cefzil (cefprozil)
Duricef or Ultracef
  (cefadroxil)
Dynabac (dirithromycin)

E.E.S., E-Mycin, Eryc, Ery-Tab,
  Erythrocin, Ilosone, or PCE
  (erythromycin)
Lorabid (loracarbef)
Pen-Vee K (penicillin V)
Suprax (cefixime)
Vantin (cefpodoxime)
Zithromax (azithromycin)

Over-the-Counter Drugs

You can get a variety of lozenges and sprays to soothe a sore throat without a prescription. Your options include:

Cepacol Sore Throat Lozenges
Cepacol Sore Throat Spray
Cepastat Sore Throat Lozenges
Halls Cough Drops
N'Ice Sore Throat and Cough
  Lozenges

Sucrets
Vicks Chloraseptic Cough &
  Throat Drops and Lozenges
Vicks Chloraseptic Sore Throat
  Spray
Vicks Cough Drops

Over-the-counter painkillers such as Tylenol (acetaminophen), Advil (ibuprofen), and aspirin may also provide some relief. (Avoid aspirin, though, when treating sore throat in a child. If the problem is caused by a virus, aspirin could trigger a serious illness called Reye's syndrome.)

Herbal Remedies

Over the years, a wide assortment of herbs have been found effective for easing the pain of a sore throat. Usually, they are taken as a soothing tea. Possibilities include:

Agrimony	Couch Grass	Onion
Anise	Dill	Peppermint
Balsam	Echinacea	Pine Oil
Balsam of Peru	English Oak	Potentilla
Bilberry	English Plantain	Radish
Blackberry	Galangal	Rhatany
Blackthorn	Garlic	Rose Flower
Brewer's Yeast	Iceland Moss	Sage
Caraway	Jambolan	Sandalwood
Cardamom	Japanese Mint	Slippery Elm
Chamomile	Knotweed	Tormentil
Chinese Cinnamon	Larch	Usnea
Cinnamon	Marigold	White Nettle
Cloves	Mustard	Witch Hazel
Coffee Charcoal	Myrrh	

Nutritional Support

Science is finding evidence to support the use of chicken soup as a remedy. Hot liquids—including chicken soup—break up congestion, relieve sore throat, and increase the flow of nasal secretions. Researchers also have found that chicken soup is capable of reducing the inflammation that causes many cold symptoms, such as sore throat. It is thought that the hundreds of biologically active compounds found in the vegetables used in the soup may be the "good guys."

Alternative Treatments

Alternative medicine offers little relief for sore throat. However, *hyperthermia* treatments may help combat the underlying infection. A typical treatment requires a 20-minute, full-body immersion in water heated to between 101 and 108 degrees Fahrenheit. It is thought that the temperature will kill heat-sensitive germs without damaging the surrounding tissue.

Sprains and Strains

The Basics

Sprains occur when ligaments (the tissues that hold bones together) are suddenly stretched or torn. Strains involve similar damage to the muscles or the tendons that connect the muscles to the bones.

Usually the result of a fall or a twist, most sprains happen around joints such as the knees or knuckles; the ankle is the most common site. Strains are more common during sports and exercise. Both types of injury typically cause pain, tenderness, and swelling in the damaged area. Movement may be difficult.

With rest, a muscle strain may heal in as little as 1 to 2 weeks. Recovery from a sprain takes longer, usually 4 to 8 weeks (and even more if the injury is really severe). An elastic bandage is often needed to protect the damaged tissue from additional stress. A severe sprain or strain may require a splint.

Call Your Doctor If . . .

■ Bruising, swelling, or pain gets worse.

■ The fingers or toes near the injury become cold, numb, or blue.

Seek Care Immediately If . . .

■ You experience severe pain.

What You Can Do

■ Keep ice on the injury for 15 to 20 minutes each hour for the first 1 or 2 days. Put the ice in a plastic bag and place a towel between the bag and your skin.

■ After the first 1 or 2 days, you may put heat on the injury for the next 48 hours to help relieve the pain. Apply the heat for 15 to 20 minutes every hour. You may use a heating pad (set on low), a whirlpool bath, or warm, moist towels.

■ For 48 hours, keep the injury lifted above the level of your heart whenever possible. This will reduce pain and swelling.

■ Your doctor will tell you how long to rest the injured area. Then slowly start using the joint as the pain allows. If you have a sprained ankle, use crutches or a cane until you can stand on the ankle without suffering pain.

■ If you are given an elastic bandage (ace wrap), keep wearing it as long as your doctor recommends. Take it off at least once a day. If you have numbness or tingling below the injury, the bandage is too tight. Take it off and rewrap it more loosely.

■ If you are given a plaster splint:
- Wear it until your doctor says you may take it off or until your follow-up visit.
- Do not push or lean on it. This could cause it to break.
- Do not get it wet. You may take it off to shower.

■ If you have an air splint:
- You may adjust the inflation to make it more comfortable.
- You may take it off at night and when bathing.

■ To prevent sprains and strains, warm up your muscles and ligaments before you exercise. Gently stretching your muscles is one good warm-up; your doctor can show you others. Before heavy exercise, wrap weak joints with support bandages.

What Your Doctor Can Do

Your doctor may order an x-ray of the injury to make sure you have not broken a bone. You'll be given an elastic bandage or a splint as needed to promote healing.

Prescription Drugs

While the pain remains severe, the doctor can prescribe a variety of pain-killing pills. Typical medications include:

DHCplus (acetaminophen with dihydrocodone)
Dilaudid (hydromorphone)
Hydrocet, Lorcet, Lortab, Vicodin, or Zydone
  (acetaminophen with hydrocodone)
Kadian, MS Contin, or MSIR (morphine)
Levo-Dromoran (levorphanol)
OxyContin, OxyIR, or Roxicodone (oxycodone)
Percocet or Tylox (acetaminophen with oxycodone)
Percodan (aspirin with oxycodone)
Talwin Nx (naloxone)
Toradol (ketorolac)
Tylenol with Codeine (acetaminophen with codeine)
Ultram (tramadol)
Vicoprofen (hydrocodone with ibuprofen)

Over-the-Counter Drugs

As the pain subsides, a nonprescription painkiller should provide satisfactory relief. Your options include:

Actron	Bufferin	Orudis KT
Advil	Excedrin	Panadol
Aleve	Excedrin, Aspirin-	St. Joseph
Alka-Seltzer	Free	Tylenol
Ascriptin	Goody's	Unisom with Pain
Ascriptin, Enteric	Motrin IB	Relief
Bayer Aspirin	Nuprin	Vanquish
BC Powder		

Herbal Remedies

If you want to avoid over-the-counter drugs, there are two herbs that can help with the pain: Japanese mint and white willow.

Nutritional Support

During recovery, be sure to eat an ample, balanced diet. Don't skimp on meat and dairy products, which help to supply the proteins and amino acids needed for healing.

Alternative Treatments

Magnetic Field Therapy: Advocates of this type of therapy say that it's especially good for muscle and joint pain. While the use of small magnets for this purpose is generally considered safe, its effectiveness is still under dispute.

Myotherapy: This specialized form of deep muscle massage is said to quickly relieve any sort of muscle-related pain, including the pain caused by sprains.

Reconstructive Therapy: This form of treatment seeks to stimulate the growth of healthy tissue with a series of injections directly into the damaged joint. Injections usually contain the anesthetic lidocaine, an irritant such as sodium morrhuate, dextrose, phenol, minerals, amino acid supplements, and B complex vitamins. They have been found effective in several clinical trials.

Strep Throat

The Basics

This painful infection is named for its cause—the streptococcal bacteria that invade and inflame the throat. These germs spread easily from person to person in the home, at school or day care, or at work. Smoking, fatigue, and exposure to cold, wet weather increase your chances of catching the illness.

Typical symptoms include pain, swelling, redness, and, perhaps, a tickle or lump in the throat; plus swollen glands in the neck. You may also develop fever and a headache. People with a severe case often drool or have trouble swallowing and talking. Children with the infection may be fussy and cry frequently. Due to the pain of swallowing, they may refuse to eat or drink.

Unlike colds, flu, and many of the most common childhood ailments, strep throat can be cured with antibiotics. See your doctor for a diagnosis. If the problem is strep, it can be relieved in 2 or 3 days. Get treatment even if the sore throat begins to go away on its own. An untreated strep infection can lead to ear infections, sinus infections, and the dangerous disease known as rheumatic fever, which can permanently damage the heart.

Call Your Doctor If . . .

- You develop a high temperature, or your fever lasts more than 48 hours.
- You have large and tender lumps in your neck.
- You get a rash, a cough, or a pain in your ears.
- You cough up green, yellow-brown, or bloody sputum.

Seek Care Immediately If . . .

- You develop any new symptoms such as throwing up, really bad headache, stiff neck, chest pain, shortness of breath, or trouble breathing or swallowing.
- Your throat pain gets worse and you start drooling, or notice changes in your voice.
- A child with strep becomes increasingly sleepy, is unable to wake up completely, or grows irritable.

What You Can Do

- To ease the pain in your throat, suck on hard candy or cough drops. Adults and children over 8 years of age should gargle with 1 teaspoon of salt in 8 ounces of warm water or strong tea (warm or cold). Younger children can be given a teaspoon of honey or corn syrup several times a day. (Do not give honey to children under 1 year of age.)

■ Using a cool-mist humidifier in the sickroom also may help.

■ For swollen and tender lumps in the neck, apply a moist, warm towel to the area several times a day for 30 to 60 minutes. To prevent burns, keep the compresses warm but not hot.

■ Over-the-counter medicines such as acetaminophen and ibuprofen can help relieve fever and pain

■ If your doctor has prescribed antibiotics, be sure to finish all the medication. If you stop treatment too soon, some bacteria may survive and cause additional problems.

■ Do not smoke or drink alcohol. Try not to cough, clear your throat, sing, or talk a lot.

■ Try to get as much rest and sleep as possible.

■ Don't share food or drinks with anyone until your treatment is finished. Get a new toothbrush.

■ You may return to work or school 24 hours after starting antibiotics.

What Your Doctor Can Do

To check for strep bacteria, the doctor will swab a sample from the back of your throat and send it for analysis—a procedure called a throat culture. If the test reveals strep, you'll be prescribed an antibiotic to get rid of the germs.

Prescription Drugs

Several antibiotics have proven especially effective for strep throat. Included are:

Ceclor (cefaclor)
Duricef (cefadroxil)
E.E.S., Ilosone, or PCE
 (erythromycin)
Keftab (cefadroxil)

Omnicef (cefdinir)
Spectrobid (bacampicillin)
Suprax (cefixime)
Tao (troleandomycin)

Over-the-Counter Drugs

To ease the pain of sore throat, there are a variety of nonprescription lozenges and sprays:

Cepacol Sore Throat Lozenges
Cepacol Sore Throat Spray

Cepastat Sore Throat Lozenges
Halls Cough Drops

N'Ice Sore Throat and Cough
Lozenges
Sucrets
Vicks Chloraseptic Cough &
Throat Drops
Vicks Chloraseptic Sore Throat
Lozenges
Vicks Chloraseptic Sore Throat
Spray
Vicks Cough Drops

To relieve fever and pain accompanying strep throat, the following nonprescription painkillers may help:

Actron	Bufferin	Orudis KT
Advil	Goody's	Panadol
Aleve	Motrin IB	St. Joseph
Bayer	Nuprin	Tylenol
BC Powder		

Herbal Remedies

A tremendous variety of herbs are soothing to the throat. All of the following are considered at least somewhat effective:

Agrimony	Couch Grass	Onion
Anise	Dill	Peppermint
Balsam	Echinacea	Pine Oil
Balsam of Peru	English Oak	Potentilla
Bilberry	English Plantain	Radish
Blackberry	Galangal	Rhatany
Blackthorn	Garlic	Rose Flower
Brewer's Yeast	Iceland Moss	Sage
Caraway	Jambolan	Sandalwood
Cardamom	Japanese Mint	Slippery Elm
Chamomile	Knotweed	Tormentil
Chinese Cinnamon	Larch	Usnea
Cinnamon	Marigold	White Nettle
Cloves	Mustard	Witch Hazel
Coffee Charcoal	Myrrh	

Nutritional Support

Drink 8 to 10 large glasses of water each day. If your throat is too sore to eat solid food, drink milk, milk shakes, and soups. Resume a normal diet as soon as you feel better.

Alternative Treatments

Hyperthermia: Advocates say this style of treatment can destroy heat-sensitive germs and rid the body of toxins. One approach calls for a 30-minute soak in water heated to 108 degrees Fahrenheit. Do-it-yourself hyperthermia is not advisable due to the extremely high temperatures it requires. See a naturopathic physician if you want such treatments.

Stress

The Basics

This turn-of-the-century buzzword gets the blame for a breathtaking range of ailments, yet it's very difficult to pin down. What seems stressful to one individual may not bother another at all. And some folks seem to thrive on pressure, while others just get sick.

Technically, any source of stress is called a stressor. These stress-building events range from minor, daily annoyances to major changes in your life. Sickness or death of a friend or family member causes great stress. So do conflicts with your spouse or partner; moving; having a baby; dealing with money problems; and trying to do more than you have time for. Getting fired puts you under major stress, as does starting a new job or retiring. Joyous occasions as well as difficult ones can be stressful, but difficult ones take a greater toll.

When confronted with a stressful situation, your body responds with a chain of biochemical reactions that can affect your entire system. Any real or imagined emergency sets in motion a series of changes designed to enable you to fight or flee the danger. Responding to triggers from the brain, the adrenal glands release adrenaline and other hormones into your bloodstream. Immediately, your heart rate and blood pressure increase, your pupils dilate, and you feel a heightened sense of alertness.

A string of stressful problems, even if minor, can cause your body to build up a response that's as dramatic as a reaction to a serious threat. And if it continues, this unrelieved stress will keep your body in a constant state of alert that can seriously affect your health. Emotional stress has been known to intensify allergies, promote chronic high blood pressure, and foster serious heart ailments.

People under stress are typically anxious, tense, and moody. But physical reactions to stress are highly individual. You may also experience:

- Skin disorders, such as hives or acne
- Digestive disorders, such as stomach pain or diarrhea
- Wheezing
- Stuffy nose
- Changes in your period
- Headaches
- Back and neck pain
- Fatigue
- Difficulty sleeping
- Trouble having sex

Stress can affect your body's immune response and make you more vulnerable to illness. Clinical studies show a relationship between stress and lower resistance to infection. For example, people under stress are more prone to contract common colds.

Call Your Doctor If . . .
- You feel your problems are getting the best of you and you can no longer deal with them on your own.

Seek Care Immediately If . . .
- You feel an urge to hurt yourself or someone else.

What You Can Do
- Talk things over with your family and friends. Sharing your concerns and worries will help relieve tension.
- Don't blame yourself if things don't always go right.
- Learn what things make you feel tense, and either avoid them or learn how to deal with them better.
- Deal with your problems one at a time. Trying to take care of everything at once may seem overwhelming. List the things you need to do and then start with the most important one.
- Do not use alcohol or drugs to relieve stress. They do not solve the underlying problems—and they can quickly become habit-forming.
- Organize your house or your workspace. Get rid of things you don't need.
- Exercise at least 3 times a week. Exercise helps to reduce tension.
- Take a short time-out period when you feel stressed out during the day. Close your eyes and take some deep breaths.
- Try some of the alternative treatments listed below. These tried-and-true techniques will help you relax and limit the effects of stress.

- Take good care of yourself. Eat a balanced diet and get plenty of sleep.
- Make time for fun. Take a break from your daily routine to relax. Take a walk, a vacation, a nap, or an educational course.
- Join a support group or attend workshops on the issues that are causing your stress.

Insomnia is one of the most common signs of stress. Follow these do's and don'ts if you have problems with sleeplessness:

Do:

- Eat dinner early; make it light on fat and heavy on complex carbohydrates.
- Check with your doctor to see if your medications are a problem. Over-the-counter cold remedies and diet pills can cause wakefulness.
- Try a glass of warm milk.
- Set yourself a regular sleep schedule. Go to bed and arise at the same time every day.
- Take a warm relaxing bath a couple of hours before bedtime.
- Use relaxation exercises.
- Aim for a peaceful evening. Save conflicts with family members for the daylight hours.
- Leave yourself some "wind-down" time for an hour or two before you go to bed.

Don't:

- Drink alcoholic beverages in an attempt to get sleepy. You'll only disrupt your sleep pattern.
- Read, work, or watch television in bed. If you can't sleep, get up and go to another room.
- Have a heavy meal close to bedtime.
- Let a night or two of insomnia upset you. Worrying about sleep only makes it harder.

What Your Doctor Can Do

There is no instant cure for excessive stress. Your doctor may suggest meditation or muscle relaxation exercises to relieve the problem, or refer you for counseling in stress-management techniques.

Prescription Drugs

Medications can't relieve stress, but they can ease some of the more troubling symptoms it causes. Doctors sometimes prescribe antispasmodic drugs such as Donnatal and Bentyl, or low doses of antidepressants, to ease spasms in the digestive tract. Your doctor can also prescribe a medication such as Zantac, Tagamet, or Pepcid to reduce the amount of acid your stomach produces because of stress.

Over-the-Counter Drugs

You can relieve the effects of stress on your digestive system by using Mylanta, Maalox, or a nonprescription version of the acid-blocking drugs Zantac, Tagamet, and Pepcid. For headaches and insomnia, you can take a remedy such as Bayer PM, Excedrin P.M., Tylenol PM, or Unisom with Pain Relief.

Herbal Remedies

A wide variety of herbs will help relieve stress-related indigestion and insomnia. Turn to those profiles for a complete list.

Nutritional Support

Stress prompts some of us to overeat or snack on junk food. Yet this kind of diet can actually intensify the level of emotional stress you experience. There's no substitute for a well-balanced diet to help your body handle the ravages of stress. Keep your blood sugar at a constant level by eating smaller meals supplemented with healthy snacks, and by eating complex carbohydrates.

While researchers have yet to prove a connection between psychological stress and the need for vitamin supplements, nutritionists often recommend a diet high in antioxidants, including vitamins C, E, beta-carotene, and B-complex. Long periods of stress may deplete protein, calcium, potassium, zinc, magnesium, vitamin A, pantothenic acid, vitamin E, and linoleic acid. No amount of vitamins, however, can relieve the symptoms of stress.

Whether you take nutrient supplements or not, follow these tips for a healthy diet:

Include . . .
■ Raw fruits and vegetables
■ Complex carbohydrates
■ More fish and poultry
■ A good breakfast every day
■ Low-fat foods

Be sparing with . . .
- Refined sugar
- Salt
- Alcoholic and caffeinated beverages
- Fatty and fried foods

Alternative Treatments

The following alternative treatments for stress generally attempt to improve your ability to relax your body and focus your mind:

- *Alexander Technique* is a treatment that seeks to reduce stress-related disorders by encouraging you to shed ingrained and inappropriate muscular reactions, allowing healthy natural reflexes to take over.
- *Aromatherapy* uses highly concentrated essential oils extracted from healing herbs as a comforting ritual to reduce stress, enhance relaxation, relieve anxiety, and provide respite from insomnia.
- *Aston-Patterning* is a program of physical training and massage designed to relieve muscle tension and reduce stress.
- *Biofeedback* is a painless electronic training technique that captures information about your body's involuntary response to stressors, then relays it back to you so you can learn to modify these previously unwitting reactions.
- *Guided Imagery* seeks to make beneficial physical changes in the body by repeatedly visualizing positive images.
- *Hellerwork* is a combination of deep tissue massage and movement reeducation. Its goal is to help you get in touch with different parts of your body, and the emotions that affect it, in order to correct abnormal muscle tension.
- *Massage Therapy* uses systematic manual application of pressure and movement to the soft tissues of the body to relieve symptoms of anxiety, tension, insomnia, and stress.
- *Meditation* promotes relaxation by emptying the mind of all outside distractions. It has been practiced for centuries and is frequently recommended today as an excellent way to ease stress.
- *Qigong* is a Chinese discipline of exercises used to reduce stress and anxiety. By alleviating tension, it also may combat insomnia and relieve headaches.
- *Reflexology* is based on the belief that the foot is a microcosm of the entire body and pressing on various reflex points along the foot can

relieve symptoms elsewhere in the body. Proponents say it's especially helpful for stress-related symptoms.

■ *Relaxation* exercises use special breathing techniques to reduce symptoms of stress. Slow, deep breaths help you calm down and become more peaceful.

■ *Rolfing* uses vigorous, deep-tissue massage to provide relief from stress. Rolfers apply slow, sliding pressure with their knuckles, thumbs, fingers, elbows, and knees; this type of treatment can cause some pain.

■ *Sound Therapy* uses low-pitched, slow, soft music to calm or sedate, induce sleep, and reduce tension.

■ *Yoga* uses an age-old set of exercises that combine prescribed postures, breathing, and meditation to promote relaxation and reduce stress.

Stroke

The Basics

Stroke is one of the most dreaded of all medical emergencies. But thanks to recent advances in medicine, it no longer need be a catastrophe.

A stroke occurs when a blood vessel serving the brain either bursts or gets blocked. Deprived of the oxygen that the bloodstream normally supplies, cells in the affected area of the brain quickly become damaged or die, leading to a loss of function in the parts of the body that the cells control. The longer the blood supply is disrupted, the greater the likelihood of lasting damage.

Symptoms may appear in the first few minutes after a stroke, or may take hours to develop. Either way, you need to seek treatment as soon as possible, since the ideal window for successful treatment of a major stroke is only the first 6 hours after symptoms occur. Left untreated, the symptoms will continue, often ending in permanent disability.

A major stroke is likely to cause paralysis on one side of the body. (Only one side is affected because each side of the brain controls the other side of the body.) A stroke in the left side of the brain can also lead to problems with speech and language. A stroke in the right side typically causes problems with perception and behavior. Any stroke, regardless of the side, is likely to cause memory problems and mood swings.

The risk of stroke is highest among people with high blood pressure, diabetes, or high cholesterol. Smokers and overweight individuals are also in greater danger.

Call Your Doctor If . . .

When recovering from a stroke, you develop any of the following problems:

- During exercise, you suffer chest pain that continues when you rest.
- You have trouble with any of your therapy or exercises.
- You develop pressure sores on your skin.
- You have a high temperature.
- Your blood pressure is high.

Seek Care Immediately If . . .

Because fast treatment is crucial, it's important to remember these warning signs of stroke. **Call 911 or 0 (operator) immediately** to get to the nearest hospital if you or someone you're with experiences one or more of the following:

- Sudden weakness or paralysis in an arm, hand, or leg, occurring on one or both sides of the body
- Sudden numbness on one side of the face or body
- Sudden blurred vision in one or both eyes
- Difficulty in speaking or understanding simple statements
- Sudden severe headache
- Difficulty swallowing
- Dizziness, loss of balance, or an unexplained fall

What You Can Do

To reduce your risk of a stroke:
- If you have high blood pressure, keep it under control. High blood pressure is the single most important factor contributing to stroke. It not only promotes clogging of the arteries, but also puts unneeded strain on blood vessel walls.
- Adopt a low-fat, high-fiber diet to keep your arteries clear. Most strokes (80 percent) are caused by a clot lodged in a fat-clogged artery. If you're overweight, a low-fat diet will also help you shed pounds.

- Get regular exercise. It improves circulation and helps keep your blood pressure in check.
- If you're a smoker, try to quit. Smokers face triple the odds of a stroke. For smokers with high blood pressure, the risk can be as much as 20 times greater than for nonsmokers.

To speed recovery from stroke:

- If your doctor recommends daily aspirin, be sure to take it regularly. It helps thin the blood so blood clots won't form. Do not take other painkillers such as acetaminophen or ibuprofen instead. They do not have aspirin's blood-thinning properties.
- Check your blood pressure regularly. You may want to buy a blood pressure cuff. Ask your doctor to show you or a family member how to use it.
- You may not be able to feel hot and cold as well as you did before the stroke. To keep from burning yourself, test the water carefully before bathing.
- You may need to put in special ramps and side rails in your home to help you get around safely.
- Arrange any therapy sessions your doctor orders for the time of day when you have the most energy. Work closely with the therapists. To assure maximum recovery, you must perform the exercises as faithfully as possible, according to a step-by-step recovery plan.
- With your doctor's permission, exercise daily. It will protect your general health and reduce the chances of another stroke.

What Your Doctor Can Do

Treatment is aimed at restoring the brain's blood supply as quickly as possible. If the stroke is due to blockage by a clot, the doctor can use clot-busting drugs and blood thinners to reopen the artery. A blockage in one of the two carotid arteries serving the brain may call for an operation (a carotid endarterectomy) to remove the buildup of fatty plaque. If the problem is due to an aneurysm (a bulging blood vessel that is bleeding or likely to rupture) surgery to clip the artery may be in order.

Once the crisis has passed, the doctor may prescribe physical, occupational, and speech therapy to help bring physical and mental function back to normal. You can expect the most dramatic improvement in the first few months after the stroke, but even though the rate of recovery may be slow, continued efforts will yield further gains.

Prescription Drugs

The clot-busting drug Activase (alteplase) is now accepted therapy for clot-induced strokes, if it can be given within 3 hours of the onset of symptoms. Other clot-busters are used on an experimental basis. They include Abbokinase (urokinase), Eminase (anistreplase), and Streptase (streptokinase).

Heparin, an intravenous drug that prevents additional clots from forming, may be given along with a clot buster when you arrive at the hospital. Later, to help provide long-term protection once the crisis is past, you may be given blood-thinning pills such as Coumadin (warfarin), Plavix (clopidogrel), or Ticlid (ticlopidine).

If you are afflicted with dangerously high cholesterol levels, there are two cholesterol-lowering drugs that experts now agree can lower your risk of stroke: Pravachol (pravastatin) and Zocor (simvastatin).

Over-the-Counter Drugs

Daily aspirin is recommended for some—but not all—victims of clot-induced stroke. Check with your doctor before using it. If there is any danger of internal bleeding, it may not be appropriate.

Herbal Remedies

There are no herbs that can remedy a stroke. However, herbs that fight clogged arteries can reduce your risk of one. For more information, see the entry on clogged arteries.

Nutritional Support

A low-fat diet is imperative if you've suffered a clot-induced stroke—and a good preventive measure for anyone with high cholesterol levels. See the entry on clogged arteries for details.

If high blood pressure is a problem, you'll probably need to cut back on salt. See the entry on high blood pressure for more information.

Alternative Treatments

Do NOT seek alternative therapy when faced with a stroke. Your best hope lies in getting to a hospital as quickly as possible. When *recovering* from a stroke, however, you may find that some of the following can aid your rehabilitation:

Acupuncture: This form of treatment relies on insertion of tiny needles at designated points on the skin to promote beneficial changes inside the body. Some researchers feel it's capable of speeding rehabilitation and limiting damage after a paralyzing stroke.

Alexander Technique: Aimed at bringing the body's muscles into natural harmony, this type of exercise boosts strength and mobility, and is sometimes recommended to improve functioning in people with stroke.

Feldenkrais Method: With an emphasis on improving the patient's patterns of movement, this method is often used as supportive therapy for people recovering from neuromuscular disorders such as stroke.

Hypnotherapy: Hypnosis uses the power of suggestion to help people control emotions, habits, and even the body's involuntary responses. It has been known to provide relief from spasms and paralysis.

Sound Therapy: Carefully selected music has beneficial effects on a wide variety of problems—including the difficulty with walking sometimes caused by stroke.

Substance Abuse

The Basics

It's estimated that 17 percent of Americans over the age of 18 will have a substance abuse problem at some time in their life. It can begin as early as childhood, or surface only in the later years. While scientists still don't understand why some people are more prone to substance abuse than others, recent studies suggest that there may be genetic similarities among people afflicted with the problem. It also appears to be associated with other psychological disorders such as depression.

The "substances" that invite habitual misuse or dependence include a broad range of legal and illegal products. Among the most widely abused are alcohol; prescription medications such as narcotics (used for pain), benzodiazepines (for anxiety and insomnia), amphetamines (for attention deficit disorder and excess weight), and barbiturates (sedatives); and illegal drugs such as cocaine, heroin, marijuana, hallucinogens, or inhalants.

Although abusers often become physically dependent on a substance, a psychological dependence (addiction) can be just as damaging. Sustained misuse of alcohol or drugs can destroy physical health and quality of life. It interferes with the ability to function effectively, maintain a normal family life, and hold a job—and can ultimately lead to life-threatening medical problems.

Even in the face of severe family, career, or legal difficulties, someone who has grown dependent on a substance tends to continue using it, while, for the most part, denying the problem. Nevertheless, for anyone who can no longer control their use of medications, drugs, or alcohol, there's no question that a problem exists.

Call Your Doctor If . . .

- You need the substance daily to function normally.
- You have tried, but failed, to stop using the substance.
- Your problems are getting the best of you and you can't seem to deal with them on your own.
- You have driven while intoxicated.
- You have done something to obtain or use the substance that you would not ordinarily do.
- You cannot fight the need to take more drugs or alcohol.

Seek Care Immediately If . . .

- After overcoming a habit, you start abusing again.
- You pass out, have a seizure, or suffer hallucinations.
- You have chest pain, sweating, or trouble breathing.
- You get a severe headache, stomach pain, or a numb, prickly, or burning sensation in your arms or legs.
- You feel confused, very nervous, or suicidal.

What You Can Do

- It's a cliché, but still true: First, you must admit you have a problem. Then you need to ask for help from someone you trust.
- Don't try to quit all at once on your own. With many substances—particularly narcotics, sedatives, and tranquilizers—you will need medical help to get through a gradual withdrawal period.
- Tell your doctor exactly how much of the substance you are taking—and if you are taking any other medications. Be honest. The doctor needs the complete picture in order to plan the most effective treatment.
- While undergoing treatment, don't smoke or drink coffee. They can make you nervous and increase your withdrawal symptoms.
- Support group meetings and counseling can help you quit. Take advantage of both.
- Stay away from anyone who uses the substance or encourages its use.

■ Find new things to do. Get out of the house every day. Go for walks outside.

■ Eat a healthy diet, drink plenty of fluids each day, get plenty of rest, and, with your doctor's approval, start an exercise program.

■ Remember that the best insurance against developing a dependence on "recreational" drugs is to completely avoid them.

What Your Doctor Can Do

Any substance abuse problem must be evaluated by a doctor to determine the extent of the problem and the best course of treatment. Long-standing abuse can cause a variety of physical problems, so your physician will probably want to do a standard medical exam before embarking on a treatment program. Hospitalization for withdrawal under medical supervision may be necessary. The doctor might also recommend a stay at an inpatient drug and alcohol center, where you can spend three weeks or more in a drug-free, therapeutic environment designed to help you establish a new pattern of behavior. At a minimum, you'll probably be referred to a counselor to address the psychological aspects of recovery, and enrolled in a program that offers regular meetings with a support group.

Prescription Drugs

Depending on the source of your problem, your doctor may prescribe medication to reduce the symptoms of withdrawal and block the physical cravings that can result in further substance abuse.

For acute alcohol withdrawal, a tranquilizer is the usual prescription. Typical choices include Librium (chlordiazepoxide), Serax (oxazepam), Serentil (mesoridazine), Tranxene (clorazepate), Valium (diazepam), and Vistaril (hydroxyzine). To quell the craving for alcohol, ReVia (naltrexone) may be prescribed. Antabuse (disulfiram) discourages a relapse by causing a severe reaction, including nausea and vomiting, whenever you take a drink.

If narcotic abuse is the problem, methadone can ease withdrawal. ReVia is prescribed to block the effects of narcotics. The oral drug Orlamm (levomethadyl) both relieves withdrawal symptoms and prevents a narcotic high.

Over-the-Counter Drugs

There are no over-the-counter drugs capable of relieving substance abuse.

Herbal Remedies

No herbs are known to have an impact on substance abuse. However, St. John's wort can be helpful for the depression and anxiety that often accompany this problem.

Nutritional Support

Poor nutrition often accompanies substance abuse, so it's important to build up your diet with plenty of proteins, fresh fruits and vegetables, and complex carbohydrates (whole grains, rice, beans). Avoid junk foods and highly processed sugary or fatty foods that provide little in the way of nutrition. Take a good quality, well-balanced multivitamin and mineral supplement each day.

Alternative Treatments

Acupuncture: This ancient Chinese therapy relies on hair-thin needles inserted at special acupoints on the skin to redirect the flow of a hypothetical vital force called qi. Although researchers have yet to find a physical reason for acupuncture's effect, it has been used successfully to ease withdrawal from drugs and alcohol.

Biofeedback: Using special monitoring equipment to report physiological reactions, this special form of training allows people to gain control over otherwise involuntary physical responses. Some people have found it helpful in overcoming drug or alcohol dependence.

Hypnotherapy: For those who are susceptible to the relaxed, trance-like state induced by hypnosis, its enhanced powers of positive suggestion can help break an unwanted substance habit.

Syphilis

The Basics

This common sexually transmitted disease can be dangerously deceptive. Although it may seem to go away without treatment, unless it is cured with antibiotics it will return later, spread, and attack almost any part of the body including the skin, heart, blood vessels, and brain. The early symptoms present an opportunity for a quick, easy cure. Ignoring them invites severe complications many years later.

The disease is caused by a type of bacteria called *Treponema pallidum*. It is spread by vaginal, oral, and anal sex, and sometimes by heavy kissing. You are at greatest risk of getting syphilis if you or your partner have multiple or casual sex partners. From one act of unprotected sex with an infected person, you have a 30 percent chance of getting syphilis.

Syphilis has three stages, each with different symptoms.

■ During the first stage (usually 3 to 4 weeks after infection), a red sore appears on the mouth, penis, rectum, vagina, or, sometimes, another part of the body. It usually doesn't hurt, and many people don't even notice it. Even though this sore disappears on its own within 1 to 2 months, the infection will remain. During this stage, the germs can be spread to others during sex.

■ The second stage occurs about 6 to 12 weeks after infection. A small, red, scaly rash appears on the skin, mouth, and sex organs. Many people also have swollen glands, headache, fever, upset stomach, a stiff neck, and fatigue. The disease remains contagious during this stage.

■ The third stage, which may take place years later, can produce a variety of symptoms. Skin sores and bone pain are especially common. If the infection spreads to the brain, the victim may lose the ability to think clearly. Other symptoms include loss of balance, lack of feeling in the arms or legs, and even paralysis. Some people have heart problems. By this stage, the disease is no longer infectious.

Call Your Doctor If . . .
■ During or after treatment, you have a high temperature, a new rash, sore throat, swelling in a joint, or any new symptoms.

Seek Care Immediately If . . .
Although treatment should never be put off, syphilis is unlikely to cause an emergency.

What You Can Do
■ It is important to follow your doctor's instructions carefully. Syphilis usually can be cured in the early stages, but only if you take antibiotics exactly as prescribed. Remember that the symptoms can clear up on their own, so an improvement doesn't necessarily mean the germs have been eradicated. If any remain, the infection will return unexpectedly after many years in hiding.

■ A few hours after beginning antibiotics, you may get a fever, severe chills, headache, upset stomach, and muscle aches. The rash may get worse. These symptoms last about 24 hours. Rest in bed. Take over-the-counter painkillers such as aspirin, acetaminophen, or ibuprofen to reduce the fever and ease the pain.

■ As many as 13 weeks can pass between the initial infection and the first symptoms. Tell anyone with whom you've had sex during the past 3 months that you have syphilis. They may be infected and need treatment.

■ Don't have sex until your doctor tells you the infection is cured. This usually takes at least 2 months. After that, use a condom for protection against syphilis and other infections.

■ If you are pregnant, discuss the situation with your doctor. A pregnant woman can pass syphilis on to her baby before it is born, and the infection can cause birth defects or even death.

What Your Doctor Can Do

A shot of penicillin is the best treatment. If you are allergic to penicillin, the doctor can prescribe an oral antibiotic. A blood test will be done at three months to see if the infection is gone, and again at 6 months. A spinal tap to test cerebral spinal fluid for syphilis will probably be conducted one year after treatment.

Prescription Drugs

If you need to take oral antibiotics, the doctor can prescribe one of the following:

Achromycin V (tetracycline)
Declomycin (demeclocycline)
Doryx, Monodox, or
  Vibramcyin (doxycycline)
Dynacin, Minocin, or Vectrin
  (minocycline)

E.E.S., EryPed, Ery-Tab,
  Erythrocin, Ilosone, or PCE
  (erythromycin)
Terramycin (oxytetracycline)

Over-the-Counter Drugs

Nonprescription painkillers can ease some of the symptoms that accompany treatment with antibiotics, but they have no beneficial effect on the underlying infection.

Herbal Remedies

In bygone days, people attempted to cure syphilis with a variety of herbs. None, however, really work.

Nutritional Support

There are no dietary measures that will help in this situation.

Alternative Therapies

To make certain that you're rid of this problem—and not just between stages—there's really no alternative to antibiotics.

Tension Headache

The Basics

A simple tension headache usually lasts a few hours and has no other symptoms. Among the many culprits are tension, stress, eye or muscle strain, depression, allergic reactions, changes in sleeping patterns, colds and flu, alcohol, caffeine, certain foods and medicines, and weather changes. Variations in hormone levels during a woman's monthly cycle can also be at fault. Sometimes the cause is unknown.

Pain from a tension headache is typically steady rather than throbbing, and affects both sides of the head. In addition, muscles in your neck or head may feel tight. You may wake up with a headache and be unable to get back to sleep. Tension headaches can occur at any age and often run in the family.

Most people have an occasional tension headache, but some people suffer them chronically. To be labeled chronic, the headache must occur more than 15 times per month.

Call Your Doctor If . . .

■ Your headache gets worse or lasts longer than 24 hours.
■ You develop a high temperature.
■ You need to take medicine frequently to relive headache pain.

Seek Care Immediately If . . .

■ Your headache is different from or significantly worse than any headache you've ever had before.
■ You feel confused or drowsy.
■ Your neck feels stiff.
■ Your temperature becomes extremely high.
■ You have eye problems such as sensitivity to light or blurred or double vision.
■ You start to vomit.

What You Can Do

To relieve a tension headache:

■ Try stretching and massaging the muscles in your shoulders, neck, jaw, and scalp.

■ Take a hot bath.

■ Rest in a quiet, darkened room. Place a warm or cold wet cloth (whichever feels better) over the aching area.

■ Get a good night's sleep. It's often the best way to relieve a headache.

To prevent tension headaches:

■ Don't skip or delay meals. Drink plenty of liquids.

■ To help your doctor diagnose the problem, keep a headache diary containing all the circumstances that surround your headaches, such as the time of day, what you ate and drank, what medications you took, who you were with and what you were doing, and how the headache felt.

■ Learn to relax.

What Your Doctor Can Do

You can treat a simple tension headache just as effectively as the doctor, who usually will just recommend over-the-counter pain relievers. However, if a tension headache keeps recurring or becomes chronic, you should see the doctor to make certain that there's no serious underlying cause. To check for abnormalities, he will probably do a routine medical exam, order blood tests, and have some pictures taken with an x-ray, a CAT scan, or an MRI. He may also want an *electroencephalograph (EEG)* to check electrical activity in the brain.

Prescription Drugs

Prescription pain relievers are generally not needed for true tension headaches. However, if over-the-counter remedies fail to do the job, the doctor can prescribe a combination product such as the following:

Esgic-plus or Fioricet (acetaminophen, butalbital, caffeine)
Fioricet with Codeine (acetaminophen, butalbital, caffeine, codeine)
Fiorinal (aspirin, butalbital, caffeine)
Fiorinal with Codeine (aspirin, butalbital, caffeine, codeine)
Phrenilin or Sedapap (acetaminophen, butalbital)

If these products don't work, some doctors turn to prescription nonsteroidal anti-inflammatory drugs such as Naprosyn, Anaprox, Ponstel, Meclomen, Tolectin, and Toradol.

If you suffer from chronic tension headaches, your doctor may suggest you take medicine *prophylactically* to help prevent them from starting. The major prescription drugs used to prevent chronic tension headaches are *beta-blockers* such as Tenormin, Lopressor, and Inderal; *calcium channel blockers* such as Cardizem, Dilacor, and Procardia; *antidepressants* such as Elavil and Zoloft; *serotonin antagonists* such as Sansert; *anticonvulsants* such as Tegretol, Depakote, and Dilantin; and *ergot derivatives* such as Cafergot and Sansert.

Over-the-Counter Drugs

Nonprescription remedies for headaches are numerous. Here are some of the leading brands:

Actron	Excedrin	Pamprin
Advil	Excedrin, Aspirin	Panadol
Aleve	Free	St. Joseph
Alka-Seltzer	Excedrin P.M.	Tylenol
Ascriptin	Goody's	Tylenol PM
Bayer	Midol	Unisom with Pain
Bayer PM	Motrin IB	Relief
BC Powder	Nuprin	Vanquish
Bufferin	Orudis KT	

Special formulas are also available for children, including:

Children's Advil
Bayer Children's Chewable
Junior Strength and Children's Motrin
Panadol Children's
Junior Strength Tylenol

Herbal Remedies

Japanese mint and white willow are considered all-purpose pain relievers. Cayenne, applied as a cream, can help relieve the muscular tension that accompanies these headaches.

Nutritional Support

About one-quarter of headache sufferers say that certain foods trigger their head pain. Many foods contain substances that can provoke the release of the *neurotransmitters* (chemical messengers in the brain) implicated in causing headaches.

Tyramine is a leading culprit. It's found in chocolate, aged cheese, vinegar, organ meats, alcoholic beverages (especially red wine), sour cream, soy sauce, yogurt, and yeast extracts.

Nitrites are another common offender. They are especially common in smoked fish, bologna, pepperoni, bacon, frankfurters, corned beef, pastrami, canned ham, and sausage.

Monosodium glutamate is also a well-known trigger. It crops up in dry roasted nuts, potato chips, Chinese food, processed or frozen foods, soups and sauces, diet foods, salad dressings, and mayonnaise.

Other troublemakers include high doses of vitamins (particularly vitamin A and niacin), and a lack of water (dehydration). For some people, citrus fruits, dairy products, soybeans, wheat products, onions, fatty foods, seafood, and artificial sweeteners (aspartame, NutraSweet) cause or worsen headaches. Alcoholic and caffeinated beverages are also frequent offenders.

If you're prone to headaches, you might also want to try taking a magnesium supplement on a regular basis. (Check with your doctor first if you have a kidney problem.) In one study of 3,000 women, 80 percent found that magnesium helped. The recommended dosage is 200 milligrams daily. You may need to take it for a couple of months before you begin to feel the benefits.

Alternative Treatments

Acupressure: This traditional Chinese therapy seeks to remedy illness through the application of deep finger pressure at points located along an invisible system of energy channels called meridians. It often relieves muscle tension and headaches.

Acupuncture: This therapy focuses on insertion of tiny needles at points along the Chinese meridians. It frequently proves effective for all types of pain.

Aston-Patterning: A combination of physical training and massage, this form of treatment is designed to relieve the muscle tension that can contribute to the headaches.

Biofeedback: The technology-assisted exercises of biofeedback help people gain control of involuntary reactions. It has helped many victims of both migraine and tension headache.

Chiropractic: This technique for manipulation of the joints often relieves muscle spasms, and is sometimes used for headaches.

Environmental Medicine: Practitioners of this discipline focus on ridding the body of harmful toxins. They can help you identify dietary and other environmental triggers.

Feldenkrais Method: These treatments aim to correct counterproductive movement patterns. Relief of chronic headaches is one of their chief applications.

Hypnotherapy: Using the power of suggestion, hypnotherapists can relieve all types of pain—including headache—if you prove to be susceptible.

Magnetic Field Therapy: This controversial form of treatment uses small magnets to relieve pain, including (occasionally) headaches.

Massage Therapy: This relaxing manipulation of the soft tissues eases the muscle tension that may contribute to headaches.

Meditation: By clearing and calming the mind, meditation promotes relaxation and relieves tension. Many find it helpful for headaches.

Myotherapy: Like regular massage, this form of deep muscle massage helps to relieve almost any sort of muscle-related pain, including tension headache.

Osteopathic Medicine: Manipulation by an osteopath often relieves back, neck, and joint pain, and may be helpful for some types of headache.

Qigong: These slow, disciplined Chinese exercises relieve tension, thereby combating tension headache.

Reflexology: Some people find that pressure on specific points in the foot can help relieve their tension headaches.

Transient Ischemic Attack

The Basics

A transient ischemic attack, often called a ministroke or TIA for short, is an early warning sign you ignore at your peril. Like the majority of major strokes, a TIA is caused by a glob of fatty plaque or a blood clot that becomes lodged in an artery leading to the brain, interrupting the supply of oxygen-rich blood the brain needs to survive. In a stroke, this blockage is severe and protracted, ending in permanent damage. TIAs differ in that the obstruction is mercifully brief, usually subsiding within a few minutes and sparing the brain from lasting injury.

Harmless as a TIA may be, however, in roughly half the people who suffer this type of attack a full-blown stroke follows within a year. (For about 20 percent, disaster strikes within a month.) It's therefore extremely important to seek care even if stroke-like symptoms pass within seconds. Chances are that you'll need blood-thinning medications to avert a more serious attack later on.

Be especially alert for signs of a TIA or stroke if you have a chronic condition such as high blood pressure, high cholesterol, hardening of the arteries, or diabetes. These problems make TIAs (and stroke) more likely. Smokers and overweight individuals are also in greater danger.

Call Your Doctor If . . .

- You think you may have had a TIA in the past (see the symptoms below).
- You've been prescribed a blood-thinning drug and find that you are bruising easily or have blood in your urine.

Seek Care Immediately If . . .

You have any of the symptoms of stroke, even for a minute or two. Possible warning signs include:

- Sudden weakness or paralysis in an arm, hand, or leg, occurring on one or both sides of the body
- Sudden numbness on one side of the face or body
- Sudden blurred vision in one or both eyes
- Difficulty in speaking or understanding simple statements
- Sudden severe headache
- Difficulty swallowing
- Dizziness, loss of balance, or an unexplained fall

Because you could be in the process of having a full-fledged stroke, call **911 or 0 (operator) immediately** to get to the nearest hospital.

What You Can Do

To reduce your risk of TIAs and stroke:

- If you have an artery-damaging condition such as high blood pressure or diabetes, be careful to keep it under control. Follow your doctor's lifestyle recommendations and be sure to take all medicines exactly as directed.
- Adopt a low-fat, high-fiber diet to help keep your arteries clear. If you're overweight, a low-fat diet will also help you shed pounds.
- Get regular exercise. It improves circulation and holds back the chronic conditions, such as high blood pressure and heart disease, that increase the odds of a stroke.

■ If you're a smoker, try to quit. Smokers face triple the odds of a stroke. For smokers with high blood pressure, the risk can be as much as 20 times greater than for nonsmokers.

■ If your doctor recommends daily aspirin, be sure to take it regularly. It helps thin the blood so blood clots won't form. Do not take other painkillers such as acetaminophen or ibuprofen instead. They do not have aspirin's blood-thinning properties.

What Your Doctor Can Do

Aspirin or a stronger blood-thinning drug is the usual treatment for anyone who's suffered a TIA. However, if one of the carotid arteries serving the brain has become severely obstructed, an operation called a *carotid endarterectomy* may be necessary to remove the buildup of fatty plaque.

Prescription Drugs

Heparin, an intravenous drug that prevents additional clots from forming, may be given when you arrive at the hospital. Later, to help provide long-term protection, you may be given blood-thinning pills such as Coumadin (warfarin), Plavix (clopidogrel), or Ticlid (ticlopidine).

If you are afflicted with artery-clogging levels of cholesterol in your blood, there are two cholesterol-lowering drugs that experts now agree can reduce your risk of stroke: Pravachol (pravastatin) and Zocor (simvastatin).

Over-the-Counter Drugs

With its blood-thinning effect, aspirin is typically considered the first line of defense for most—but not all—victims of TIA. Check with your doctor before using it. If there is any danger of internal bleeding, it may not be appropriate. The usual dosage is 650 to 1,300 milligrams a day.

Herbal Remedies

Herbs that fight the buildup of arterial plaque may help to reduce your chances of TIAs or stroke. For more information, see the entry on clogged arteries.

Nutritional Support

A low-fat diet is imperative if you've suffered a TIA—and a good preventive measure for anyone with high cholesterol levels. See the entry on clogged arteries for details.

Alternative Treatments

Any alternative regimens that tend to fight high cholesterol should offer some degree of protection from TIAs—if followed faithfully over the long term. In particular, consider the following:

Orthomolecular Medicine: This type of therapy places vitamins and minerals in the role of medications. A form of the B-complex vitamin niacin is considered especially beneficial against high cholesterol.

Vegetarianism: By omitting meat, a vegetarian diet automatically eliminates the primary source of artery-clogging fat and cholesterol. Vegetarian diets also tend to be high in artery-clearing fiber.

Ulcers

The Basics

An ulcer—known medically as a peptic ulcer—is an open sore in the digestive tract. Most ulcers are found in the stomach and at the top of the small intestine. When stomach acid comes in contact with an ulcer, it becomes quite painful.

The most common symptom of an ulcer is pain in the upper abdomen (the area around the stomach), especially when the stomach is empty. The pain may be relieved by food, only to worsen again one and a half to three hours after eating. The pain sometimes wakes people in the middle of the night. Other possible symptoms include nausea, vomiting, and burping.

Most ulcers are caused by a bacterium called *H. pylori.* Once the ulcer is established, excess stomach acid makes the situation worse. Smoking, drinking, and consuming too much caffeine also play a role in the development of an ulcer, as does excessive stress.

Most ulcers can be treated at home and heal in 1 to 2 months. If your ulcer starts to bleed, however, you will probably have to go to the hospital. If you lose too much blood, you may need surgery, and possibly a blood transfusion.

Call Your Doctor If . . .

■ Your stools are black, bloody, or tarry-looking.
■ You have diarrhea or constipation. (These conditions can be caused by antacids.)
■ Your symptoms do not improve in a few weeks.

Seek Care Immediately If . . .

■ You vomit blood or material that looks like coffee grounds.

■ You have severe abdominal pain.

■ You have cold skin, begin to sweat, and feel weak or faint.

What You Can Do

■ Your doctor will probably prescribe several different drugs that have to be taken at different times each day. Be sure to follow the directions exactly. Don't stop taking the medicines on your own, even if you're feeling better.

■ You can use over-the-counter antacids, but take them only as directed by your doctor. Antacids can interfere with the absorption of other medications, so be sure to ask your doctor or pharmacist how to space out the doses.

■ Antacids and some acid blockers are available without a prescription. It is okay to use these medications for occasional heartburn, but if you feel the need to use them on a daily basis, you should seek the care of a physician. Left untreated, ulcers can cause serious problems. Over-the-counter products are useful for controlling pain, but they will not cure the infection that causes the ulcer.

■ Be sure to tell your doctor about every prescription and over-the-counter medication you are taking, even if you take it only occasionally. Some medications can cause ulcers. Nonsteroidal anti-inflammatory drugs (NSAIDs) such as ibuprofen and naproxen are the most common culprits. Taken to relieve arthritis, fever, menstrual cramps, pain, and swelling, they can trigger a bleeding ulcer without any warning. If your doctor suspects one of these drugs is causing a problem, he can prescribe a drug called misoprostol to counteract the NSAID's ulcer-causing effect or switch you to a less ulcer-prone medication such as Celebrex.

■ If you smoke, try to quit. Smokers are more likely to develop ulcers—and their ulcers take longer to heal and are more likely to recur.

What Your Doctor Can Do

Your doctor will perform several diagnostic tests to determine the cause of your stomach pain. You may need to have a test called an upper GI. This is an x-ray of your stomach and intestines. Before the pictures are taken, you'll need to drink a chalky liquid that helps to outline the stomach. You may also have to undergo an endoscopy so the doctor can examine the inside of your stomach. In this procedure, a tiny camera is attached to a tube, then passed through your mouth and into your stomach.

Several different types of medication are available to treat ulcers. Antibiotics are used to fight the infection that causes them. You may need to take several different brands for several weeks. Acid blockers are used to restrict the production of acid in your stomach. They relieve pain and help the ulcer heal. Antacids are used to neutralize stomach acid and ease the pain. If you suffer excessive blood loss from a bleeding ulcer, a transfusion may be needed. A perforated or bleeding ulcer may require surgery.

Prescription Drugs

There are two prepackaged drug regimens for curing *H. pylori*–induced ulcers. One, called Helidac Therapy, combines two antibacterial drugs (metronidazole and tetracycline) with an antacid (bismuth subsalicylate). The other, dubbed Prevpac, includes two antibiotics (amoxicillin and clarithromycin) and an acid blocker (lansoprazole).

Other drugs used in the treatment of ulcers include:

Axid (nizatidine)	Pepcid (famotidine)	Tagamet
Carafate	Prevacid	(cimetidine)
(sucralfate)	(lansoprazole)	Zantac
Cytotec	Prilosec	(ranitidine)
(misoprostol)	(omeprazole)	

Over-the-Counter Drugs

A wide variety of nonprescription antacids and acid blockers can help relieve ulcer pain:

Alka-Mints	Maalox	Rolaids
Alka-Seltzer Gold	Antacid/Anti-Gas	Tagamet HB
AlternaGEL	Mylanta AR	Titralac products
Amphojel	Mylanta products	Tums
Axid AR	Nephrox	Tums
Basaljel	Pepcid AC	Antigas/Antacid
Di-Gel	Phillips' Milk of	Formula
Gaviscon	Magnesia	Zantac 75
Maalox		

Herbal Remedies

The only truly effective herbal remedy for ulcers is licorice root (or more specifically, the glycyrrhizic acid that licorice contains). It reduces inflammation and protects the stomach lining from the harmful effects of gastric acid, thus promoting healing.

Nutritional Support

Bland ulcer diets are a thing of the past. Spicy foods and citrus fruits rarely do any harm. You should, however, take pains to avoid items known to trigger acid production. These include refined sugar, alcohol, tea, and coffee.

You might also consider taking a zinc supplement. Zinc promotes wound healing; and animal studies have shown that it can prevent the release of chemicals that weaken the lining of the digestive tract.

Missing meals and eating irregularly can make your symptoms worse. Try to avoid having an empty stomach. Eat several small meals at regular times during the day.

Alternative Treatments

Biofeedback: This treatment program is designed to teach patients how to control otherwise involuntary bodily functions such as digestion. With sensors leading from various parts of your body to a small computer, the biofeedback therapist will put you through a set of mental and physical exercises aimed at bringing digestive acid under control. This form of treatment won't eliminate the *H. pylori* bacteria responsible for most ulcers, but it may relieve pain and speed healing.

Urinary Incontinence

The Basics

Though rarely discussed openly, involuntary urination is a surprisingly common medical problem. It plagues one in 10 people over age 65, and at least 10 million people in all. Despite its prevalence, many victims are too embarrassed to seek help—a serious mistake, since research shows that 8 out of 10 could benefit from therapy.

Incontinence is neither a disease nor a normal part of growing older. It is a symptom of something else gone awry. There are two broad types: *transient,* a temporary problem that results from an illness or medication and which is usually easily eliminated once diagnosed, and *chronic,* a stubborn disorder which nevertheless yields to treatment most of the time. Age-related changes in the lower urinary tract make both forms more likely in our later years. Women are twice as prone to the problem as men.

Chronic incontinence, the more intractable of the two varieties, is not a single disorder. In fact, doctors have identified seven types:

Stress incontinence is a tendency to leak urine when laughing, sneezing, coughing, or lifting. The problem in this case isn't with the bladder but rather with the urinary canal (the urethra) or pelvic muscles. It is extremely common in women after pregnancy and childbirth.

Urge incontinence, also known as overactive bladder, is marked by an overwhelming need to urinate before you can get to the bathroom. This type originates in the bladder itself and can be caused by inflammation or disorders of the nervous system.

Reflex incontinence is the diagnosis when urination occurs completely without warning. Causes include nervous system problems or bladder tumors.

Overflow incontinence is characterized by periodic leakage of small amounts of urine. It develops when the bladder cannot empty completely, either because of a failure of the muscles to contract properly or because the urethra is partially blocked. In men, this type of incontinence is usually the result of an enlarged prostate (a gland that surrounds the urethra).

Functional incontinence is not a urinary problem *per se.* In fact, the urinary system is working fine, but the individual is unwilling or unable to get to a toilet when necessary. Severe arthritis, weakness, and dementia are among the major culprits.

Mixed incontinence is a label for situations in which several of the above problems are at work.

Total incontinence, the rarest of the types, is the complete loss of control and continual leakage of urine. It is usually the result of an injury, malformation, or hole (fistula) in the bladder.

Call Your Doctor If . . .

■ You are having any problems with urinary control. Don't let embarrassment stop you. *Remember: the condition is common and can almost always be treated.*

Seek Care Immediately If . . .

Fortunately, incontinence is not a medical emergency.

What You Can Do

The first step in treatment is getting a diagnosis. If your doctor is not experienced in treating incontinence, consider seeing a gynecologist, urologist, or geriatrician.

Before your appointment:
- Keep a record of when you go to the bathroom and when you have leakage for at least 4 days prior to your visit. Note what you were doing and the time of day when leakage occurred. Also jot down what you typically eat and drink.
- List or bring to your appointment all the medicines you are currently taking, including over-the-counter remedies. Also make a list of any questions you want to ask and be sure you understand the answers provided.

After your diagnosis:
- If the doctor prescribes exercises or biofeedback training, be patient and pursue the treatment faithfully. These therapies won't provide an instant cure, but they can pay off handsomely over the long term.

What Your Doctor Can Do

First the doctor will gather a medical history and conduct a thorough examination. Because the pelvic muscles or nervous system could be at fault, he's likely to do an abdominal, rectal, and neurological exam, as well as a pelvic exam for women. He'll probably order a urinalysis and various blood tests, and may perform a bladder catheterization, passing a sterile tube into your bladder to see whether it's emptying properly. Depending on what he finds, he may then conduct a variety of more specialized tests. Although none are dangerous or particularly painful, don't hesitate to ask for a full description of each if you have any concerns.

Once the cause has been identified, the doctor can choose the best form of therapy. There are five major types:

Behavioral techniques such as biofeedback and bladder training help people become aware of—and learn to control—the body's ordinarily involuntary responses. These treatments are especially helpful for urge incontinence.

Muscle training strengthens and trains the pelvic muscles either through special exercises or by electrical muscle conditioning with a device placed in the vagina or rectum to cause sphincter muscle contractions. The treatments help relieve urge, stress, and mixed incontinence.

Medications are available for urge, stress, mixed, and overflow incontinence. They work by either preventing the bladder from contracting or strengthening the sphincter that shuts off the outlet.

Bladder catheterization is often the best treatment for overflow incontinence that doesn't respond to medication and can't be fixed surgically. There are two methods: *indwelling* (the tube is left in place) and *intermittent* (the tube is inserted and removed each time you void).

Surgery is the last resort for most incontinence problems, but sometimes proves helpful for urge or overflow incontinence due to an enlarged prostate. Remember, however, the operation itself leads to continued incontinence about 10 percent of the time.

Prescription Drugs

Medications for urge incontinence include:

Anaspaz (hyoscyamine sulfate)   Propantheline
Bentyl (dicyclomine)   Tofranil (imipramine)
Detrol (tolterodine)   Urispas (flavoxate)
Ditropan (oxybutynin)

For overflow incontinence, the doctor is likely to prescribe one of the following:

Cardura (doxazosin)   Minipress (prazosin)
Catapres (clonidine)   Proscar (finasteride)
Flomax (tamsulosin)   Urecholine (bethanechol)
Hytrin (terazosin)

Over-the-Counter Drugs

Nonprescription drugs are the preferred remedy for stress incontinence. They include:

Dexatrim (phenylpropanolamine)
Primatene (ephedrine)
Sudafed (pseudoephedrine)

Check with your doctor, however, before using these products for incontinence.

Herbal Remedies

Prostate enlargement, a leading cause of overflow incontinence, can sometimes be relieved by the following herbs:

Pumpkin Seed	Saw Palmetto
Pygeum	Stinging Nettle

Nutritional Support

Certain dietary items seem to cause incontinence problems for some people. Although there's little medical research proving a definite connection, you might want to experiment with elimination of the following foods from your diet to see if it makes a difference:

Alcohol	Tomatoes and tomato-based
Carbonated soft drinks	products
Caffeinated beverages	Spicy foods
Decaffeinated coffee and tea	Natural and artificial sweeteners
Milk and milk products	Chocolate
Citrus fruit and juices	

Alternative Treatments

Biofeedback is a training technique that helps you become more aware of, and gain control over, the body's ordinarily involuntary responses. More than 80 percent of people treated with biofeedback for urge, stress, or mixed incontinence achieve improvement or a complete cure.

Myotherapy, a form of deep muscle massage, is said to help with certain types of incontinence, but has never been validated through controlled clinical trials.

Reflexology endeavors to relieve symptoms throughout the body by pressing on various reflex points along the foot. Several small research studies have found the technique helpful for incontinence, although it has never been verified in major clinical trials.

Urinary Tract Infection

The Basics

These unpleasant infections develop when bacteria travel up the urinary duct *(urethra)* and gain a foothold in the bladder. They're annoying, painful, and even frightening, but at least they're easy to cure. A fast dose of antibiotics usually does the trick—provided you get treatment promptly. If you allow the bacteria time to migrate further up the urinary tract and settle in a kidney, you'll find that the problem becomes not only more painful, but more difficult to treat.

Urinary tract infections (UTIs) attack women more often than men. Sexual intercourse, pregnancy, diabetes, or a past UTI increase a woman's chances of an infection. Wiping back to front after a bowel movement also increases the odds. Among men, the problem tends to occur when an enlarged prostate gland cuts off the flow of urine, causing it to stagnate and allow bacteria to multiply. For either sex, delaying a needed trip to the bathroom tends to raise the odds of infection.

Symptoms include a frequent need to urinate with inability to pass more than a small amount, pain and burning on urination, and dribbling or leaking during the day and while sleeping. After urinating, you may still feel the urge and may need to urinate often during the night. Urine may develop a foul odor or become blood-specked. If the infection reaches your kidneys, you may also suffer back pain, fever, chills, nausea, and vomiting.

Call Your Doctor If . . .
- You have a high temperature.
- You see blood in your urine.
- Your symptoms do not improve after a few days of treatment.
- You develop nausea, vomiting, diarrhea, or a rash.
- You develop any new or unexplained symptoms. They may be related to the medication you are taking.
- Your symptoms (especially fever) return after you finish treatment.

Seek Care Immediately If . . .
- You start vomiting and can't keep down any fluids or medicine.
- You are unable to urinate.

What You Can Do
- Take antibiotics for as long as directed. Do not stop when your symptoms subside. If you give up treatment too soon, some bacteria may survive and re-infect you.
- Get plenty of rest, especially if you have a fever.
- Drink 6 to 8 large glasses of water a day to help flush the infection out of your system.
- Urinate often, as soon as you have the urge, and try to completely

empty your bladder each time. Also, urinate before and after sex. If UTIs are a particularly recurring problem, try washing your vaginal area after sex with a hand-held shower attachment.

- If you wear a diaphragm, make sure it fits properly; pressure from the rim of a diaphragm can lead to UTIs. If you've lost or gained more than 10 pounds, have your diaphragm refitted.
- Be sure you and your partner keep your genital and anal areas clean at all times. Both of you should wash your hands before foreplay and sex. If your partner is uncircumcised, he should always clean under the foreskin before sex. If you have anal sex, be sure your partner uses a condom, discards it, and washes his penis before vaginal entry.
- Women should remember to wipe front to back after a bowel movement. It's also best to wear underwear and pantyhose with cotton crotches; nylon-crotch underwear and tight jeans create a moist environment in which bacteria can grow. For the same reason, change into dry clothes as soon as possible after swimming, particularly if you were in a chlorinated pool.
- To minimize irritation, use a mild laundry detergent and make sure that your clothes, nightwear, and sheets are well rinsed. Do not use a public laundry to wash your underwear since soap and detergent deposits can accumulate in the washers. If you don't have your own washing machine, sterilize underwear by boiling it in a pot.
- For pain, try holding a heating pad or hot-water bottle against your abdomen or on the urethral area. If your genital area is warmer than the urine waiting to be released, it won't burn as much when you urinate.
- If you have a kidney infection, also called *pyelonephritis,* be sure to keep your follow-up visit with your doctor to make sure the infection is cured. Persistent kidney infections can lead to permanent damage or even kidney failure.

What Your Doctor Can Do

Your doctor will have your urine tested for bacteria and prescribe antibiotics to fight the infection. If the doctor needs to find out exactly which bacteria has invaded, he will order a urine culture, which takes 24 to 72 hours to provide results.

Prescription Drugs

For this type of infection, the most commonly used antibiotics are:

Amoxil, Trimox, Wymox
  (amoxicillin)
Bactrim or Septra
  (trimethoprim/
  sulfamethoxazole)
Ceftin, Kefurox, or Zinacef
  (cefuroxime)
Cipro (ciprofloxacin)
Floxin (ofloxacin)
Gantanol (sulfamethoxazole)

Keflex (cephalexin)
Macrodantin (nitrofurantoin)
Maxaquin (lomefloxacin)
Noroxin (norfloxacin)
Omnipen (ampicillin)
Penetrex (enoxacin)
Suprax (cefixime)
Trimpex (trimethoprim)
Trovan (trovafloxacin)

For pain, your doctor may prescribe a drug that relaxes the bladder, such as Prosed and Urised (methenamine) or Urispas (flavoxate). He can also prescribe the local anesthetic Pyridium (phenazopyridine).

Over-the-Counter Drugs
Acetaminophen (Tylenol), ibuprofen (Advil, Motrin, Nuprin), or aspirin can be taken for fever and pain.

Herbal Remedies
A number of herbs have been found effective against urinary tract infections. They include:

Asparagus Root
Barberry
Bearberry
Birch
Couch Grass
Dandelion
Goldenrod

Horseradish
Horsetail
Java Tea
Juniper Berry
Lily of the Valley
Lovage

Mate
Nasturtium
Parsley
Restharrow
Sandlewood
Stinging Nettle

Nutritional Support
Drinking cranberry juice and taking vitamin C helps make the urine more acidic, which discourages bacterial growth. As an alternative to drinking cranberry juice, try grinding fresh cranberries with honey and eating them with plain yogurt.

While highly acidic urine will help kill the bacteria, it also stings more when you urinate. If your primary objective is to relieve the pain, you can *reduce* the urine's acidity by drinking a pint of hot or cold water mixed with 1 teaspoon sodium bicarbonate (baking soda). If bicarbonate makes you queasy, try potassium citrate. Some people even take commercial antacids, such as Rolaids and Tums, to relieve the burning of urination.

For some people, taking 6 to 8 tablets of dolomite every few hours seems to provide relief. Avoid caffeine and alcohol during treatment; they irritate the bladder. It may also help if you cut back your intake of refined starches and sugars, vegetable fats, onions, beans, and chocolate.

Alternative Treatments

If you suffer from repeated UTIs, you might want to try one of the following alternative health regimens:

Juice Therapy: High in concentrated nutrients, fruit and vegetable juices are ideal for keeping your immunity high and fighting off all kinds of infections.

Naturopathic Medicine: More of a philosophical approach to health than a particular form of therapy, naturopathic medicine offers a wide variety of natural, noninvasive remedies for stubborn minor ailments such as UTIs.

Vaginal Infections

The Basics

Vaginal infection and inflammation, known as *vulvovaginitis* or *vaginitis,* is the most common gynecological disorder in the United States today. Its symptoms include unusual mucus discharge, odor, pain in the vagina during intercourse, and itching, irritation, or pain in the external genital area (the vulva). Fortunately, while vulvovaginitis is uncomfortable, it is essentially harmless and responds to simple treatment.

Bacteria, yeast, and protozoa cause vaginal infections. The healthy vagina is home to a variety of these microscopic organisms. Normally, they live harmoniously in an acidic environment that prevents the overproduction of any one species and repels foreign invaders. A number of factors, however, can upset the body's balance, allowing an infection to develop. Antibiotics, birth control pills, frequent douching, pregnancy, menopause, tampons, tight or non-breathing pants, excess weight, and diabetes all can encourage a vaginal infection.

There are three main types of vaginal infections. Each tends to produce a distinctive type of discharge:

- *Yeast infection* or candidiasis is marked by a thick, white, cottage cheese-like discharge, itching, and irritated skin. Women with diabetes and those taking antibiotics are more likely to develop this type of infection. Most women will have at least one yeast infection at some point in their lives. (For full discussion see the entry on yeast infections.)
- *Trichomonas,* caused by a tiny one-celled parasite, produces a thin, yellow, foul-smelling discharge. The infection is usually transmitted sexually. Its most striking symptoms are vulvar and vaginal burning and itching. The burning may be most apparent after intercourse. There may be vulvar swelling and frequent, uncomfortable urination. In men, this infection rarely produces symptoms, and many women are also asymptomatic.
- *Bacterial vaginosis (BV),* sometimes called nonspecific vaginitis, produces a thin, gray or white, foul-smelling "fishy" discharge. The odor may seem the strongest in the shower or after you have sex. Other signs may be mild itching and irritation of the vagina and vulva. Bacterial vaginosis accounts for 40 percent of all vaginitis-related visits to the doctor. For most women, BV is more a nuisance than a significant health threat. However, it has been linked to pelvic inflammatory disease and premature births.

Call Your Doctor If . . .
- Your symptoms become worse or continue for more than a few days.
- You have vaginal bleeding after your period.
- Your symptoms come back after treatment.
- You have any problems that you suspect are related to the medicine you are taking.

Seek Care Immediately If . . .
Vaginal infections do not require emergency treatment.

What You Can Do
- Keep your genital area clean and dry. Take showers instead of tub baths. Use plain, unscented soap. Heavier women, frequent exercisers, and those who wear pantyhose may need to wash more often to keep the bacteria count to a minimum.
- Don't use feminine hygiene sprays or powders, and don't douche more than twice a month. If you douche, use plain water or a water and vinegar mixture. During treatment, don't douche at all unless your doctor recommends it.

■ Don't have sex while you are being treated. Otherwise, the infection could be passed back and forth between you and your partner.

■ To discourage growth of yeast and bacteria, use underpants and pantyhose that have a cotton lining in the crotch.

■ After urination and bowel movements, wipe from front to back to prevent the spread of germs.

■ Avoid activities that make you sweaty, especially during hot, humid weather.

■ Be sure that your clothing "breathes"; avoid tight garments and fabrics containing a high percentage of synthetic fiber.

■ Use condoms and a spermicide to prevent sexually transmitted infections.

What Your Doctor Can Do

Your doctor will examine your vulva, vagina, and cervix for signs of infection; check the appearance of any vaginal discharge; and note any tenderness in the uterus and ovaries. A sample of the vaginal discharge may be tested to confirm the cause of the infection. Based on the findings of the examination, your doctor will prescribe medication.

Prescription Drugs

If a bacterial infection is at fault, your doctor will prescribe an antibiotic application such as Cleocin Vaginal Cream (clindamycin), Metrogel Vaginal Gel (metronidazole), or Sultrin (triple sulfa cream). For *Trichomonas* infections, the treatment is metronidazole taken orally (Flagyl, Protostat). To prevent reinfection your sexual partner should be treated as well.

Over-the-Counter Drugs

Although most yeast-infection remedies can be purchased over the counter (see separate entry), you will definitely need a prescription medication for bacterial vaginosis or trichomoniasis.

Herbal Remedies

There are no herbs capable of curing bacterial infections or trichomoniasis.

Nutritional Support

Although good nutrition builds overall resistance, there are no specific dietary measures you take to prevent or cure either bacterial infections or trichomoniasis.

Alternative Treatments

Nothing in the world of alternative medicine has been judged effective specifically for these problems.

Varicose Veins

The Basics

Fortunately, these annoying blemishes seldom pose any danger to life or limb. They usually appear in the legs (though they can occur in other parts of the body) as snakelike, bluish streaks that swell and bulge under the skin's surface. They are more common with advancing age, but can strike in youth as well, most commonly during pregnancy. Up to 50 percent of all women eventually get them.

Varicose veins develop when blood flow slows or backs up. About two-thirds of all people who have them have a close relative who has them too. Some risk factors may be inherited, such as missing or malfunctioning valves within the veins, or unusually stretchy veins. Taking hormones adds to the risk, as does excess weight. Jobs that require long periods of standing can make matters worse. Varicose veins can cause aching, burning, tingling, or fatigue, but even when they are painless, nobody likes the way they look.

Call Your Doctor If . . .

■ The skin around your ankle itches, looks brownish, and starts to break down.

■ You develop pain, redness, tenderness, itching, and hard swelling in your leg.

■ Leg pain begins to cause you great discomfort.

Seek Care Immediately If . . .

Varicose veins hardly ever cause an emergency.

What You Can Do

■ Avoid prolonged standing or sitting with crossed legs. Rest with your legs raised above heart level as often as possible during the day.

■ Don't wear tight garters, jeans, or other garments that cut off circulation to the groin or legs.

■ Try wearing elastic or support hose—the therapeutic kind sold in pharmacies, not the standard support pantyhose sold in department stores. Look for graduated compression stockings, which are tightest at the ankle and looser higher up the leg.

■ Walk as much as possible to keep blood flowing.

■ Raise the foot of your bed with 2-inch blocks.

■ Avoid constipation—preferably with a high-fiber diet—or take a stool softener. Straining can worsen this condition.

■ If you get a cut in the skin over the vein and the vein bleeds, lie down with your leg raised and press on it with a clean cloth until the bleeding stops. Then have a doctor take care of the wound.

What Your Doctor Can Do

The most widely used remedy for varicose veins is *sclerotherapy*. The vein is injected with a chemical that causes it to wither and eventually be reabsorbed into surrounding tissues. The treatment can be performed in a physician's office, though several visits may be required for complete removal. When performed by an experienced doctor, this procedure is effective and low-risk, but beware of "mills" dedicated to nothing but varicose vein treatment. These practitioners, some of them none too skilled, have given something of a bad name to varicose vein therapy.

Major varicose veins can be surgically tied off and removed, a procedure called *stripping*. After stripping, smaller veins nearby are eliminated with sclerotherapy. The results are usually satisfactory, although there's no guarantee that other varicose veins won't show up elsewhere. The newest techniques for surgical removal require only a few tiny incisions and stitches, and leave only minor scars. These operations can be performed under local anesthesia as same-day outpatient surgery. Be suspicious, however, if offered laser therapy. Lasers are generally effective only for tiny capillaries, not big veins.

Prescription Drugs

Aside from the vein-withering shots given in the physician's office, there are no medications for varicose veins.

Over-the-Counter Drugs

No over-the-counter remedies will affect this condition.

Herbal Remedies

While they won't eliminate varicose veins, the herbs horse chestnut and sweet clover are said to improve poor circulation in the veins.

Nutritional Support

Eat a high fiber diet (lots of whole-grain breads and cereals) to prevent constipation and unnecessary straining.

Alternative Treatments

Advocates of *hydrotherapy* still recommend it for circulatory disorders, though it has fallen out of favor among mainstream physicians. Despite its potentially beneficial effect on circulation, however, it's unlikely to clear up varicose veins.

Whooping Cough

The Basics

Highly contagious and potentially dangerous in any child under 2, whooping cough is not a disease to dismiss lightly. In severe cases, thick sputum plugs the air passages, while long spells of coughing leave the victim starving for air. Infants stricken with the disease must sometimes be hospitalized.

Known medically as *pertussis*, whooping cough is a bacterial infection of the air passages and lungs. It is spread by droplets sprayed into the air when an infected child sneezes or coughs.

The ailment begins like a cold, with sneezing, watery eyes, runny nose, listlessness, loss of appetite, and a nighttime cough that gradually gets worse. After 10 to 14 days, severe coughing spells set in. Typically, the child will cough 5 to 15 times in row, then inhale with a whoop. During the spell, the child's face or nail beds may turn red, blue, or white from lack of oxygen. The coughing is often intense enough to cause vomiting. In infants, choking spells may follow the coughs.

Improvement usually begins within 4 weeks. Coughing spells become less frequent, vomiting subsides, and the child begins to look and feel better. Full recovery can usually be expected by the seventh week, but cases have been known to last as long as 3 months. The disease sometimes progresses to pneumonia. Ear infections are a common complication.

Call Your Doctor If . . .

■ The child has a high temperature.

■ The child begins tugging on his ears or complains of ear pain—both signs of ear infection.

■ Vomiting lasts more than a few hours.
■ The child is not drinking liquids.
■ Coughing spells continue to get worse.
■ The cough is interfering with the child's sleep and rest.

Seek Care Immediately If . . .
Call **911 or 0 (operator)** for help if the child develops any of these signs of an emergency:

■ Trouble breathing.
■ Sucking in of the skin between the ribs with each breath.
■ Blue or white lips or fingernails.

What You Can Do
■ Keep the child in a quiet, darkened room, as free as possible from other activities. Any disturbance can set off a coughing spell.
■ Do not let anyone smoke around the child. The smoke can make the breathing problems and coughing worse.
■ Do NOT give cough medicine unless it is suggested by your doctor. Coughing helps keep sputum from clogging the lungs.
■ During coughing spells, put the child on his or her tummy with the head to one side. This is a safe position because it will prevent choking if the child vomits. Raise the foot of the crib or bed. This will help drain the lungs. You can also hold the child in a sitting position. Help older children sit up and lean forward during a coughing spell. This makes it easier to cough and bring up sputum from the lungs.
■ The child may need to have postural drainage to loosen sputum in the lungs. In this procedure, the child's head will be tilted lower than the feet while a nurse gently taps the child's back. The coughing will temporarily increase after each treatment.
■ To help loosen the sputum in the child's lungs, use a cool mist humidifier in the sick room. Place it out of reach by the bed. Fill it with cool water. Direct the mist stream toward the child's face.
■ Your child needs rest and plenty of liquids. Switching to smaller, more frequent meals may help prevent vomiting after coughing spells. Try for 6 small meals daily. Wait a short while before giving the child food after a coughing spell.

What Your Doctor Can Do
The doctor can give your kids a vaccine that prevents whooping cough in 70 to 90 percent of all that receive it. It's part of the DTP series

of shots that begin shortly after birth. (DTP stands for diphtheria, tetanus, and pertussis.) There's also a chance of preventing a severe case of the disease by giving the child erythromycin immediately after exposure to the germs. Later, however, antibiotics can't help.

If the disease becomes so severe that the child can't breathe, a stay in the hospital may be necessary. There, the child can be given oxygen and excess mucus can be suctioned from the lungs.

Prescription Drugs

Given before symptoms appear, erythromycin sometimes can stop the illness. Recommended brands are E.E.S., EryPed, Ery-Tab, and PCE. No other prescription drugs are used for this illness.

Over-the-Counter Drugs

Remember that for this disease it's usually unwise to give any sort of cough medicine, whether prescription or over-the-counter.

Herbal Remedies

Again, it's best to avoid suppressing the cough, even with natural herbs.

Nutritional Support

If vomiting is severe, it can leave the child dehydrated. Give as much liquid as possible.

Alternative Treatments

There's really nothing that an alternative medical practitioner can do for this problem. Seek conventional medical care, especially if the illness becomes serious.

Wounds

The Basics

Any tear, scrape, or cut in the skin is considered a wound. There are three main types:

- *Abrasions* are wounds in which the outer layer of the skin has been rubbed or scraped off.
- *Lacerations* are cuts through the skin.

■ *Puncture wounds* are cuts made by round, sharp objects such as needles or nails.

Virtually all wounds cause pain and bleeding. Bruises and swelling are likely as well. It usually takes 2 to 4 weeks for a wound to heal.

Your two most important goals when treating a wound are to stop the bleeding and prevent infection.

■ First, try to stop the bleeding. Applying pressure to the site and elevating the wound above your heart will help. If the wound is large, deep, or keeps on bleeding, you may need to have it closed with sutures (stitches).

■ Once the bleeding has stopped, turn your attention to preventing infection. Keep the area around the wound as clean as possible. You may need a tetanus shot if you have not had one in the past 5 to 10 years. If an infection does take hold, call your doctor without delay. Certain wound infections can be very dangerous and require rapid treatment with potent antibiotics.

Call Your Doctor If . . .
■ Bleeding in the wound area won't stop or gets worse.
■ You develop a high temperature.
■ You notice any signs of infection. These include increasing pain or soreness, swelling, redness, pus, a bad smell, or red streaks coming from the injured site.
■ You develop numbness or swelling below the wound.
■ You cannot move the joint below the wound.
■ The wound is slow to heal.
■ You have a chronic medical condition such as diabetes.

Seek Care Immediately If . . .
■ The wound is bleeding profusely.

What You Can Do
■ Keep the wound and bandage clean and dry. If the bandage gets wet and you need to change it, unwrap it slowly and carefully. If it sticks and starts to hurt, use water to loosen it gently. Pat the area dry with a clean towel before putting on another bandage.
■ If possible, keep the wound lifted above the level of your heart for 24 to 48 hours. This will promote healing and ease the pain and swelling.

■ Clean the wound gently 3 to 4 times a day:
- Flush the wound thoroughly with clean water. Wash the area around the wound with soap and water or a cotton swab dipped in a mixture of half water and half hydrogen peroxide.
- If you have a mouth or lip wound, rinse your mouth after meals and at bedtime. Ask your doctor what mixture to use. Do NOT swallow the mixture.
- If you have a puncture wound, soak it briefly 3 to 4 times a day.

■ If you have a scalp wound, you may wash your hair gently after you get home. Then keep your hair dry until the day you are to have your stitches removed, when you may wash it gently again.

■ Do not go swimming or soak the wound for long periods.

What Your Doctor Can Do

If the area around the wound is dirty, or if any foreign objects (such as gravel) are found in it, the doctor will need to clean it out. If the wound will not stop bleeding, has jagged edges, or is located where it may leave an unwanted scar, it may require stitches.

Over-the-counter painkillers are usually sufficient to ease the pain of a simple cut. For more severe pain, the doctor may give you a prescription pain medication.

Prescription Drugs

There are two prescription ointments used to clean out dead tissue from serious wounds: Panafil and Granulex.

Over-the-Counter Drugs

To prevent infection, you can choose among four nonprescription product lines:

Neosporin   Betadine
Bactine   Polysporin

To cleanse minor wounds inside the mouth, use a product such as Orajel Perioseptic.

Herbal Remedies

The following herbal remedies are considered useful in the treatment of wounds and burns:

Balsam of Peru	Marigold	Slippery Elm
Chamomile	Poplar	St. John's Wort
English Plantain	Shepherd's Purse	Witch Hazel
Horsetail		

Nutritional Support

For optimal wound healing, the body needs an adequate supply of zinc. Unless your diet includes lots of meat, poultry, seafood, and whole grains, you may want to consider taking a zinc supplement.

Alternative Treatments

Oxygen Therapy: Oxygen plays a key role in every cellular process: It supports the immune system, destroys toxic substances, fuels metabolism, and promotes new cell growth. Hyperbaric oxygen therapy— in which patients inhale 100 percent oxygen under pressures of up to 2 atmospheres—is now considered standard treatment for serious wounds that refuse to heal.

Yeast Infections

The Basics

Yeast infections, also called vaginal candidiasis (can-dih-DYE-ah-sis) are a common cause of discharge, itching, and swelling in the vagina. The infections are not serious, and with treatment usually go away in less than 2 weeks. However, they often come back.

The infections are caused by a type of yeast or fungus called *Candida albicans.* This yeast is a normal inhabitant of the mouth, vagina, and rectum, and becomes a problem only when it grows out of control.

The main symptom of a yeast infection is a thick, white discharge from the vagina that may look like cottage cheese and has a bad smell. Swelling, redness, and itching around the vagina are also common symptoms. If your urinary opening is inflamed because of the infection, you may have to urinate more frequently than usual, and urination may be uncomfortable. If the infection is severe, the vulva may swell and fine breaks, called fissures, may appear. Inflammation of the vulva and vagina, combined with the dryness of the discharge makes intercourse painful.

A number of factors can foster a yeast infection. Normally, the vagina contains harmless bacteria that limit the growth of the fungus.

Anything that kills these bacteria, such as feminine hygiene sprays and antibiotics, will allow the fungus to multiply. Clothing (such as nylon and Lycra) that traps heat and moisture can also change the normal balance of organisms in the vagina. Other factors that make this type of infection more likely include pregnancy, diabetes, use of birth control pills, and a diet containing large amounts of sugars, starch, and yeast. Any condition that undermines the immune system, such as AIDS, will also make you more susceptible.

Call Your Doctor If . . .
■ Your symptoms get worse or last more than a few days.
■ You have vaginal bleeding after your period.
■ Your symptoms come back after treatment.

Seek Care Immediately If . . .
Yeast infections do not require emergency treatment.

What You Can Do
While treating the infection, remember that it's best to:
■ Avoid sex until your symptoms are gone.
■ Avoid douching.
■ Wear a sanitary napkin if you are using a cream or suppository. Do not use a tampon because it will absorb the drug.

To prevent future infections, follow these simple guidelines:
■ Wear clean cotton underpants or pantyhose with a cotton crotch.
■ Keep the vaginal area clean and dry.
■ Take showers instead of tub baths. Use plain, unscented soap.
■ Don't use feminine hygiene sprays or powders or bubble bath, and don't douche more than twice a month.
■ Limit your intake of sweets and alcohol.
■ Take antibiotics only if absolutely necessary.
■ Try substituting another form of birth control for the Pill.
■ Wipe from front to back after urinating or having a bowel movement.

What Your Doctor Can Do
To diagnose a yeast infection, the doctor will take a case history, perform a pelvic examination, and examine a few drops of vaginal discharge under a microscope. If the diagnosis is unclear, the doctor may order a vaginal culture. The infections can be treated with either prescription or nonprescription antifungal medications.

Prescription Drugs

Yeast medications taken by mouth are available only by prescription. They include ketoconazole (Nizoral) and fluconazole (Diflucan). For use in the vagina, the doctor can also prescribe a high-strength form of clotrimazole (Mycelex) and various forms of terconazole (Terazol).

Over-the-Counter Drugs

A number of yeast medications are now available over-the-counter: butoconazole nitrate (Femstat), clotrimazole (Gyne-Lotrimin, Lotrimin, Mycelex), miconazole nitrate (Monistat), and tioconazole (Vagistat). These medications come in suppository or cream forms. Some require only a single dose, while others call for 3-day or 7-day treatments. Be sure to check the package directions and use these medications exactly as directed. Use all of the medication called for by the instructions, even if your symptoms disappear. Otherwise the infection may flare up again.

Some women make up their own vaginal suppositories to treat yeast infections with boric acid. You can buy boric acid powder in the eye-care section of most drugstores. Pack it loosely into size "0" capsules (available at some pharmacies and most health food stores). To treat a current yeast infection, insert 1 capsule as deeply into your vagina as possible in the morning and again at bedtime for 5 to 7 days.

If you have frequent yeast infections (three or more a year) that can't be prevented by lifestyle and hygiene changes, your doctor may recommend using preventive doses of antifungal medications. Preventive regimens call for inserting an antifungal suppository one or more times per menstrual cycle or inserting a boric acid capsule twice weekly beginning one week after menstruation until the next period begins.

Herbal Remedies

Fungal infections such as candidiasis can be treated with pau d'arco, a medicine made from the bark of a South American tree. Pau d'arco contains potent antifungal compounds called naphthaquinones.

Nutritional Support

Eating large amounts of sugars, starch, and yeast has been associated with an increased risk of yeast infection. If you have frequent infections, you may want to decrease the amounts of these foods in your diet.

Alternative Treatments

The world of alternative medicine offers no remedies for yeast infections. Your best course is to take the preventive measures outlined above and use antifungal medications when a flare-up occurs.

Disease and Disorder Index

Printed in the United States
by Baker & Taylor Publisher Services